TO

Halli 12/25/2020

FROM

 This information presented in this book is for educational purposes only. This information does not replace the advice of a qualified medical professional or diagnose or treat any medical condition and should not be relied on as such. If you have any concerns or questions about your health you should always consult with a physician or other health-care professional. Do not avoid or delay obtaining medical or health related advice from your health-care professional because of something you may have read in this book. The use of any information provided in this book is solely at your own risk.

For my parents: Edgar and Dahlia Greene

And for Ari.

Table of Contents

PART 1:

A NEW PARADIGM

Your body is a gift.

You didn't design it. You didn't make it. It is yours to use.

The purpose of your body is to give you ***time and freedom.***

When your body stops working your time is up. When your body ceases to be young or healthy you lose your freedom. Freedom with your body is expressed by enjoying the energy, health, and vitality you need to live life to the fullest. Allowing you to do **all** you need to fulfill your greater purpose is the purpose of your body.

Freedom and health are one. Without health you have no freedom. Never has this been more true than today.

Today a new world is upon us. It has new rules. Having real health, defined by real immunity, is at the top of the list. Without real health, without immunity, you will not have real freedom in the world going forward.

Ironically, if the purpose of your body is freedom, for most people, over time, **the body becomes a kind of prison.**

Our bodies become a cage. They imprison us with bars made from declining energy, restricted mobility, excess body fat and disease states like cancer. Eventually the body even restricts your identity. There is a power **everyone** desires - the power to keep the body young and healthy. It is a power that gives you the ability to control the things time steals; health, energy, weight, vitality and **youth.**

The purpose of this book is to give you the most valuable commodity in existence.

More **time.**

Specifically, the purpose of this book is to give you **more time in a healthy, youthful body.**

I know some very wealthy people. They can buy anything they want. The one thing they can not buy is more time. More time in a younger body is the most valuable asset you can have. As you make your way through this book, don't lose sight of this. For this reason, I am going to ask much more of you.

You were meant for more. It's time to stop settling for less.

We live in a time where until now we could extend life seven to ten years with meds and machines. Ironically living 7 to 10 years longer with meds and machines is hardly the life anyone wants to live.

A new era is upon us. The biological commonalities of the leanest, healthiest, longest lived humans are being uncovered. I call these Peak Humans and their biological states are Peak Human Physiology. The discovery that changes the game is many of these states *can be accessed by anyone.*

THE NEW PARADIGM OF IMMUNE CENTRIC AGING AND HEALTH

A new possibility has arrived. Something far richer than 7 to 10 years with meds and machines is now available. For the first time it is possible to lengthen your window of youth - significantly. You just have to **opt in.** The key, however, is **not** found in what we think of as fitness or weight loss. Instead the key is a new paradigm. The new paradigm is based on learning to control **immune mechanisms** to replicate the same physiological states found in the leanest, healthiest, longest lived humans - peak human physiology. In practice this means using various techniques, hacks if you will, to replicate peak human physiology in your own body. This is not fitness. It's not bodybuilding. It's not weight loss. It's something new. You don't have to give up those things, but they will rest on a new foundation and live in a new reality. In this new reality, learning how immunity works and how to control it for fat loss, health and anti-aging are the new must haves.

Peak human physiology can be quantified. It refers to very specific things. Here are 5 examples.

Peak Human Immune Cells.

The masses face an inevitable process known as *inflammaging.* Inflammaging refers to accelerated aging driven by signals from immune cells reacting to cellular junk. You are going to learn how to "steer" populations of immune cells away from inflammation and aging. You will learn how to drive immune cell types towards the kind that not only reduce inflammation but promote living longer and better. You are going to learn how to control immunity to obtain real health in the new world.

The Healthy Fat Cell Mix:
New science tells us **healthy fat** is as important as low body fat. The Obesity Paradox is a new revelation that many overweight people are in fact super healthy. Eric Esch, better known by his stage name Butterbean, was considered a sideshow event in the world of boxing. At 425 pounds, he looked out of shape, but fans loved to see one of his thunderous knockouts. Unknown to almost everyone but boxing insiders, Eric had a metabolic edge. He was the healthiest fighter in the game. For virtually every measure of health, Eric's blood work would always come back with the best markers in every category. Eric had healthy fat. Healthy fat not only determines whole body health, it also controls aging. Healthy fat is composed of a specific mix of immune cells. The configuration of immune cells in health fat exerts vast control over stem cells, collagen fiber types, and immune signal states. You're going to learn what healthy fat is and how to replicate it.

The Peak Human Enterotype:
An enterotype is a specific profile of gut bacteria. Peak human physiology has commonalities of bacteria species in the gut, what could be called a Peak Human Enterotype. We can rapidly alter gut bacteria species to affect things like energy, cravings and fat metabolism.

Even more important than all the fitness stuff, we can actually reduce your risk for cancer and even influence how long you live! And it's easy. And I have done it longer and with more people than anyone in the world, as you will soon see.

You will learn how to load the Peak Human Enterotype.

Peak Human Gene Activation:
The leanest, longest lived, healthiest humans have certain genetic advantages. Some of these are inherited. Many, however, are things anyone can literally *switch on.* Learning how and when to activate specific genes that control aging on a regular basis will become part of your daily routine. It will be like brushing your teeth. You won't even think about it. It will just be part of how you live life.

Peak Human Cell Maintenance
Our cells have critical maintenance functions that decline with age. These are things like timekeeping and data storage. As these functions decline you age faster. For example, one of these functions is taking out the cellular trash. Young cells are clean. Old cells are

dirty. Peak Humans maintain cellular housekeeping longer. The good news is cellular housekeeping is switchable. You're going to learn how to take out the trash at a cellular level. It's going to keep you younger, much longer. And again, it's easy!

Keeping the body young is our new meta paradigm. Hacking Peak Human Physiology is our new currency.

Historically speaking, massive progress in any area of endeavor is not the result of some increment of an old way of thinking. Massive shifts in progress come when an entirely new way of thinking is introduced. Big shifts result when we put on a new filter. We stop doing things the old way. In a sense this book is like new wine. You can't put it into the old wineskin of the existing paradigm(s).

When you put on a new filter many things we thought were true will turn out to be false. It is when a given body of thought yields to something outside the old thinking that we see big progress. That's what is in store for you.

If you look at the world of fitness, there is a very disturbing trend. A number of iconic figures in the business of health, fitness, and weight loss, i.e., *really fit people,* are dropping dead very young. They look good. They are lean. One after another they are dropping dead before 60. Many before 50. In the modern era we have separated health and long life from the equation.

Real health is missing.

It seems paradoxical that being fit can often be very unhealthy and lead to a much, much shorter life! Health is identified as the most important value for the body by people over 40. The value placed on health by people over 40 is often motivated by personal experience. Someone you know gets cancer or diabetes or has a heart attack. And yet, many aspects of the modern paradigm of fitness and weight loss are in fact **extremely unhealthy.** What we call weight loss and fitness often compromises long term health. We will explore this at length. You will learn how appearance often has nothing to do with immunity. If immunity is the new measure, then we need to re-examine what we automatically associate as being healthy. Many things in the pursuit of health actually *compromise* immunity!

Brenton is a famous fitness guy. I have changed his name. He is rich. He's fit. He's in very poor health. Recently he was hospitalized with a life threatening condition related to decades of steroid use.

Charles Poliquin was one of the most prominent thought leaders in fitness. His Poliquin research certification was a prized credential sought out by many trainers and nutritionists in the field of fitness. He epitomized the look of fitness and the ethos of hormone replacement. The fitness world was shocked by his death at age 57 from a heart attack.

Fitness icon Mandy Blank was always in shape. At 42, she seemed to have the body every woman is striving for. Her death surprised everyone. How could an icon of the paradigm of fitness and health die so young?

If the people who exemplify the solution are dying young can we expect any better?

And it's not just fitness.

As the CEO of gaming retail giant GameSpot, Paul Raines was known for being resilient. He guided the company through many challenges. Under his leadership GameSpot morphed from a retail-based gamer to a digital game company. Paul exuded a youthful countenance. He played video games four hours a week. He ate healthy. Despite all that, he sadly passed away at age 53 from cancer.

Fifty Something: The New Epidemic of Dead.
We have an epidemic of successful people, CEO's, executives, fitness icons and famous people, dropping dead in their 50's from heart attacks, cancer and stroke.

There is something wrong with this picture. Enter something different and better.

THE IMMUNE CENTRIC PARADIGM FOR AGING AND HEALTH

The current paradigm is all about the short term. But virtually every strategy in today's marketplace has significant long term consequences that are never spoken of. Some examples we will cover:

- How a single episode of fat loss or weight loss can spawn a lifetime of chronic weight cycling. The cause? Changes mediated by immune cells.

- How alterations to immune cells from weight cycling can promote long term inflammatory signaling issues.

- How short sighted eating fads can cause temporary improvements in things like gut dysbiosis, but may promote long term immunity problems.

- How working out too much over the long haul can deplete satellite stem cells in muscle and promote fibrosis resulting in "used up" muscles.

- How eating, workout and hormone replacement regimens can drive excess growth signaling and result in shortened life span.

The word *hacking* implies some kind of trick or shortcut. Really it means taking into consideration **time.** *Time and results,* are the essence of hacking. We are going to change the way you go about solving the problems you really want solved. In the process your will learn that much of what you believed to be true was *never really true.*

WHY SHOULD YOU LISTEN TO ME?

So who am I and why should you listen to me? First, a few things you might find interesting. I work out on average about once a week. It's been that way for over a dozen years. I also eat anything and everything I want anytime I want. I don't eat strict but I do **eat for function.** I don't do any meal prep. Most of what I eat is on-the-go healthy fast food. It's something of an ongoing joke with anyone who knows me. This is me on an average day.

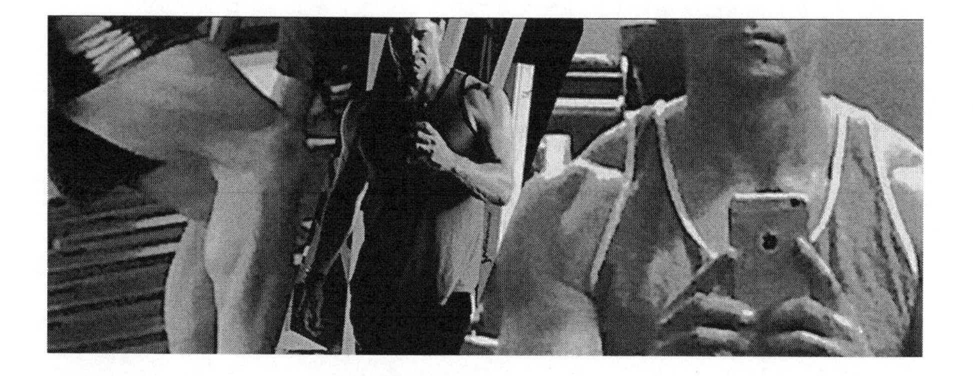

As of this writing I am 55. I don't take steroids or any kind of hormone replacement, TRT, SARMS, GH or any substances like that.

Never have. If you are not over 50, let me tell you, the difficulty of achieving this without steroids, GH or other drugs or peptides is several orders of magnitude more challenging. Many would say it's impossible. You have found the real, real deal.

I said this is new. It's the pursuit of a **young body by learning to control immunity.** You can take a bunch of substances and workout a lot. You will look like an old person who works out a lot and takes hormones and peptides. A young body is something **entirely different.** Young bodies can do things old bodies can't. They are supple, pliable, and full of energy. There is even a simple test. It is the dividing line between a young body and an old one. You can do it right now.

THE YOUNG BODY TEST:

On a moments notice, go from zero to an all out sprint without getting injured.

All healthy kids and teens can do this.

As we go from teens to 20's, 30's and 40's, there comes a line where you can't do this. The simple reason is you are *getting old*. At 55, I do this routinely. I do it for a very good reason. The ability to go from zero to an all out sprint is the one exercise **tied to survival** for almost all mammals. It's why the young survive and the old perish. Before we are done this is something you may even be able to do.

KEY IDEA: Your body has a set of "programs" that tap into survival.

Your "survival wiring" is the most powerful force at work in your body. Any time you tap into the bodies survival programming you get the highest reward for the least effort.

MY RESUME: YOUR ADVANTAGE

Today there is a gut biome expert on every corner. If you go way back to 2006 there **were none. In 2007** I published one of the first, if not **the very first,** article on the gut biome based on Dr. Jeffrey Gordons ground breaking 2006 research that began the gut biome era. You can see it here on my site lookcut.com with the dates from Google.

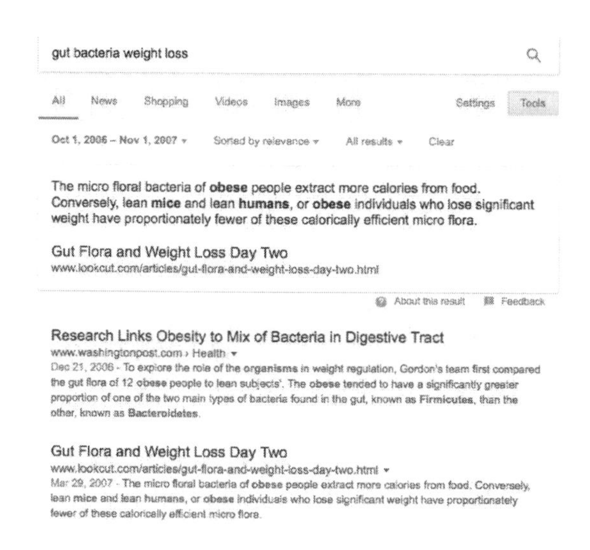

I immediately began experimenting on myself in 2007. I had some astounding results. By using very specific food as substrate for key bacteria I went from 229 lbs to 212 in **7 days!** And I did it with **zero exercise!** It was not by choice. I didn't have the energy. The grumpy countenance below was me on Day 7. My body fat was measured in

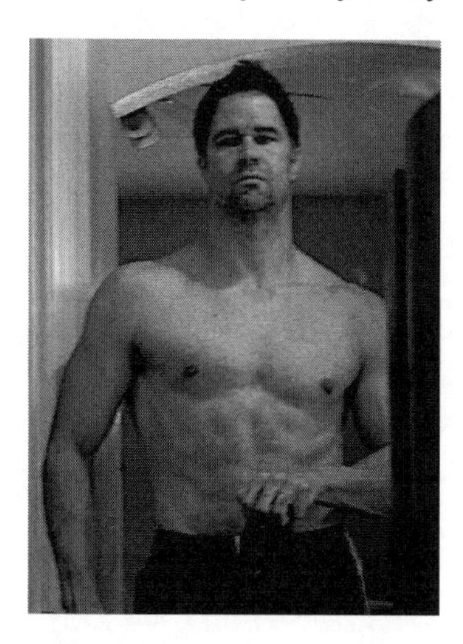

water at **6.7 %.** I knew I was on to something.

My results spawned the creation of the **worlds first** nutrition program (and even to this day the only) based on the gut biome.

This was in my VEEP Nutrition System launched in 2009. I had three advantages. Number one I was first. There were no other gut gurus. **Not a single one.** No one had heard of the gut biome. Number two I had a software used by thousands of people. Number three, I could implement new science protocols and harvest data overnight. These three advantages allowed me to rapidly refine the application of what worked. I jumped ten years ahead. For example, by 2010 I was introducing radical and unheard of new ideas like targeting the gut bacteria via a special protein called ***FAIF,*** or ANGLP4. It's called Fasting Induced Adipose Factor. It controls fat loss. This protein is only now, ten years later, being discovered by what are considered *the* most cutting edge podcasts. It's barely at the awareness stage. Yet I have had it at the application stage for ten years! Here is the proof, from a 2010 facebook post you can look up today.

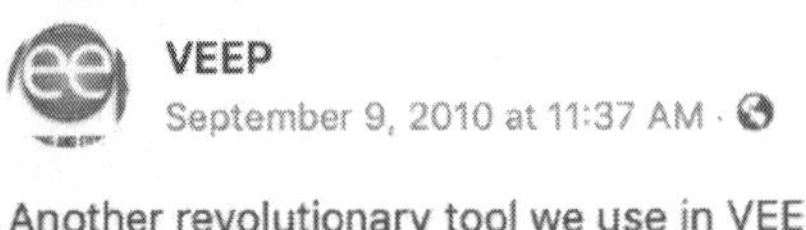

Another revolutionary tool we use in VEEP is to use FOOD to stimulate FAIF - fasting induced adipocyte factor - a protein triggered by certain gut bacteria that increases fatty acid uptake in cells.

I have amassed the **worlds largest known body** of outcomes targeting the gut for body composition.

By 2013 I had developed functional protocols for symptoms of Parkinson's, dairy intolerance and other issues. These were protocols that could seemingly do the impossible literally overnight. This book is the first time I have ever released most of this IP to world apart from the walled garden of my VEEP System.

For example, one of those outcomes from my VEEP system was Andrea. Weighing 322 lbs, and on twenty two medications all at once, Andrea was given five years to live by her doctor. She went on the Dr. Phil Show and was placed on my VEEP System by the show's trainer, my good friend Robert Reames. She hurt her leg in the first month and could not exercise. At month four they gave her a blood test. Shockingly, all her blood parameters were normal. They gave her a second blood test. Her bloodwork was normal. At month four, she was taken off all twenty two medications!

From twenty two meds to none in four months!

There is no drug in existence capable of doing that! This is the power of food used to target **functional outcomes.**

My work has been featured on several Dr. Phil storylines, hospital utilized, used by large employers and entities like the YMCA. I have consulted with billion dollar nutrition companies on concepts like fasting mimicking years before anyone else, designed foods for PhD's to mimic fasting. I have shown consistently shown a track being many years ahead of the field.

For example, in 2015 I introduced the concept stimulating testosterone by targeting the bacteria L.Reuteri in an article published in Muscle and Fitness. This broke the concept to the fitness world. Predictably, within a year of publication several supplement companies were selling L.Reuteri for testosterone. There is just one problem. They did not understand this is something you can not supplement for, which is why I don't sell one myself. I could have made a lot of money. The quick buck has never been what I was after. The purpose, all these years, was one thing - to solve the problem of the body we all face.

If it's popular today I have been doing it at least 20 or 30 years.

- Olympic lifts. Late 70's.
- HIIT Training. Early 80's (there was no word for it then)
- MCT's: Late 80's.
- Keto: Early 90's.
- Fasting and time restricted eating: Mid 90's
- Eating fresh, whole, organic: Late 90's.

Having done those things for many years is a huge advantage for you. I know where all those roads end. In the early 90's I was eating one meal a day in the evening. (Sound familiar) I was ripped to the bone for nearly five years. And then the uncontrolled eating started. Years of time restricted eating had so disrupted the control points over food intake it took nearly 10 years to fix. One of the major reasons you read this book stems from long term negatives I experienced from short sighted protocols. That experience has taught me a biological truth.

The long term effect of anything often opposes the short term effect.

I routinely get asked where I learned all this stuff. "Where did you get all this knowledge?", "Are you a doctor, did you go to med school, how do you know all this?" The answer is really simple.

You can't fake 50,000 hours.

So here is your advantage. **You will jump 10 years ahead.** You will be where the herd will be in 10 years. Over and over, what you will get in this book is not anything you have heard. Examples....

- How if you don't already have cancer long term sustained Keto diets may possibly even ***promote cancer onset.***

- How Intermittent Fasting disrupts REM sleep and activates the bodies starvation defense mechanisms.

- How not one but three different genomes interact to dictate your bodies active operating state.

Revolutionary changes in a way of thinking often come from outside the existing body of thought. The unique proposition here is the things you are about to learn came by way of replicating the real world habitat, not the fitness ecosystem. This unique perspective, the perspective of what it takes to sustain results over time, under real circumstances, is about to change everything. It is what has been missing.

RESTORING THE GUT LINING PART 1

Think of a series of legos. You learn one simple thing. It's easy to do and has great power. Each one builds upon the next. Before you know it, its like you have a black belt in Jiu-Jitsu. That's how you will hack into Peak Human. It is much easier than what you have been doing. By the time we reach the end of the book you will be well equipped to do something that seems impossible - hack into Peak Human physiology, eat anything, anytime, and do it all on the go with no meal prep to keep your body younger, longer. Let's begin.

YOU NEED:

A bag of apples.

THE TO DO:

Day 1-3: Eat skins of two apples,
Day 4-11: Eat skins of four apples,

When to take: mornings.

WHAT IT DOES:

There is one very specific bacteria most responsible for the health of your gut lining. It is called Akkermansia Mucinilpha. It is very difficult to feed directly, meaning, to provide what it needs to thrive. Apple skins are one of the only ways to feed Akkermansia. This is the first of several moves that will allow you to hack into real health via controlling specific immune cells.

IMMUNE 101: INTERLEUKINS

Real immunity is specific. It's not the result of random happenstance, The things you need immunity from work a certain way. A proper approach to real immunity is not a shotgun approach. There are key players. Until you know what they are and how to control them, you can't have real immunity which means you won't have real health. There are three core components to immunity. These three components are **immune cells, immune signals and membrane linings**. Lets meet one of the key players, Interleukin 6.

INTERLEUKINS

Simply put, interleukins are signal molecules. They function as intermediaries between immune cells. Some interleukins seem to be critically involved in inflammatory immune reactions. One of these, Interleukin 6, deserves special attention.

INTERLEUKIN 6

Interleukin 6 is key player in the onset of inflammation, arthritis, cancer, and viral attack. Covid 19 onset involves a massive recruitment of interleukin 6.

HACKING INTERLEUKIN 6: STEP 1

We need Interleukin 6. It's essential. But there are times we need to lower it. One example is with Covid 19. Reducing Il-6 recruitment at the start of Covid 19 onset is an emerging strategy. A first step, or rather a simple baby step to lower IL-6 in the serum, is eating more blueberries and billberries. Increasing blueberry consumption will begin to lower IL-6. Its not a panacea. Its just a simple first step. We will add to this several other steps. Before we are done, you will have a complete picture of how to steer immunity by controlling immune cells, immune signals, and membrane linings.

Chapter 1

The New To Do

THE NEW TO DO

I have a younger brother. If not for the fact he was born with Down's Syndrome we might have been almost twins. We have the same dark hair and blue eyes. He is a very special soul. About a year ago I noticed he was starting to have symptoms of Parkinson's; tremors, a downward progression in his demeanor, and a lack of energy. The progression of symptoms became very rapid . Within a year he went from his normally happy, ebullient personality to a catatonic rigor. I brought him home with me for a week to work on his health. He was in pretty bad shape at the start. He couldn't walk twenty yards without collapsing. He was barely able to support his own weight. He was sleeping just a few hours a night, and dealing with severe depression. His tremors at times would take over uncontrollably.

He wasn't a candidate for exercise. He could barely walk. I am sharing this with you to help you understand just how much is really possible. I set about doing many of the things you will learn herein. In a short seven days my brother went from full blown Parkinson's onset to the following.

- He had 100 percent amelioration of Parkinson's symptoms. **100 percent. No tremors. No shaking. None**

- He went from collapsing after walking twenty yards to being able to walk half a mile and go up and down a flight of stairs unaided several times per day.

- His old personality was ninety percent restored. He went from being catatonic much of the time to being engaged, talkative and vibrant.

- He went from sleeping five hours per night to sleeping twelve.

By day four he was feeling so good we took him to Trader Joe's. He broke away and bolted down one of the aisles in an energetic sprint (it was really a fast paced run/walk but for him it was a sprint). He could barely walk a few days earlier.

Let me recap. Seven days total. **100 percent asymptomatic of Parkinson's.**

Not possible you say? **It is possible.** I have it recorded on video.

I am a very private person. This is not something I share easily but I wanted to share this to demonstrate a new premise to you.

It's possible to keep the body younger and drive real health by focusing on a few master mechanisms.

You see, in seven days what happened with my brother was a radical alteration of his physiology. In short, I swapped the physiology of Parkinson's and replicated a Peak Human physiology into his body. The results were astounding. Just like Andrea's story from the Dr. Phil Show storyline, and even my own radical fat loss drop in 2007, things that seem impossible were not only very possible, but much easier than you might think, and mostly without exercise. I'm not advocating that you don't exercise. **You absolutely, 100 percent, must exercise.** The point I'm making is what is possible apart from exercise by focusing on a few key master mechanisms, things like immune populations, the gut biome and signal pathways form a new paradigm.

This is not the old stuff you are used to. This is something new. And it has everything to do with what you will learn in the next couple of chapters. To do this you have to understand what goes into a Peak Human physiology, what the parts are, and then how to map those things on to your body.

The key is knowing **what** to do. I am talking about a power. The power I speak of is **the power to *control* your body.** Control over your body comes down to one word.

DO.

It all comes down to what you ***do*** at any given moment.

When you decide to make a change it all comes down to a decision to start doing stuff. Toward that end, in your journey you have acquired a ***to-do*** list. The list contains the boxes you check. Whatever your list, I suggest all along there has been something missing. The first thing missing has been the right focus. Focus is the thing you are aiming for. The second thing missing has been **what, when and how***.* It's knowing the right things to do, at the right time and in the right way.

I won't sugar coat it. You will still have to **do stuff.** But keeping the body younger longer **is different.** It's not the same to-do list. **It's**

different stuff. You only have so much time. Where you put time has a return on investment. Some things just matter much, much more than others. Let me give you a couple of quick to-do's so you get the basic idea.

Right now, at this exact moment, the most important thing is you keep breathing. Continuing to breathe, in the next 5 minutes, is much, much, more important than what you eat, any exercise you do, or any supplement you might take.

Maybe that sounds ridiculous, but with a bit of thought it really isn't.

Think about something, to varying degrees, **most of us** either don't get enough air, or stop breathing altogether every night. It's called apnea and hypoxia. As we age and the airway begins to contract, the jaw and face structure loses bone mass. Our blood thickens and clumps. Poor circulation, apnea and hypoxia during sleep are common. A funny thing happens wherever we see chronic or intermittent hypoxia. **We find cancer.** Just being fit does not solve it. Lots of fit people suffer from chronic hypoxia. In fact, many fit people, may be **more cancer prone.**

Your body has a couple of proteins it makes when tissues are oxygen starved. One of them is called HIF-1, or hypoxia inducible factor one. HIF-1 is a sensor. It senses oxygen levels in cells.

HIF-1 has what can be called duality. It can be bad or it can be good. HIF-1 works in conjunction with a master mechanism that can control your rate of aging. In that sense it's good. On the other hand, it is also connected to driving cancer. In that sense it's really bad.

As you get older, a condition called **pseudo hypoxia** can take place. Pseudo hypoxia happens when cells accumulate the HIF-1 protein. This means, even though you are breathing and oxygenating the body during the day, your cells are signaling oxygen starvation! This is one of the ways HIF-1 can drive cancer. For starters, clearing the body of excess HIF-1 is a promising way to mitigate things like breast cancer.

A powerful way to keep the body young is to clear excess accumulation of HIF-1.

Once again, the trick is that HIF-1 can also be good. In certain tissues at specific times and conditions you want to make it. At other times you want to suppress it and clear it. For example, you want to make this protein right after working out. It helps you recover from exercise and make better gains. You can actually induce more of it via simple *hypoventilation training* during exercise. You also want to make it in the dermis of your skin. It helps skin regenerate and profile younger.

Where you don't want to make HIF-1 is during sleep with intermittent hypoxia. Too much of HIF-1 from intermittent hypoxia, particularly in your brain, disrupts sleep. In turn this promotes obesity and cancer, and can disrupt the heart's pacemaking mechanism, known as the carotid.

HIF-1: THE GOOD AND BAD
Good: Post workout .
Good: Fasting.
Good: The dermis.
Bad: During sleep.
Bad: Obesity or overweight.
Bad: Age related accumulation.

Lets look at a couple of quick and easy to-do's in this new way of thinking that help on both ends of HIF-1.

INDUCING MORE HIF-1 POST WORKOUT

Whatever your workout, at the end, do your last two sets or exercises using hypoventilation. Hypoventilation means you hold your breath for varying periods.

THE WHAT: Hypoventilation to stimulate HIF-1 and aid workout recovery.
THE WHEN: One or two sets at the end of your workout.
THE HOW: One set or exercise with high lung volume. One with low lung volume.

High Lung Volume: Take in a full breath and perform the exercise while holding your breath.

Low Lung Volume: Empty your lungs *half way* by exhaling as you normally would. Then perform the last exercise while holding your breath.

This simple technique adds hypoxic stress during exercise. It increases HIF-1 at the end of your workout. This will help you recover better. It's not a panacea. However it is one of a series of small 5% improvements that take little to no time. This is the essence of the **new to-do.**

CLEARING HIF-1 DURING SLEEP

THE WHAT: Niacin + Zinc
THE WHEN: At bed time for 2 weeks
THE HOW: After 2 weeks use ketone bodies at bed for 1 week. Zinc and niacin help clear HIF-1 in different tissues. Ketone bodies like Beta Hydroxybutyrate do the reverse, but in a very healthy and therapeutic way. This is a preliminary step for other to-do's coming later. It's not something you need to do all the time, but once or twice a year this helps clear excess HIF-1.

Are you starting to get this? This is a different to-do list and a different way of thinking. You just got 2 very small to-do's that take literally no time.

If you continue with me down this path it will rewrite all your to-do lists. You will get a different set of boxes to check. I could spend 30 minutes today training my biceps. Alternatively I could spend 2 minutes to prevent sleep hypoxia. If my time was short, what would you choose to do? At the very least it makes you think doesn't it?

THE CORE IDEA

There is one idea everything you **do** from here on out is based on.

It is the idea of a very small change played out over many years. The course correction from one small thing becomes massive over time. And then, stacking a handful of these small changes the net difference in ten, twenty, or thirty years and beyond, is life altering. Everything to come is based on this one idea.

YOU DON'T HAVE TO DO WELL TO DO AMAZING

Odds are you are **not** going to put into practice everything you learn in this book. The good news is **you don't have to.** Each of the key to-do's in this book is, by itself, a radical life change. If you implement just one, such as the Integrated Interval, or the 2 Day Immunity Core Pattern, or learning to spin down inflammaging, or learning how to recolonize your gut on cue, and any one of a dozen other to-do's, you will create a small daily change that becomes life altering over years and decades. Some will implement two things. A smaller number will implement three of the to-do's. For those who can adapt three to-do's from this book profound life change awaits you. A very few, **the outliers,** will do everything in this book to the letter. The outliers will achieve a radical jump into peak human physiology and massively extended lifespan and window of youth. Wherever you land, remember, you don't have to do well to do amazing. Just **one simple item** from this book adapted into your life will create powerful life changing results long term.

PROBABILITIES DRIVE OUTCOMES

You are going to hear me talk a lot about probabilities. The reason is probabilities drive predictable outcomes. I said real health is missing. One reason why is t**he math is missing.** We have invented all sorts of modern contrivances to explain why we do what we do; emotional eating, smart choices, commitment, and many others. What no one has really done is simply looked at the math. You are going to get beyond contrivances. You will see that all along, powerful underlying probabilities, have been driving the outcomes we see en masse and in your own life. This book is a first in the sense that the entire work has been designed around beating the previously undefined probabilities we all face over time. You are going to get much better odds.

THE IMMUNE FOUNDATION

Much of the rest of the book depends on you understanding **one big word.** It's not that hard to get. The word is really two words. *Macro* and *phage*. We are all familiar with macro. It means big. Phage means *eater.* Put together the word is **macrophage**. It means "big eater."

A macrophage is an immune cell. Macrophages keep everything clean. They eat stuff and do housekeeping. Mostly they eat cellular debris, but they also eat pathogens. When tissues need repair macrophages show up and do a lot of the heavy lifting.

There are different types of macrophages. Some reduce inflammation, some promote it. Most of what you really need to know about how to control your body will revolve around learning to control these things. Before we are done, "macrophage" will be a **word you use every day.**

KEY IDEA: If you can learn to "steer" and control macrophages, you can control immunity, health and aging.

Colorful analogies help us remember things and depolarize our brains from the fear state that big words trigger. For simplicity, let's call the inflammatory macrophages the **Red Team**. Red means they *inflame.* Let's call the anti-inflammatory macrophages the **Blue Team.** Blue means they *cool* things down.

OUR MACROPHAGE MEME
Inflammatory Macrophages: The Red Team
Anti-Inflammatory Macrophages: The Blue Team

Just like HIF-1, macrophages have duality. They can be good or bad. While the Red Team/Blue Team analogy is an oversimplification, it holds in most of the cases we will concern ourselves with.

The Red Team has a proper role. We need them. They are the killers. They show up at the onset of injury. Injury can be physical, like when you break a leg or tear a muscle, or pathogenic, like when you get an infection. Interestingly, the red macrophages tend to be where we find the hypoxia protein HIF-1.

The Red Team are first responders. They recruit inflammation and initiate an exact sequence of biochemical events and signals that engage the healing process. But eventually we need them to go away. The Blue Team are the healers. They are the clean up crew. The Blue Team needs to come in and clean things up and clear infection. That's the problem. With age, large populations of the Red Team become ever present.

Obtaining real health to keep your body young can be viewed as a balance of immune cells. You will see how this holds true tissue by tissue, from your blood to your gut to your body fat. When your body as a whole gets too many of the Red Team and too few of the Blue Team:

- You can't lose weight.
- You tend to have a weak immune system
- You tend to be cancer prone.
- You age faster than you otherwise would.

As the Red Team dominates, responding to aging as if it were a system-wide injury, inflammatory signals propagate and your body falls apart much faster.

NEW IDEA: STEERING IMMUNE CELLS
Coming up with ways to help your body "steer" towards the Blue Team or rebalance the killers vs the healers, is almost entirely the future of pharmaceutical drugs for many conditions. As it turns out steering macrophages is something you can actually do everyday yourself.

KEY IDEA: *Obtaining real health and aging slower involves understanding how to **shift and rebalance** macrophage populations.*

Learning how to shift populations of macrophages toward those that reduce inflammation is the center of The Immunity Code. This will become as important to you, if not even more important than your diet or exercise. It's that critical. **And it's a new to-do.** Once you learn how to steer macrophages, in particular macrophages in key tissues, such as your fat mass and your gut lining, and your lungs, you will get your first oar in the water to control the things that control your susceptibility to things like COVID and the decline of the body and even aging itself.

Hif-1 and macrophages - these will form the basis of your new paradigm for health. With these two mechanisms, you can understand a new way of thinking about how you care for your body. With these two mechanisms, you can understand everything else.

For example, at the end of the last chapter you learned about Interleukin 6.

KEY IDEA: One of the ways we control interleukins is by controlling macrophages.

Are you getting this?

If not, take another read of this last section. It may seem daunting at first, but keep in mind what we are talking about - **the most important consideration in the new world** - your health. You are going to have to put in some effort.

STEERING MACROPHAGES 101:

The way we steer macrophages is **tissue by tissue.** The same macrophages can work very differently in different tissues. Order of operations matters here. A lot. We start with the most important tissues and work our way through the body. Here is the order of operations we will do in this book by order of importance.

1. The Gut Lining:
2. Body Fat Mass:
3. The Blood
4. The lungs
5. Gums
6. Brain
7. Organs
8. Cells at large

Our goal by the end of the book is three things. Our first goal is to give equip you with an immunity centric approach to health and aging. Next is to give you a new and better to do list. And finally, to give you key abilities that give you a power you don't currently have to control your body.

An order of operations is like baking a cake. The sequence matters. This entire book is one giant to-do list in **order** of operations. One to-do may seem to have no connection to the next one but like the steps to bake a cake **they are connected!** You will discover how and why chapter by chapter.

ABILITIES BEAT LIFESTYLE

You hear a lot of talk about the "healthcare crisis." Every day another company springs up to solve the healthcare problem. Yet the obvious solution, ***which is just to stay healthy,*** seems to elude the great mass of people over time.

Why?

Why does the simple solution - staying healthy - elude the great mass of people over time?

On the part of you the consumer, it's not for lack of trying. **You keep trying, repeatedly.** Despite the body transformations, before and after pics, despite all the healthy choices, when you widen the window far enough, even people who devote themselves to looking fit suffer the same problems: heart attacks, cancer, mobility issues and shortened life spans.

You want real change? Don't focus on lifestyle. Focus on acquiring **abilities.** This is *not about a lifestyle.*

This is a book on acquiring *abilities.*

Abilities are power. Abilities are skills and skills solve real problems. The purpose of every to-do in this book is to *build abilities.* There are 3 meta-abilities you must acquire. Each is like a super power. At first, you are going to think you have these all figured out. As we progress, you will discover we are in virgin territory with each.

THE 3 POWERS.

You need three abilities, or rather 3 powers. You need to learn how to eat, how to age slower, and how to lose fat without triggering weight regain. I call these the three powers because having them is like a superpower. Each is something new, and breaks new ground and changes the way you think about what is on your to-do list.

Here are the three powers.

THE FIRST POWER: LEARNING HOW TO EAT

Learning ***how*** to eat is perhaps the most critical skill you will ever acquire in order to control your body. How to eat is not focusing on macro's, or dieting, or any diet, or even a dietology (a dietology is when you merge a diet with your highest beliefs of what is good and right). In fact learning how to eat is not anything you know. Learning **how** to eat is 100% virgin territory. It involves things such as sequencing meals, timing, combinations of foods and amounts for specific **functional outcomes.** What is a functional outcome? You have already begun. You have begun eating to restore the gut lining and spin down Interluekin 6. This is something entirely new. It is the ***what,*** the ***when*** and the ***how.*** "What, when and how", is what you have always wanted to know. "What, when and how", give you control over your body in the real world.

THE SECOND POWER: HOW TO CONTROL YOUR FAT

We are going to spend a lot of time talking about body fat. The reason is **body fat is central to immunity.** Because body fat is central to immunity it's central to aging. This makes body fat a bigger conversation than the old fitness approach. Everything you knew about body fat will be deconstructed, overturned and washed away. A new era will begin. You will have a new emphasis. Up until now the focus was losing fat. Going forward the emphasis will be controlling fat to control immunity. Control of fat is a much higher order with far more reaching benefits. Body fat is also co-equal with the gut lining and the blood in steering immune cell populations. Conversely, losing body fat, or rather, the way we have been coached to lose it, is a massive driver of the long term problem. You are going to learn that losing body fat at a cellular level is creating injury. You will gain the power to **steer the health** of your fat. This is the power to be one and done with fat loss in order to steer immune cells to keep you younger longer. It will change your life for the better forever.

THE THIRD POWER: HOW TO AGE SLOWER

You are going to learn how to actively take control of some of the most powerful components that affect your rate of aging. You will learn how to literally command your body to age at a slower rate on any given day. Far from hype this is real science applied in powerful ways. You will acquire very useful abilities.

- The ability to steer immune cells toward healthy populations.
- The ability to amplify fasting. Amplified fasting is the next step in anti aging.
- The ability to steer the bacteria in your gut toward maximum immune function.
- The ability to activate signal pathways that govern immunity, youth and aging.
- The ability to turn on key anti-cancer mechanisms on a regular basis.
- The ability to make insulin function better to slow aging.
- The ability to stay lean on the go with no meal prep.
- The ability to spin down whole body inflammation to age slower.

The three powers, how to eat, how to age slower, and how to control body fat, will give you real health. You will gain access to freedom in the new world, which going forward, will depend heavily on your health.

With each chapter, as you complete the different to-do's, you will build an inventory of easy to do, non-time intensive actions that all work together. A funny thing is going to start to happen.

You are going to begin to feel amazing.

You are going to find the energy of youth flowing again. You are going to find a vitality filling your body. And it's going to be easy.

TO-DO: STEERING MACROPHAGES 101

Begin Restoring the Gut Lining by Restoring Akkermansia Mucinilpha

Add this on to what you learned at the end of the last chapter. This is the first major step in learning to control immunity by steering populations of macrophages.

YOU NEED:

Some baby formula with HMO on the label (Human Milk Oligosaccharides) or you can order pure HMO on our website. You can get these in single serving canisters or if you have the powdered stuff it will work fine. The key is it says "HMO" on the label.

WHAT THEY ARE

HMO's are specialized carbohydrates. They are the main carbohydrate in mothers milk. They stimulate Bifidobacterium longum and other key strains of Bifidobacteria. They also drive immunity in the gut.

THE TO DO:

Day 6-8: Skins of 4 apples, and 1 gram HMO powder or 1 serving baby formula
Day 9-12: Skins of 4 apples, 1 gram HMO powder or 1 serving baby formula.

You don't have to worry about exacting precision here with each day and the amount of apple skins and HMO. The basic idea is to start very small. You build up dosing as you go. Our bodies are all different, and dosing will vary by individual.

When to take: Mornings before breakfast.

WHAT IT DOES:

The carbohydrate present in HMO helps steer immunity in the gut by driving macrophage types. We are steering macrophages in the most important tissue where they get compromised by restoring the gut lining. This will selectively feed very specific bacteria that promote the Blue Teams. You will feel this immediately. You may begin going to the bathroom more frequently. In later chapters, you will learn more about why and how this works as part of steering macrophages. For now, enjoy the benefits of more energy, better digestion and improved cognition.

Chapter 2

The Map of Peak Human

A simple way to think of aging is deterioration.

Aging is deterioration.

The really important question is what specifically is deteriorating? As we go through this book the answer may often surprise you. Generally speaking, aging is not any one thing. It's a number of interconnected things that seem to converge around immunity. Aging is marked by a **decrease** in some things and an **increase** in other things.

Here are some of the most important things decreasing with age.

- Energy production declines.
- Blood viscosity declines.
- Circadian rhythm declines
- B vitamin production declines.
- Membrane permeability and voltage signaling within your cells declines.
- Mitochondrial number and efficiency decline.
- Cellular maintenance and housekeeping declines.
- Bifidobacteria levels decline.
- Stomach pH declines.
- Cellular reserves of anti-oxidants decline.
- Key proteins that regulate growth decline.

At the same time these things are decreasing other things are increasing. Here are some of the most important.

- Inflammatory macrophages increase.
- Blood coagulation increases.
- DNA damage increases.
- Levels of cellular free radical damage increase.
- Errors when reading and copying DNA increase.
- Inflammatory signals increase.
- The number of non-dividing cells increases.
- Immune cell receptors fueling inflammation increase.
- Pools of iron both inside and outside your cells are increasing.

The decline of some things and increase in others mean one thing - there is a general level of deterioration.

Again, **It isn't any one thing.**

The fact it's not any one thing is at odds with the non-stop programming of the marketplace. The marketplace wants you to buy into something that never was and never will be true - that aging is due to one thing.

According to the marketplace, it's just the molecular lifespan clock in each cell - the telomeres, or it's a pill that reverses aging. But we just listed many things that contribute to the sum of the problem, not one thing.

So stop believing aging is due to one thing. It's not.

That being said, the fact many things are at work, does not mean everything is equal. And that brings us to the really interesting question.

Is there an order of operations to slowing aging?

What are the most important things, in order, to keep the body young? Now that is a really important question don't you think? In recent years, new research has peeled back the interconnected causality of not just aging, but virtually every disease, with shifting populations of immune cells.

IMMUNITY AND AGING: THE CRUX VARIABLE HIDDEN IN PLAIN SIGHT

New science of the last decade has uncloaked a simple, obvious master accelerator of the aging process.

Changes in immune signals accelerate aging.

In many ways, aging is biochemically identical to an injury. Many of the exact same systems kick in to deal with both.

A new way to look at aging is to view it as a problem of immunity.

The immune system is doing the exact same things it would do with a localized injury, but across the whole body. Have you ever had an area of your body stay constantly inflamed, as in say a skin disorder? You may have noticed the inflamed area just looks older than the areas that are not inflamed.

Recently Usain Bolt, the greatest sprinter the world has ever seen was quoted as saying, "My body is saying it's time to go. Every morning I wake up, I'm in a little pain here, a little pain there."

As of this writing Usain is facing his 31st birthday. He's a young man by most standards, except the elite standard of being the worlds fastest human, where even now, at his young age, his cells are already beginning the immune shift toward the inflammatory macrophages and he is starting to feel it.

If you break down the actual thing that Usain is feeling, the thing causing the aches is inflammation. *Inflammation,* mediated by immune cells like the Red Team is the **signal** telling Usain Bolt that it's time to retire. .

Inflammaging is the new word for when inflammation accelerates aging.

INFLAMMAGING: WHEN INFLAMMATION ACTS LIKE A VIRUS

Inflammaging is the idea that signals from inflammation essentially act like a virus. Here is how it works.

JUNK ACCRUES:

As we age, cellular junk along with cells that no longer divide begins to *increase.* At the same time a number of very important maintenance functions *decrease*. The inflammatory "signal noise" from the cellular junk is interpreted by your body's defenses as a system wide injury. To deal with the injury the Red Teams multiply. In effect, the Red Team **responds to aging like its one giant injury.**

THE BLOOD CATCHES FIRE

The blood is the transport system for inflammatory signals. In essence, your blood works like a river to ferry inflammation signals across the body. Inflammatory signals are downloaded into what amount to cellular jump drives. These jump drives, called exosomes, spread via the blood. Just like a virus, they download inflammatory signals into cells and organs in other parts of the body. It gets worse.

With age, the blood itself becomes a pro-inflammatory medium.

The blood becomes like an oil spill on a river that catches fire. The mechanism is *old blood.* Young blood has a balance between red blood cells and different types of immune cells. With age production of blood changes. As we age the blood becomes imbalanced. The makeup of blood shifts. You have fewer red blood cells and more immune cells. The blood itself works to spread inflammation across the body.

As the "fire" gains intensity, the decline of the system as a whole accelerates. This establishes a foundational idea for our journey together.

KEY IDEA: Immunity and aging are one. They are two sides of the same coin.

TELOMERE LENGTH EXPOSED

Returning to the idea that aging is one thing, I have studied aging a long time. I have looked at many theories by the worlds most well credentialed experts for many years. The thing is, they don't agree. There are many theories as to why we age. Some of the older theories have to do with free radical damage and the mitochondria. There are also several newer theories. One is called Network Theory. Its the idea that a network of cellular defense mechanisms control aging. Another is called Remodeling Theory.

THE IMMUNE HYPOTHESIS OF AGING

Remodeling theory is an immune centric theory of aging that says our immune system makes trade offs in aging. The theory is our bodies balance immunity defense vs declining cell function. The immune defense of older populations becomes overworked trying to repair increasing populations of cells that have issues. It's a compelling theory. In light of recent data showing the Covid-19 virus has its highest mortality rate in older populations with declining immunity, the notion of aging and immune function has been thrust upon us all.

In fact, many of the most popular and over-subscribed theories on aging are starting to show cracks.

One such idea is the notion telomere length drives aging. This is the one thing we should focus on, says both the marketplace and many authorities as well. Yet, several recent studies say otherwise. Most notable, was a 2015 study in the *Journal of eBioMedicine* on populations living longer than 100 years of age in Japan. This study demonstrated that inflammation has **a much more powerful effect on the aging process** than telomere length. In very long lived individuals telomere length has far less of an impact on aging than inflammation. Going further, the marketplace now tells us we can know our real biological age via DNA methylation markers that estimate telomere length. Yet several recent studies have found that specific types of sugar proteins in the serum, called glycans, are **far more accurate predictors of biological age than methylation.** Specific types of serum *glycans* are linked to inflammaging and immunity. The reason is they **predict inflammation and immunity.** What this newer data indicates is that runaway inflammatory signals are the most powerful factor to accelerate the aging process and potentiate many disease states up to and including cancer. The word for this is **inflammaging.**

The driving mechanism behind inflammaging is shifting populations of immune cells.

IT'S NOT ALL BAD

Ironically, inflammaging itself may not necessarily be bad! Like everything else, it has duality. It can be both good and bad. It seems the longest lived humans have inflammaging in a chronic low grade state. What makes them unique is they have adapted several mechanisms to offset the effects of inflammaging that most people do not possess. These mechanisms seem to potentiate long life. A key focus in this book is the "switchability", or "acquirability" of those defense mechanisms, via controlling immune centric mechanisms. Toward that end, learning to steer and control macrophage populations and other immune centric **abilities and toolsets** will be part of your new skill set. Another example is the anti-oxidant catalase. Super long lived people just seem to make more of this anti-oxidant than the rest of us. One technique, or hack, will center around conditioning the fitness of key cellular mechanisms to produce catalase.

If you feel you are getting old overnight pay extra close attention to this next paragraph. In the last chapter I laid out the order of operations for steering immune cell populations via controlling macrophages. At the top of the list was the gut lining. Here is why.

THE BODY FAT/GUT LINING AXIS

The largest concentration of macrophages in the entire body is in the gut lining, just below the cells that line the gut. This layer is called the Lamina Propia. Generally speaking, **immunity begins where your inner body meets the outside world.**

Apart from the gums, the place the outside world most often meets your body is the gut lining. The gut lining is the **first** incursion point for shifting populations of macrophages.

The gut lining is a thin 2 sheet layer of mucus. The top layer is like a kelp forrest. Protective bacteria live in, what is, on their scale. an ocean, and forage here. These bacteria are called **commensal.** Commensal refers to when two different species live together and benefit one another, like humans and dogs. Dogs are commensal with humans. Commensal bacteria in your gut are like guardian pets. They keep the creepies out. The most important bacteria in this layer is called Akkermansia Mucinilpha (not by coincidence, the very first thing I had you target). As we age, because no one ever taught you "what, when and how", regarding this bacteria - what it is, what it does, when to feed it and how, you accidentally starved it out. In turn this wore down your gut lining. Picture a kelp forrest where the water recedes and exposes the kelp to the sun and the fish die. That's analogous to what happens to the gut lining. Not to worry, we can bring it back.

When the gut lining is worn down, cell wall fragments of bacteria, let's call them LPS for short (we don't need the big word here, the abbreviation will do), penetrate into the Lamina Propia, where the macrophages reside. When the outer world penetrates into the macrophage defense layer, **it's an injury.** You may not feel it, but it is an injury nonetheless. This injury, like all injures, causes an **immune reaction. Interleukin 6** becomes hyper activated. This causes a shift in macrophage populations. In turn, immune signals shift toward the kind that make you susceptible to disease. After penetrating the gut lining, LPS and other bad bacteria can penetrate into the bloodstream.

NEXT: LPS FINDS YOUR FAT

Once in the blood LPS has an affinity for your body fat and causes proliferation of the Red Teams in your body fat. This causes all sorts of problems. The first, and least of our problems when this happens is weight gain. It's easier to gain weight and harder to lose it. There is a word for this - **macrophage infiltration.**

By the way, if you Google "macrophage infiltration weight loss", history repeats. Just like in 2007, when I published the first article on the gut, history repeats, this time with macrophages. Once again **the only non research publication in the world** on this topic is written by me - dated 2017 in Google. With Covid-19, you can bet that In five years, just like the gut is today, there will be a macrophage guru on every corner. But you are ahead of the curve just by reading this.

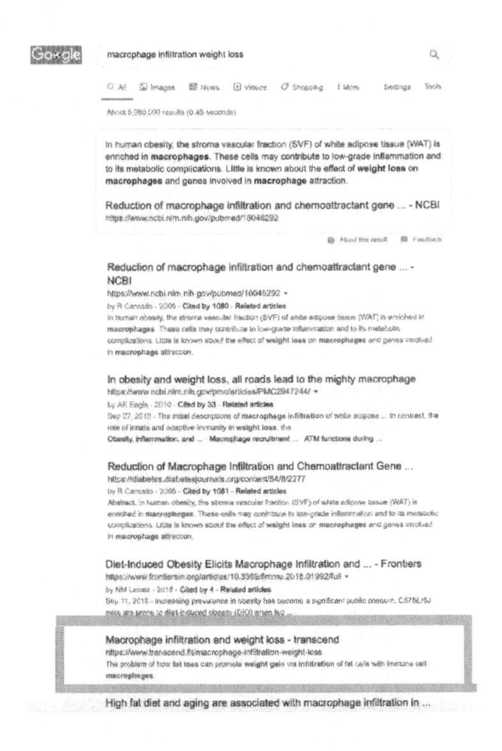

In the last chapter I laid out the idea that **fat loss is an injury.** Injury provokes an immune response. The body's response to injury is the Red Team shows up. There is a vast problem most people suffer from that is almost totally unrecognized. It is the combination of a compromised gut lining, leading to body fat already infiltrated by Red Team, and then on top of that we add fat loss, which itself is an injury. What I am doing here is laying a new foundation to understand something unprecedented. We will spend nearly a quarter of the book on this. It is the idea that we have been creating **repeated untreated injuries** from the modern era of weight loss and fat loss. These untreated injuries accumulate over time. What you think of as a weight gain problem is in fact a problem of immune centric mechanisms.

Body fat works something like a megaphone. It magnifies inflammatory signals. The reason is partially due to the sheer number of cells involved. This gives body fat more strength, i.e., "volume", than other tissues. With age the immune signaling of your body fat becomes compromised. When this happens, **the immune status of your fat can in essence be "downloaded" into other cells.** Your inner organs in particular are at risk. As we age body fat shifts from under the skin to the organs and the inner body cavity. If you struggle with the upper distended gut this is you.

That's a much simplified but generally accurate big picture of the **Body Fat/Gut Lining Axis.** As a concept it gives us cause to rethink a few things

RETHINKING EVERYTHING 101:

- Immune cell populations in our body fat are a key control point of total health and aging.
- We can not address body fat without addressing the gut lining.
- The idea of simply losing body fat is an outdated notion that often drives the problem long term. **Controlling body fat** is a much more up to date and comprehensive idea.

Have I given you a lot to think about? As you progress through the book I urge you to grab on to one simple idea.

Forget what you know.

Before we are done I promise you, you **will** rethink everything and you will see clearly an order of operations.

TOWARD A MAP OF PEAK HUMAN PHYSIOLOGY

I've shown you a list of the most important things that are **decreasing** and things that are **increasing as you age.** The emphasis is on learning to steer and control types of immune cell populations.

What is very interesting is from the two lists I started this chapter with is we can construct a couple of profiles. We can construct the profile of an **older, faster physiology.** An older, faster, physiology is the one your were doomed to prior to picking up this book. It is the physiology most people fall into - a state of accelerated aging.

We can also construct a profile of **younger, longer physiology.** The younger, longer, physiology is one that you can begin to replicate. It represents a **Peak Human** state of physiological advantages. Something profoundly interesting is many, if not most, of the items in our list are things that are specific and measurable. We have even begun. the process of stack ranking which things matter most, such as immune populations.

In short, we can build a map.

What do maps do? They tell you how to get where you want to go. They tell you the shortest route. They also keep you from getting lost. Have you ever been moving forward toward a destination only to reach a dead end? It's frustrating. You lose time. A map can show you that many possible forward routes are ultimately dead ends.

THE MAP OF A PEAK HUMAN PHYSIOLOGY

You need a map. It's what you have always needed. A map gives us the turn by turn steps we need. So here it is- the worlds first map of Peak Human physiology.

- Sleep 7 to 8 hours per night.
- Regular activation of youth promoting signal pathways and mechanisms.
- High levels of bifidobacteria
- Viscous blood with higher levels of specific proteins.
- Low populations of inflammatory macrophages (Red Teams)
- Cellular energy production is relatively high.
- Cellular membrane voltage is higher and membranes are permeable.
- Reservoirs of molecules within cells to offset free radical damage are high.
- Fat mass is extremely healthy, with the right mix of macrophages and collagen fibers
- Gut lining is intact with high populations of Akkermansia.
- Circulation is excellent and key circulatory markers are high.
- Immune cell receptors that represent youth dominate.
- Immune cell receptors that represent age are minimal.

Those are the generalities of what a map would need. But only specifics solve problems. Now let me give you the specifics. None of the following will make an ounce of sense to you right now. By the time you finish this book, however, each of the following points will be a clear goal in your mind and you will understand each perfectly. There will be a couple of words you are not familiar with here. Don't get intimidated. By the end of the book you will use them every day.

THE SPECIFIC MAP

- High levels of Akkermansia Mucinilpha in the gut lining.
- High levels of Bifidobacteria in the gut.
- High levels of the metabolite Butyrate in the gut.
- High levels of anti-inflammatory macrophages in the body fat.
- Low levels of body fat.
- High levels of proteins found in young blood.
- Low levels of the blood clumping protein fibrinogen
- Regular activation of the AMPK pathway.
- Low levels of the immune cell receptor CD38.
- High levels of NAD+.
- Low levels of the hypoxia protein HIF-1 in cells.
- High levels of melatonin production.

Like settings on a dial, this is what you need. This is how you stay young.

That's the map.

This is what you have always needed, a clear map. If you can get your body to replicate all this, you can stay younger much, much longer. The map is specific. It's even measurable. And the best part is it's immediately actionable. And it totally and forever changes your idea of what being "off track" is. It charts a new course, one you can take action on right now.

For the rest of your days on this earth, this map will be your guide to Peak Human physiology and staying younger, longer. If you follow this map, I absolutely, positively guarantee you will maximize your youth, your energy, your health, and your time on this planet.

For the rest of this book we will concern ourselves with why these things matter and how to make obtaining each one of these points easy and doable at every stage of your life even when you have zero time.

TO-DO: STEERING MACROPHAGES 201

Driving cross reactions with Bifidobacteria and Akkermansia

Continuing on from the 101 lesson, add this now.

YOU NEED:

Red phenol powder. This is a powdered mix of red fruits - raspberries, grapefruit, apples, and many others. You can get it on our site or there are several commercial brands. You can even find this at WalMart. It's not expensive. Organic is always better.

WHAT THEY ARE

Specialized color pigments that are a key food source for Bifidobacteria.

THE TO DO:

- Day 12-15 : Skins of 4 apples, 2 scoops HMO powder, 1 scoop red phenol powder.
- Day 16-20: Skins of 4 apples, 2 scoops HMO powder. 2 scoops red phenol powder
- When to take: Take 1 scoop red powder in the morning and 1 after lunch. As previously noted, you don't have to be exacting on the dosing presented here at each day. Just get the main idea - you are starting small and building up.

WHAT IT DOES:

The red phenol powder is a great food source for Bifidobacteria. It will drive what are known as "cross feeding reactions." In other words, you feed Bifidobacteria what it needs, and Bifidobacteria will feed Akkermansia and other bacteria. Many of these bacteria produce a special fat called Butyrate. Butyrate gets its name from butter. Think "Butter-ate." Butyrate actually steers macrophages in the gut lining to the anti-inflammatory Blue Team macrophages. We are quietly and quite easily sealing and healing the gut as we go.

INTERLEUKIN 10

Interleukin 6 is a key inflammatory signal involved in activation of your bodies immune defenses. Opposing Interluekin 6 is another signal molecule called Interleukin 10. Interleukin 10 is like the opposing force to Interleukin 6. The two very often have opposing functions in key tissues.

INTERLEUKIN 10, MACROPHAGES & MEMBRANES

Interleukin 10 is a key player whenever membranes are disrupted. You have begun targeting the gut lining with these first few sets of to-do's. Whenever key membranes get disrupted Interleukin 10 is the key signal molecule involved in doing the repair.

Interleukin 10 steers macrophage populations. When Interleukin 10 is present in the gut lining, it recruits the Blue Team.

With these last two exercises, you are specifically targeting Interleukin 10 and the Blue Team macrophages in the gut lining. The net result, is to seal and heal the gut.

Interestingly, when the gut lining is breached, it is Interleukin 10's opposite, Interleukin 6 that is the tip of the spear to signal the gut to open up.

Interleukin 10 is like a command to seal and heal the gut. Interleukin 6 is like a command to open the gut and allow pathogens in the body.

Chapter 3

Defining the Problem

Simon spent several years building a successful company in a non-fitness industry. He cashed out, chilled out, pigged out and got really fat.

Simon decided to get in shape. He did the 90 day transformation. You know the schtick. You devote lots of time to working out and diet. Oh, and he took lots of growth hormone and steroids. It all worked. He looked good.

People started asking Simon what to do to get in shape. His newfound passion landed him in the fitness business. He came out with a supplement line. It sold well. The young, the old, men and women - they all fed on his advice about getting healthy and in shape.

Simon would give clean advice to consumers about getting healthy and eating right. Behind the scenes he was on growth hormone, testosterone and a few other things. When asked about steroids he would get visibly angry and deny using them.

For several years Simon's supplement business thrived. He was the young embodiment of "the healthy lifestyle." He walked the talk and lived the dream. His life revolved around his workouts. Eventually, however, he got married and started a family. Business and family at first started to cut into his workout time and, over time, became a full time job leaving zero energy or time for much else. He was also getting older. Several more years passed. Often, he did not have the energy to workout even when he did have the time. He had passed the young, single and carefree phase of his life into the harried, frenetic world of overseeing business and family. At times he would finish the work day mentally and emotionally exhausted only to deal with the demands of family.

As the years rolled on Simon encountered an even bigger problem than dwindling time and energy. Without the steroids, the workouts that worked so well on his young body had little effect on his old body. Once the noticeable slow down of his cellular machinery kicked in, Dad Bod drop shipped to Simon's doorstep. The only sure solution seemed to be returning to steroids. Now a family man he no longer wanted to go that route and wisely chose to put his long term health first.

Over time Simon's life looked less and less like the "fitness lifestyle" he represented and more like the busy, harried, life most people experience in our modern habitat. When the combination of age and real life pressures wiped Simon's fitness plans off the calendar he regained all his weight back and even more.

All in 16 years passed from when he first got in shape. He didn't just return to the starting line, he was behind where he started. And he wasn't just heavier. His body was now **old.**

SIMON'S PROBLEMS ARE YOUR PROBLEMS

Simon's story is highly relevant to our objective. First, it gives you **a 100 percent accurate** glimpse behind the curtains. His story exemplifies a marketplace riddled with illusion. More importantly, it shows quite accurately what happens over time for most people. Simon's 16 year journey begs a very important question.

What did Simon really solve?

The short term makes it seem like Simon conquered the problem. The long term view, however, **tells the real story**. Not only did he solve nothing, the strategy actually made things worse long term! This is Simon's 16 year journey ultra-compressed.

Fat, in shape, fatter.

Despite spending several years in great shape the larger problems of the declining body **were not solved.** The question is why? Some would say priorities and time management were Simon's downfall. Sounds good except, remember, making time to eat right and exercise was Simon's business. He was the embodiment of the strategy.

I would offer there are 3 underlying reasons why Simon's strategy failed.

1. Simon had no strategy for how the body really works.
2. Simon had no strategy for what really happens long term.
3. Immunity was nowhere in the equation.

As Simon aged and his cellular machinery declined, the reality of how his body works was not on the radar. Things like clearing hypoxia proteins, or steering macrophages, were not in the strategy. Simon's story would be very different had he understood The Map of Peak Human. His only solution was steroids. His strategy also was not designed for real life circumstances. **It fell apart under real life**

pressures. Your strategy is the same as Simon's. It's a strategy that basically has not changed for 60 plus years. Generally speaking, the strategy goes like this.

- Needing to get in shape.
- Needing to start working out.
- Needing to lose weight.
- Devoting regular time to staying in shape.
- Trying to eat a certain way for life.
- At the high level taking a ton of physique enhancing substances.

It was the dominant strategy everyone subscribed to for a long time. It sounded great. But it failed Simon long term. I mean the real long term, not 90 days or a year or a few years but 16 years. It fails most people over long periods.

THE DATA SPEAKS

- Only 12% of the US has metabolic health.
- 70% of the population on prescription meds.
- Cancer 2nd leading cause of death worldwide behind cardiovascular disease.
- 50% of US projected to be obese by 2030

The math tells the story. *Nothing was solved.*

And now a greater imperative has arrived. The primary determinant of health is no longer merely getting in shape or how you look. Going forward, the primary measure of health is immunity. We must all adapt.

This brings us to the most important question of the entire book.

How do we define and solve the real barriers to health, immunity, and the declining body?

THE HIDDEN META-SCALE SEASONS

Across my forty plus year journey I have uncovered very real patterns that play out for the vast majority of people over time. These patterns remain largely unexamined and un-illucidated, yet they are nearly universally common. These patterns are effectively large scale "seasons." They are tied to the transitions of life and involve long periods both getting in shape and, like Simon, long seasons where time constraints and pressures wipe out the time needed to "do fitness." More importantly, there is an accumulated cost to these seasons that plays out. It's mediated by fat loss, and it culminates later in life, beginning in the forties and going turbo in the fifties. These changes make it very difficult to get control of the body. One reason these patterns have, until now, been unexamined is they operate on very large time scales, usually between seven to ten years. I have seen them repeat over and over for thousands of people and heard testimony from just as many.

Simon's story shows us exactly how these large scale seasons play out. The transitions from carefree and single to family and peak earning years, and the decline of the body all factor in. I have given you the Map of Peak Human. In a sense it's like a map for how to win the World Cup for soccer. You need to get the best players, the best coaches, the strategy, etc. But the map by itself also needs **a game plan** to execute the map.The game plan is where you identify the specific problems your team must overcome.

DEFINING THE PROBLEM

If you have a problem, any problem, you will never, ever solve that problem until you do two things.

1. You must define the problem in specific detail.
2. You have to replicate the problem to see if your solution works.

Let's use the example of astronauts breaking orbit to illustrate. It's not enough to say "we need to get in orbit." Generalities don't solve problems. To get in orbit the specific barrier we must solve is exceeding escape velocity of 25,020 mph.

Defining a problem in specifics reveals what's not going to work. This is crucial. People who climb mountains know a profound life truth. Not every route up will get you to the summit. A lot of things create forward motion, but don't get you where you need to go. There are lots of solutions slower than 25,020. They all have one thing in common.

They all seem like progress but are doomed to failure.

Simon's 16 year journey was an example of a solution that seems like progress but is doomed to failure. This is what happens to everyone. Because the specific barriers you must overcome are not defined you **waste years** on solutions that *seem like progress but are doomed to failure.*

Equally important is the necessity of replicating the conditions of the problem. In our astronaut scenario, imagine if we did the first step correctly by defining the problem as needing to exceed orbital velocity of 25,020, but we never replicated the conditions of zero gravity the astronauts would face. Failure would be guaranteed because we **did not prepare for what really happens.** This is what happened to Simon. Failure was guaranteed because his strategy was not designed for what really happened in the real life ecosystem. This is what will happen to you if your strategy is not designed for the real life conditions you will face over time.

Here are the conditions you will face over time.

THE REAL LIFE CONDITIONS OF THE PROBLEM

- No time to workout.
- No time to meal prep.
- No drugs of any kind.
- High stress.
- Long hours working and commuting.
- Travel.
- Social eating.
- Family and relationship pressures.
- Long periods off track.
- Declining physiology.

And to those conditions we can now add

- Working from home for long durations.
- Seasonal viral attacks.
- Access to gyms being restricted.

These are the conditions of the problem most people face over time. These conditions crush the old strategy. They represent a level of difficulty of **a 10.** Like replicating zero gravity conditions for astronauts, a real solution for the problem of declining body has to work under these conditions or it is **guaranteed to fail.**

Simon started with a problem. He was overweight. He implemented a solution. It worked when he was single, on steroids and made his living being fit. It was a difficulty level of a 2. When his level of difficulty shot to 10 with family, business, age and all the pressures I listed, the strategy failed. Not every route up gets you to the summit. It all seemed like progress but was doomed to failure.

There are 3 barriers evident from Simon's story that everyone faces over time. Later, each of these topics will get at least a full chapter but for now here is a brief summary of each.

THE FIRST BARRIER: THE DECLINE OF THE BODY

Simon's body didn't just get old. It was used up. His declining physiology negated his efforts. It left him with dwindling energy, poor recovery, and not a lot of options outside of steroids.

You face **the exact same problem.**

Until now, everyone had the exact same strategy as Simon; get in shape, carve out more time and energy to working out, eat clean. That strategy, however, does not equip you with what you will really need long term in today's reality. It's not designed to. It's designed to get you in shape. Simon got in shape. He was in such great shape he became a fit guru. *It solved nothing.*

KEY IDEA: Getting in shape doesn't solve the long term problems you will face.

The specifics of the declining body, the decline in immunity that drives aging, are masked, not solved, by simply getting in shape.

Simon had no idea why his body was getting old. He had nothing he could specifically address. He didn't have the Map of Peak Human.

You do.

The Map of Peak Human gives you a list of specific things we will address to restore the things time subtracts. It's based on what is really true about your body.

Specific Problem 1: We need a specific map to counter the declining mechanisms of aging.

The next barrier is that of our modern habitat.

THE SECOND BARRIER: THE MODERN HABITAT

Simon's story also shows us the next barrier we must overcome. We all live in the **modern habitat.** Our modern habitat constraints time resources, subtracts key genetic triggers, adds environmental challenges, presents seasonal illness, and makes eating much easier than expending energy. The problems of the modern habitat create three specific problems we need to define.

The Problem of Time

All of us have seasons where time and energy face very real constraints. They happened to Simon. They **will** happen to you. The problem is this - **over time, time goes to zero.** There is no avoiding it. If it won't work when time goes to zero it can't work long term.

Specific Problem 2: We need a strategy that works when time goes to zero.

The Problem of Environment

The modern ecosystem works like one giant gene activator and immune system threat. Many things we need are missing and many things we don't need are present. They take a tremendous toll on our physiology. It's like a series of dials all set to the wrong positions. The problem of decline combines with immunity problems to accelerate decline. Simon needed a strategy to offset the environmental factors. You need one as well. Later, we devote a whole chapter to specific solutions to offset the modern habitat.

Specific Problem 3: We need to offset the effects of the modern habitat:

The Problem of How Humans Eat

In the modern habitat it is much easier to consume more energy than you expend it. We have all been led to think this is the problem. It's not. The real problem has to do with **how humans are hard wired to eat.**

Eating has one, and only one, constant across all of history, all cultures, and in fact, all mammals — feast and famine. To survive famine there is a mechanism ***hard wired*** into the biological machinery of all mammals, humans included. That mechanism is called **Ad Libitum eating.** To *ad lib* with food means to eat whatever. Eating whatever is the hard wired mode of eating for mammals. You, being a mammal, are included in that statement. Over 16 years, Simon had many times where family, work, life, post dieting, and other factors led to eating whatever. In the next 16 years so will you. Our modern habitat combines with modern diet practices to mimic starvation and amplify this innate, hard wired, behavior of eating whatever.

Specific Problem 4: We need a way to offset the effects of eating Ad Libitum.

THE FINAL BARRIER: THE FAT LOSS PARADOX

Unlike aging, or the modern habitat, which are readily visible, there is a third force working against you that is invisible. This invisible force is a barrier created by the solution itself. Simon was using a strategy, a system for his body. You use that exact same system. **That system itself is driving part of the problem!**

Simon believed something that is not true - that fat is just stored energy and all you have to do is lose it. He deluded himself into believing that being in great shape conquered the problem. Ironically it actually made things that much harder long term. It may sound counterintuitive but fear not. You are going to learn how the fat loss paradox works and how to counter it. You will learn how the immune system all along has been in control of fat loss.

Specific Problem 5: We need to counter the fat loss paradox.

This is the first time the real barriers of the declining body have been defined into a list of specific problems to solve. You now have a game plan for the real game you must play, and a map that tells us what matters most. We are going to apply the new science of how our bodies really work and combine it with the new realities for health and immunity we must all face to solve the specific problems that make a prison out of the body.

While new science revelations about how the body actually works are the underlying foundation of this book, and where the transformational horsepower rests, our journey together will also require a new level of reality check from you.

At the core, the problem is greater than health. We live in an era of thought compliance. The result is truth itself has gone by the wayside. We have taken the dynamics of the dysfunctional family and applied them to society at large. In the dysfunctional family you better not say what's really true. You will be attacked with shame, blame and name calling. That's the era we live in. Rent out your head to thought compliance or else. But when truth goes by the wayside we lose the ability to reason. Without reason we lose our power. We can not **learn new things without reason.** When it comes to your body and health, without reason you will chase illusions and fitness fantasy. You must shed illusions. You must get real health, the kind that lasts and protects you from disease.

Simon spent 16 years chasing an illusion. He pursued fitness fantasy. He learned the hard way that real life always crushes fantasy. When you chase illusions you will never be happy. Over 40 years I have witnessed thousands of people chase illusions of fitness fantasy only to discover 20 or 30 years later what they were chasing was never real to begin with.

The essence of immune centric health to keep your body young means changing the way you measure results. We will have one and only one standard.

If it does not work over time it does not work.

WHAT'S NEXT:
To solve the 5 specific barriers you need a new foundation for what is (and always was) really true about your body. Over the next 4 chapters we will lay the new foundation.

TO-DO: DRIVING D
Restoring Vitamin D Levels to peak human

With age we lose B-Vitamin production. At the same time serum levels of Vitamin D also decline. This one-two combo of decline has a massive negative impact on the bodies immune system. Both of these things work together. Either one, by itself, when restored to peak human levels, can be miraculous. The issues with my brother and Parkinson's had a lot to do with declining immunity from lost b-vitamin production and low vitamin D. The reason B-vitamin production declines is primarily due to loss of bacteria. You have already begun to restore those things. Now we are going to begin restoring Vitamin D.

YOU NEED:

A good vitamin D supplement, preferably in a 5,000 mcg dose, along with melatonin. Trader Joe's has a good one for less than $5.

WHAT IT IS

Vitamin D is a steroid hormone. You need it to absorb calcium in the gut. It is highly involved in regulating immunity.

THE TO DO:

THE WHAT: Generally recommended intake is between 1000-4000 i..u. of Vitamin D.
THE WHEN: At bedtime. Do this for 4-6 weeks and then stop for at least 4 weeks.
THE HOW: With Melatonin.

The Endocrine Society Clinical Practice Guideline recommends that up to 10,000 daily i.u. is safe for adults. Thirty minutes of whole body exposure in the sun will give you 15,000 i.u. of vitamin D. Taking 15,000 i.u. of vitamin D you might only absorb seventy percent of that. I personally do this at a dose of 15,000 i.u. for 4 weeks. Consult with your doctor if you have any concerns about higher dose levels or just do the generally recommended intake.

WHAT IT DOES:

Low vitamin D levels are a global epidemic. Most people are walking around with serum vitamin D under 30. Above 90 is where Peak Human physiology kicks in.

CAUTIONS

See your doctor first if you have any concerns. If you wake with a headache at any time, discontinue for at least 4 weeks.

PART 2:

NEW FOUNDATIONS

Chapter 4

New Foundations: The Core Truth of Balance

THE BIOLOGICAL TRUTH OF BALANCE

The juice fast is a favorite of alternative therapies around the world. Just the words alone sound invigorating. Juice and fasting together. What could be healthier, right? Just yesterday I read of a woman with irreversible brain damage from doing a juice fast. Three weeks of fasting on juices led to an *imbalance* of sodium and key hormones like aldosterone. The result of her juice fast was not health, but a severe medical condition.

Prior to Covid-19 we had gotten away from the most basic truth of health. The purpose of this chapter is to re-establish you in a foundation. If you want to get anywhere long term you must deal with what is really true about how your body actually works. It's just one word.

Balance.

Why does the simple solution, which is just to stay healthy, elude the vast majority over time? Truth. We have gotten away from what is really true about the single most foundational aspect of health. Balance.

I have spent thousands of hours studying the bodies biochemistry. The net takeaway of all those many hours comes down to one single word. "**Balance.**"

The core truth of how your biology works is the systems underlying your health need balance. It is an intractable, non-debatable, reality. And everyday the balance of your biochemistry and immunity can and is effected by what you do. We have an entire industry, allegedly devoted to health, that has **gone away** from this reality. With an immune centric approach to health and anti-aging, many things we think are healthy can actually compromise immunity. That reality is balance is health. Imbalance is disease.

HOW HEALTH *IS* BALANCE. IMBALANCE *IS* DISEASE.

In the science literature, there is a word for balance. The word is **homeostasis.** Use of the words "loss of homeostasis", always describes a disease or an *imbalance* driving aging and disease. Always. There is never a case where this is not true. Here are some direct quotes from scientific studies. I have used the word balance in place of "homeostasis."

- ...Chronic inflammation deregulates cellular *balance* and can drive carcinogenesis (cancer).
- ...A hallmark of aging is a decline in metabolic *balance."*
- *...*loss of *balance* in cartilage contributes to the development of osteoarthritis.
- "...Disturbance of systemic iron *balance* causes two major classes of disease."
- "...the disruption of dynamic circulatory *balance* mediated by the brain causes heart failure."

What the science literature makes perfectly clear is that ***imbalance drives disease.*** Cancer is an imbalance of tissue growth. Neurodegenerative diseases like Alzheimers or Huntington's are an imbalance of energy production in the brain. Obesity is an imbalance of energy storage. Edema is an imbalance in fluid retention. Diabetes is an imbalance of insulin production. It is easy to see that disease and imbalance are one. Life itself depends on keeping every major system in your body balanced. The need for balance is the single highest truth of your body.

Balance is the **highest truth of health.**

The woman doing the juice cleanse imbalanced fluids for 3 weeks. Super condensed, her story looks like this.

Imbalanced juice intake => brain damage.

And that's the main point of this chapter - the modern era has **gone away** from what is really true. The modern era of solutions for your body is really an **era of imbalance.**

THE ERA OF IMBALANCE

All the big trends today promote doing things that are **imbalanced!** You don't have to look far. Entire schools of thought and practice devote themselves to imbalance. One says to imbalance foods from animals, another foods from plants, another says to imbalance fats, yet another says to imbalance protein. Ironically, they are all doing the exact same thing. They all promote **imbalance** as the way to obtain health! If balance is the highest truth of health then we need to ask a *very important* question.

Will sustained imbalance of healthy things produce health or disease?

What do you think the long term result will be from seeking health via practicing imbalanced health protocols? I'll bet you have never considered this. What you are about to see is something quite shocking. You will learn that sustained *imbalance,* even from healthy things, will *always,* produce disease long term.

Always.

It may take time, sometimes years or decades, but the core truth of biology requiring balance, will always assert itself. It's how things really work.The reason has to do with the concept of **biological duality.**

BIOLOGICAL DUALITY

In Chapter one, you learned about macrophages and hypoxia proteins. You learned things are not black and white. They can be both good or bad. The reality is that *any given thing* can be both good and bad. I call this **Biological Duality.** Biological duality is the idea a given thing can at times be beneficial. At other times, stages or conditions, *the same thing* can be detrimental.

Biological duality is at the core of the need for balance. Duality is why the systems of our body require fine balance. And it governs everything. Anything can be either good or bad. It just depends on balance or imbalance of the thing in question.

What follows is a powerful example of both duality and balance. Here is how duality and balance overturn everything we thought was true about free radicals and anti-oxidants.

THE DUALITY OF ANTI-OXIDANTS AND OXIDATIVE STRESS

Thousands of products and services in the modern marketplace for health are based the idea that anti-oxidants are good and free radicals are bad. **Anti-oxidants are good for immunity right?** If it's an anti-oxidant, you should take it to help fight off infection. At least that's the prevailing belief. And what you are about to learn is this idea is not only mistaken, it has **nothing to do** with the reality of how either anti-oxidants or free radicals work.

Our purpose here is to ground you in reality.

Reality means how things really work.

Many things in the pursuit of health actually compromise immunity. Nowhere is that more true than with anti-oxidants. Here is the reality of anti-oxidants and free radicals. What you will see is balance, driven by duality is how things really work.

Think of rust. That's **oxidation.** In the body both oxygen and nitrogen can be major sources of free radicals. When either is "oxidized" our bodies essentially rust. **Reduction** is the opposite of oxidation. Anti-oxidants "reduce" free radicals. From this we get the idea that oxidation is bad, and anti-oxidants are good. The reality, however, is it simply doesn't work like that.

FACT: Oxidation can be good or bad.
FACT: Reduction can be good or bad.

HOW BALANCE RULES ANTI-OXIDANTS AND FREE RADICALS
We need minor stress from free radicals. Free radicals act as critical signal mediators. Key immune cells, macrophages, and others, rely on free radical signals for proper function and to stay in balance.

KEY IDEA: Free radicals are essential for immunity.

When you eat, when you recover from exercise, when you sleep, low level minor stress from free radicals are essential for life. This is why over reduction, i.e., too many anti-oxidants at the wrong time, can be very bad. It knocks out the vital free radical signaling we need for proper immune function. Too much reduction, meaning you take too many anti-oxidants, has even been shown to shorten total life span!

On way over reduction, meaning too much anti-oxidant activity, can effect immunity is with T-cells. T-cells are vital for healthy immunity. As we age T-cells can become **over reduced.** The net result of being over reduced, is T-cells begin to lose function. They don't work like they should. That's very bad. Over reduction, in the case of t-cells, is bad. See Appendix A: Over Reduction And Aging.

At the other extreme, sustained high levels of free radicals promote **oxidative stress.** Oxidative stress is when free radicals overwhelm the bodies anti-oxidant reserves. When imbalanced over long periods, oxidative stress can promote inflammation and disease states, including cancer. Let's look at the case of nitric oxide, a beneficial free radical.

NITRIC OXIDE AND BALANCE

Whenever you eat anything that makes insulin, which is most things, your body makes a free radical called nitric oxide. Nitric oxide is a gas. It allows blood vessels to dilate. That's good. If you have ever eaten a lot of carbs and your arms feel full shortly after, that's nitric oxide dilating blood vessels.

Generally speaking nitric oxide is really good, despite being a free radical. The problem is when nitric oxide becomes imbalanced. When imbalanced, nitric oxide out-competes the bodies natural defense against a key oxygen radical. The result produces a cancer promoting compound called **peroxinitrate.** Where you find sustained imbalances of nitric oxide and peroxinitrate, you find immune imbalance via the Red Team macrophages that drive inflammation.

Surprisingly, one of the most common ways nitric oxide is regularly imbalanced is via consumption of pre-workout drinks. Millions of fitness enthusiasts regularly consume these drinks prior to workouts. They drive nitric oxide and help workout pumps. Covid-19 presented the world a bit of a paradox for nitric oxide. Most people make too little. A little extra nitric oxide is good for immunity. But for people into the working out, the reverse is true. Excess consumption of these drinks may unwittingly compromise immunity. Too much nitric oxide steers the body towards greater populations of the inflammatory Red Team macrophages! While the occasional pre-workout drink is not an issue, the *imbalance* of these drinks merits very serious concern. See Appendix A : Why Do Fit People Get Cancer?

The example of nitric oxide helps us to see how duality and imbalance are at the core of how things really work. Even though it's a free radical, nitric oxide is mostly good. When imbalanced, it can be very bad.

TAKING ANTI-OXIDANTS: THE REALITY OF DUALITY

As you can see, we need minor free radical stress. The reality of duality is **both** free radicals and anti-oxidants can be either good or bad. It really just depends on the concentration, the tissue, the timing and the duration. The use of anti-oxidants without taking into account the tissue, the timing of use, and the duration - the what, when and how - can do more harm than good. The deciding factor for what side of the coin play will play out is *balance or imbalance*

THE OLD: Taking anti-oxidants is good.
THE NEW: The beneficial use of anti-oxidants depends on the type, the tissue and the timing.

Let's look at an example.

HOW ANTI-OXIDANTS CAN RUIN YOUR WORKOUTS
Many people take anti-oxidants with their workouts. Maybe it's that greens drink just after your workout, or maybe it's vitamin C, or Green Tea. Unwittingly, you are blunting much of the benefit to working out.

Working out creates micro muscle tissue injury. The basis of recovery from a workout involves activation of the immune system. The onset of inflammation after a workout is what triggers healing and the improvements you desire. Taking antioxidants around or right after a workout disrupts the critical signaling, much of it mediated by nitric oxide, needed to signal repair and recovery. This is especially true if you are older. A 2014 study in the *Journal of Physiology,* showed that combining the life extending phenol resveratrol with exercise **eliminated the benefits of exercise!** The culprit was most likely the anti-oxidant properties of resveratrol. This is also not to say that we can not use anti-oxidants on the right tissue, in the right timing and right way to extend lifespan. We can and we will!

What we can no longer do is operate in **ignorance of the reality of duality.**

The reality of biological duality is simply how things work.

Here is another example. In Chapter 14, you will learn about cellular housekeeping. In most cases cellular housekeeping slows aging. It's a great practice, but not always. Even cellular housekeeping has biological duality. For example, with certain types of cancers cellular housekeeping can cause them to proliferate!

Protocol: Cellular Housekeeping.
No Cancer: Generally a good practice.
Later Stages of Certain Cancers: Horrible idea.

Just now, as I write this, another example came across my Linkedin feed. Someone posted about how bile acids are good. But that's not how things work. Bile acids have biological duality. They work both ways. Bile acids can drive health but they can also be major cancer promoters! See Appendix A: The Map of Bacteria Guilds.

HOW IMBALANCED HEALTH PROTOCOLS CAN DRIVE DISEASE

What happens when healthy things are imbalanced? Do you get health or disease? Let's look at a practical question.

Does eating healthy foods always make you healthy?

You might have said yes But think again. Juice is healthy, yet the very tragic experience of the woman with brain damage after a 3 week juice cleanse shows us quite readily a core biological truth.

Healthy things, when imbalanced, produce disease!

I am saying what is, and always has been, really true. Sustained imbalances in pursuit of health, even with healthy things, eventually produce imbalance in the body. Imbalances in the body **are** disease. It's extremely easy to see. Here are some powerful examples.

Water is healthy. You need it to live. Drink too much water too fast and it will kill you.

Imbalanced water => death.

Protein is healthy. You need it to live. Eat too much and you can ferment cancer promoting compounds in the gut.

Imbalanced protein => cancer promoting compounds.

Grains are healthy. Imbalance too much of them and you can actually injure the gut.

Imbalanced grains=> gut injury.

Now what about fats? Are fats immune from duality? Can an imbalance of even healthy fats work to produce disease? The answer is yes.

Fats are not spared biological duality.

First, several studies have linked high fat diets with cancer. If you sustain an imbalanced of fat intake it can produce an imbalance in the body which can produce disease. Wait, surely Keto diets are spared duality. Keto diets, since they use the word Keto, must be only good, right?

At the back of the book in the Appendix A, we look at the Keto diet and duality. What you will see is how the reality of duality applies even to Keto Diets. You will see how long term Keto diets, which is really long term sustained imbalance of fat intake, may even promote cancer onset. See Appendix A: Can Keto Diets Drive Cancer Onset?

BALANCE AND DUALITY IS HOW THINGS REALLY WORK:
In this era, the foundational truth of how your body works, balance and duality, is absent. It is time for the most crucial of resets. The systems of your body depend on fine balance. Long term imbalances of anything can and will eventually drive disease. We will take this idea now and build upon it to snap you back to what is and always has been really true about how your body works.

TO DO: HACKING SLEEP 101 WITH THE SEATTLE PROTOCOL

Restoring peak human sleep is foundational to immunity. One poor nights sleep and you entire immune system can be compromised. Our first job is to eliminate hypoxia, or lack of oxygen during sleep. In later chapters you will see how sleep hypoxia promotes obesity, cancer and accelerated aging. The Seattle protocol is an emerging set of standards at the cutting edge of dentistry to relieve sleep hypoxia. Here is the first level. You can do immediately.

YOU NEED:

Breath rights.
Mouth tape.
Nasonex

THE TO DO:

At bedtime, apply breath rights first. Position at midpoint of nose and hold for thirty seconds. Experiment with and without Nasonex on subsequent nights. If you feel better with Nasonex use the Nasonex for fourteen nights and cease for fifteen days but continue breath rights and mouth tape.

Right at lights out apply mouth tape. You don't need to cover whole mouth just the front.

WHAT IT DOES:

We are increasing oxygen during sleep. You will notice significant improvements in energy, aches, trips to the bathroom in the middle of the night and even weight. Taking air in through the nose increases brain oxygenation while sleeping.

IMPOSSIBLE BUT TRUE SLEEP FACT: *You should not be getting up to go to the bathroom at night.*

Proper sleep shuts down the parasympathetic nervous system. In a properly oxygenated sleep state you will sleep through the night. Over excitation of the para sympathetic nervous system driven by sleep hypoxia or inadequate oxygen will wake you in the middle of the night to go urinate. Many people doing this protocol report a nearly 100 percent difference in late night bathroom runs.

TO DO: HACKING INTERLEUKIN 6 AND NF-KB FOR MAXIMUM VIRAL IMMUNITY

Previously you learned about the key immune signal modulator interleukin 6. Remember, I said you had to know the players and the teams to control immunity? You met a key player with Interleukin 6, now meet one of the key teams. The name of the team is NF-KB. Team NF-KB stands for a really long name that we don't need to worry about.

WHAT IS IS: NF-KB is a group of proteins, or rather a family of co-factors involved in several critical cell functions. For our purposes, what you need to know is NF-KB is a key regulator of the **immune response to infection.** In fact, some proposed therapies for flu like virus outbreaks like Covid 19 focus on lowering NF-KB!

HOW IT WORKS: NF-kB is at the center of mediating immune and inflammatory responses. In essence it works as a feedback look for immune and Inflammatory signals. When NF-KB is activated by say a viral infection, it acts as a coordinator for lots of genes involved in immunity and inflammation. Typically, wherever we see inflammation, or infection or cancer, we find elevated NF-KB.

HACKING NF-KB AND IL-6: When immunity is challenged, lowering IL-6 and NF-KB have been shown to be a promising approach to maximize immunity.

THE WHAT: Hacking NF-KB and IL-6
THE HOW: With CBD and Fucoidan
THE WHEN: At bedtime

CBD has been shown to have a marked effect lowering IL-6, particularly in the cells lining the vasculature of the lungs. Fucoidan is a seaweed extract with multiple pro-health properties. We will look at it extensively in Chapter 17. One of the unique abilities of Fucoidan is to suppress **both** NF-KB and IL-6. Together, with a goods nights sleep, CBD and Fucoidan are an ultra advanced and powerful way to suppress both NF-KB and Il-6 for maximum viral immunity.

Chapter 5

New Foundations: The Language of Real Health

In the first chapter we looked at hypoxia proteins. What was immediately clear, although the concept had not yet been introduced to you, was **biological duality rules the discussion.** In certain tissues, at certain times, HIF-1 is good. The dermis of the skin is a great example. Stimulating HIF-1 in the skin can rejuvenate aging skin. At other times and in other specific tissues, HIF-1 is very bad, for example, excess HIF-1 in the brain during sleep.

With just this one example, it's easy to see there is an underlying and undiscovered principle for the body at work.

That principle is *what, when and how.*

THE LANGUAGE OF REAL HEALTH

If you really think about it, the central question of all health, fitness and longevity is just one question. The one question you have always wanted to know, for anything and everything, is what to do, when to do it, and how you do it. What you really want is a framing foundation. You need a guide for the use of anything and everything. The framing foundation is **what, when and how.**

What, when and how, together form a new way of thinking. In effect these three things form a new language. It is the **Language of Real Health.** The way you drive immune centric health to keep your body young is not by dedicating hours in the gym. You don't even need to do super strict dieting. What you do need is an *order of operations.* You need to know how to do things in the right time, in just the right way; **what, when and how.**

Like settings on a smartphone the distinct physiological conditions of real heath and a younger body can literally be **switched on** if you understand what to do, when to do it, and how.

Let's use the example of words and language to illustrate.

Words are powerful. Even babies use them to good effect. "Cookie" may just get your one year old a cookie. But as powerful as words are, they are nothing when compared to powerful **speech.** Powerful speech can change the world. Powerful speech can win you that job or the heart of that special person, and even launch you into your destiny. Speech harnesses the power of words, but takes into account three all important things - ***what, when and how.*** What you say, when you say it, and how you say it is absolutely everything. People who master their choice of words, the timing, and delivery, rule the world. The same holds true for learning how to master your body. What, when and how, are what give you mastery.

The first step is to open your eyes to the truth - *you have been doing **baby talk.***

You see, the entire health, wellness, and fitness industry, as you know it, the marketplace as a whole, is stuck in **baby talk for health!** You have been unknowingly sucked into *extremely severe limitations.* The ironic and comical irony is 100 percent of what is popular today is defined only by *"what." The when and how are missing!*

You won't have to look far to see this is *dead on accurate!* The entire way of thinking today is a simplistic, black/white/good/bad, spin on "what." You want examples?

THE BABY TALK OF "WHAT" - MINUS WHEN, AND HOW

Dairy is bad. Coconut milk is good.
Carbs are bad. Fats are good.
Mushrooms are good. Roots are bad.
Fasting is good. Big meals are bad.
Plants are good. Meat is bad.
Protein is good. Carbs are bad.
Meat is good. Plants are bad.
Red light is good. Blue light is bad.
Cholesterol is bad. Antioxidants are good.
Antioxidants are bad. NAD+ is good.
Blueberries are good. Bananas are bad.

This kind of thinking is *100 percent* of what is out there!

100 percent.

Did you catch yourself agreeing with one or more of those statements? You may even feel highly charged emotionally, like I tapped into your highest ideas of right and wrong (That's called religion, by the way.)

Even if you feel highly polarized by one of those statements, reserve judgement. As we continue to unpack how your body really works you are going to be re-thinking a number of things. Timing rules the body. It dictates when and how to do anything. That's not so hard to accept is it?

Do you find tons of conflicting information and don't know who to believe?

Do you want to overcome this? Step one is to spot the baby talk. Milk bad. Blueberries good. Meat good. Plants bad. Ga ga, goo goo. Fats good. Fiber bad. **It's all simplistic baby talk for health.** It's like knowing a word, but with no idea of how, or when, to use it.

Why does the simple solution, which is just to stay healthy, elude the vast majority over time? Truth. We are stuck in baby talk. We are not dealing with what's really true about how things work. Real health begins and ends with immunity. Immunity depends on biological duality. Once you understand biological duality the lights go on. You see the baby talk for what it is. You will quickly begin asking what, when, and how, about **anything and everything.** What, when, and how, will overnight become your new language to understand anything about the body. The old paradigm of baby talk is being swept away as you read this.

EVERYTHING STARTS WITH WHEN

Let's begin with *"when."*

When it comes to your body, everything begins with when. We are circadian creatures. Our bodies work in a masterfully orchestrated 24 hour symphony of gene activation, membrane permeability, free radical balance, food inputs, and thousands of other factors. All of these things are synced to a 24 hour cycle.

Science papers are awash in a new word - *chronobiology.* Chronobiology means we can visibly observe and measure time related data points about the human body. These data points can tell us the best time to do or not do a certain thing. They can tell us when a given event is more likely to take place.

For our purposes, the first and most important place in the 24 hour cycle is what amounts to a genetic rush hour.

THE GENETIC RUSH HOUR:
As far as keeping the body young is concerned there is a Genetic Rush Hour. It's roughly around 4am. The deep stretch of the night is when production of immune cells is highest. It's when circulating

lymphocytes peak. It's when many of the most important genes that prolong life are being activated. This period of time has a very high level of importance relative to all others. The results when disrupting this period of time are highly quantifiable and measurable. Research with shift workers has shown disruption of the Genetic Rush Hour promotes a higher incidence of obesity, diabetes and cancer!

Dawn, and the hours preceding it, tap into ancestral mechanisms tied to survival. These hours are your bang for the buck period Targeting activation of your survival mechanisms during this period keeps the body young. For over 13 years I have done very specific things around this time. Among these things

Sprints.
Deadlifts.
Cold immersion.
Supplements that aid fasting like Berberine.

Notice it's not so much the activities or the items. It's not the *what. When* and *how* to do them, is equally important. What, when, and how, together, is what matters. Doing these things around dawn aids the youth preserving mechanisms that *naturally fire during this period.*

Later, we will devote an entire chapter to the decline of the daily timekeeping architecture of your body. Beyond the daily rhythm, there are larger patters that dictate "when."

THE 7 DAY CYCLE

Beyond circadian rhythms our bodies have a natural 7 day cycle. This natural 7 day cycle is bound up into all of biology. Every thing that has a body, from insects to fish to mammals, has a natural built in, hard wired seven day cycle.

It's called Circaseptan rhythm.

Circaseptan means *"about every seven days."* What you have always intuitively known - some days are better than others for certain things - turns out to be a biological fact. Some days **are** better than others for certain things.

KEY IDEA: Your body has a natural daily cycle and a natural weekly cycle.

Dr David Ellis, from the University of Lincoln's School of Psychology, was quoted in a 2015 paper saying, "The seven day weekly cycle is repeated for all of us from birth, and we believe this results in each day of the week acquiring its own character."

In 2009, when I introduced my VEEP System to the world, one piece of IP hidden under the hood was circaseptan rhythm. For over ten years, VEEP has been powered far beyond the old school simple dietary concepts about macro nutrients. All these years the big secret never revealed until now was that different days of the week **have unique nutritional requirements.** Think about it. How you eat on Sunday is very different from Tuesday. How you eat on Monday is very different from Friday. It's one reason why we have results that border on miraculous.

Once you get Circaseptan rhythms it changes everything. For example, cortisol to DHEA ratio is highest on Monday's. This proves what you already knew - **Monday's are higher in stress.** Nutrition for Monday's requires stress adaptions because stress effects immunity. The entire Monday pattern in VEEP is designed to counteract stress. There are massive amounts of dark fruits in the early AM. The purpose is to counter stress later in the day via b-vitamin production. Dark fruits are combined with whey protein. This drives production of serotonin precursors to counter stress. In the early afternoon we use EPA oil. This spins down stress induced cortisol at night. It keeps you from coming home and stress eating.

CHRONO-IMMUNOLOGY

Circaseptan rhythm is now being applied to medicine. **Chrono-immunology** is the practice of timing and dosing of treatments. It can make a 100 percent difference in effectiveness, For example, experiments with heart failure patients suggest a strong seven day rhythm. The highest likelihood of heart attack is Wednesday afternoon. Here are just a few science established facts regarding your natural seven day cycle.

- Research on heart rate variability has shown pulse rates work in a seven day cycle.
- Research on sodium balance has shown that sodium retention works in a seven day cycle directly related to cortisol. Shockingly, this works *independent* of sodium intake!

- You have a best day for sleep. It's Tuesday night. Salivary levels of melatonin secretion have a seven day cycle. Peak melatonin is Tuesday and lowest melatonin is on Saturday.

- Epileptic seizures have been shown to clearly occur in a seven day cycle.

- Cortisol to DHEA ratio is highest on Mondays. Stress and depression peak on Monday, tied to max cortisol and DHEA output in the seven day cycle.

- You have a best day for enjoyment. Plasma cortisol levels are lowest on Thursday.

Beyond seven day rhythms there are even larger time dependent patterns. The natural rhythms of **seasons** have very real effects in biology. For example, winter has a higher incidence of stroke and heart attack, blood pressure is higher, and we tend to sleep more versus summer.

KEY IDEA: Biology runs in daily, weekly and even seasonal rhythms.

WHEN IS NOT ENOUGH

When is the foundation. It's not enough. You need "how." "**How"** is what will make or break anything for the body. Let's use another speech analogy to better understand the impact of "how." Imagine you ask your boss for a raise. You wait for just the right time. You use the perfect choice of words. But instead of asking with confidence and authority in your voice, you stutter. Your voice cracks. You sound weak, unconfident and shy. Not only do you not get the raise, you get reassigned to a lesser position! You neglected **"how"** to ask. The "how" was to ask with confidence. Your voice needed the right tone, the right emotion. Let's look at some examples of putting it all together to give our bodies the power of what, when and how.

THE SYNTAX OF REAL HEALTH

I want to give you a new way to think about applying any given thing for your body. From now on, whenever you hear about any protocol for your body, things like, sunlight, protein, antioxidants, red beet root, red light, fasting or ***anything and everything,*** fill in the following blanks.

THE WAY TO USE______ ***(the what)*** *IS* ***(the when)*** *AND* ***(the how).***

As you begin to apply this syntax, *99.999 percent of the conflicting information* you have taken in will vaporize. Let's look at a few examples.

OMEGA 3's: THE LANGUAGE OF REAL HEALTH

THE WHAT: Omega 3's.
THE WHEN: During a fast
THE HOW: With Niacin. Helps to clear excess HIF-1.

The way to use Omega 3's **(the what)** is during a fast **(the when)** and together with Niacin. **(the how)**

Omega 3's during fasting potentiate and magnify the beneficial effects. They activate key organs within cells. Learning how to activate these cellular organs, called peroxisomes, is a big part of our journey. Omega 3's with niacin together, have the power to clear HIF-1 from cells of key tissues. Alone, each of these things is shown to be effective. Combined, calorie restriction with omega three's and niacin:

- Amplifies the benefits of fasting and
- Helps clear excess HIF-1
- Activates key organs within cells.

Take note; with each to-do, we are building upon basic ideas laid out in the first two chapters. Clearing tissues of HIF-1 steers the Red Team toward the Blue Team.

EXTRA VIRGIN OLIVE OIL: THE LANGUAGE OF REAL HEALTH

THE WHAT: Extra Virgin Olive Oil
THE WHEN: When you have meat
THE HOW: In small amounts not exceeding 3% of the weight of the meat.

Research shows that EVOO with meat impairs oxidation of fats. The caveat (the "how") is in small amounts. When you take EVOO in large amounts with meat the opposite happens. The EVOO **actually increases oxidation of fats in meat!** There are 96 teaspoons in a pound. Assuming you had a 16 ounce steak, that would be about two teaspoons of olive oil max.

Are you getting this? **Understanding duality is powerful.** Extra Virgin Olive Oil can work for good or bad. It depends on the timing and the amounts - what, when and how.

A BAKED POTATO: THE LANGUAGE OF REAL HEALTH

THE WHAT: Baked potato
THE WHEN:The day before a fast
THE HOW: Cooled, with butter

The way to eat a baked potato (the what) is the day before a fast (the when) cooled down and with butter (the how).

Immunity begins in the gut. Accordingly, **steering macrophages,** begins in the gut lining. Resistant starches are the preferred food source for Bifidobacteria. When you cool a baked potato, the digestible starch congeals. It becomes resistant to digestion. A baked potato the day before a fast drives Bifidobacteria production during sleep. Making Bifidobacteria while you sleep makes the bacterial metabolite Butyrate. Butyrate **seals the gut** and steers macrophages toward the Blue Team. It also mimics and amplifies fasting! We are building toward an **Amplified Fast.**

The last two chapters have begun a new foundation. You are waking up to the baby talk. Your understanding of what is really true about your body is expanding. The real truth of duality and balance are coming into focus.

Anything can be both good or bad.

Things that were once bad, like a baked potato, can be good. Things you thought were bad can actually have a functional purpose. The key is the Language of Real Health - what, when and how.

I know the big words are piling up. It may feel intimidating. Stay with it. The next major section of the book takes a break from big words. Remember, the most valuable prize of the ages - the power to stay young - is not free. It asks more of you. The fact you are at this juncture of the book is fantastic.

Next, more reality bombs. You think our human genome runs your body. In reality three different and distinct genomes run your body, not one.

TO-DO: SIGNAL AMPLIFICATION 101
Switching on hunger to switch on youth.

YOU NEED:

Ahi tuna steak, broccoli, garbanzo's (or black beans) and avocado.

THE TO DO:

This is a one-off lunch. You will have one or two seared tuna steaks with 1/2 crown of raw broccoli, 1 cup raw black beans and 1/4 avocado. You can use salsa to mix in the broccoli, beans and avocado.

WHAT IT DOES:

Your first thought might be "why the hell would I want to induce hunger?!" Here is why. One of the most powerful ways to **slow aging** is to tap into survival signals. Hunger is a survival signal. It can trigger mechanisms to stimulate growth hormone, make insulin work better, release stored fat, and even slow aging! Don't worry, I will give you ways to make this easy. This exercise will give you a tool you use later when we need to amplify fasting in order to slow aging.

THE WHAT: Ahi tuna steak, broccoli, black beans and avocado.
THE WHEN: Do this for lunch. Later we can use this at dinner.
THE HOW: Do the beans and broccoli raw.
NOTES: You will get super hungry prior to dinner. This is actually very useful. We can use this to supercharge fat burning, and many other things.

SUBSTITUTES: Vegans can substitute garbanzo beans or tofu for tuna. Cauliflower for broccoli. See substitutes for foods you don't like.

WHY THIS WORKS:

The beans and broccoli together deliver bulk to the stomach but little energy. The fibers are food for key bacteria. Avocado actually lowers insulin output. The dense protein slows gut transit time. All of these things work together to magnify hunger signaling. Normally leptin overpowers ghrelin after a meal so you don't feel hungry. These foods have the opposite effect. The stomach gets full but there is no energy.

A nice bonus is fat burning skyrockets shortly after doing this.

Chapter 6

New Foundations: The 3 Genomes

Today I saw a retail outlet installing genomic testing. What a marvel of modern technology. You can go into a drug store, get your DNA sampled, and find out what foods and nutritional habits are right for you. Amazing right? There is only one problem. The premise is flawed. It's not based on what is really true about your body.

Today, everywhere you look, entire industries and companies have sprung up based upon an idea that sounds amazing but turns out not to be true. It's the idea your human genome governs everything about you. For example, we are told the human genome can to tell you what foods to eat, if you will suffer from depression, Alzheimers, obesity, and virtually anything you need to know about yourself. The hype sounds amazing. And it's simply not the reality of how things work. Your body is **not** run solely by your human genome! The reality is your body has **three separate and distinct genomes.**

THE OLD: Your Human Genome Runs You**.**
THE NEW: Three Genomes Run You.

THE THREE GENOMES: HOW YOUR BODY REALLY WORKS:

Not one, but **three separate and distinct genomes,** working together, are what really run your body. Here they are.

- The human genome
- The gut bacterial genome
- The mitochondrial genome.

First there is the human genome. The human genome contains the genes you inherited from mom and dad.

See Appendix A: What are Genes Really?

Next, a separate genome exists inside your mitochondria. These are the tiny powers plants inside every cell. You might be surprised to know when tracing your ancestry, the DNA of your mitochondria tells just as much of your story as your human DNA.

Finally, there is the collective genome of your gut bacteria - the "microbiome." There are as many genes in your microbiome as there are in your human genome! The idea the human genome controls everything in your body **is simply not accurate.** Your human heredity exerts a lot of control over many things. The human genome is very powerful. It can tell us a lot, but there is still much, more to consider. To understand what is really true we must consider three inescapable facts.

FACT: Inside your body there are **three different and distinct genomes**.

FACT: The three genomes **interact** with each other.

FACT: The way the three genomes interact can be influenced by **external inputs.**

Three genomes run your body. This is simple fact. The distinction between one and three genomes is no small thing. You will see it's everything. It completely changes many aspects of how you approach health, nutrition and disease prevention. Here is a very small sampling of new discoveries about the three genomes and their interactions with each other.

- To date **over 116 microbial genes** have been identified connecting to aging and lifespan.
- The bacterial metabolite propionate can activate mitochondrial genes that lead to cognition decline and even autism!
- Specialized bacteria in the gut mucus layer together with the bacterial metabolite Butyrate **control human genes** involved in fat metabolism!
- The bacterial genome in the gut **influences and "talks"** to the mitochondrial genome.
- Mitochondrial genes have been correlated to specific profiles of gut bacteria.
- By increasing Bifidobacteria we can directly promote human genes that maximize longevity!
- Specific bacteria species activate several human genes involved with inflammation and potentiates several forms of cancer. One example is fusobacteria.

You can see quite readily there are three genomes at work. They operate in very powerful ways. They interact with each other. The interaction of the three different genomes defines what can be thought of as the active operating state of your body. The active operating state is highly, highly, dynamic. It depends on daily cross talk between the three genomes. The genome "cross talk" controls many aspects of your health.

Key idea: Your current biological state is defined by the interaction of the three genomes.

So great, we have three distinct and separate genomes inside our body instead of one. You might think big deal, how does that change anything?

It will change everything.

FROM CONCEPT TO PRACTICAL APPLICATIONS

The real truth sets you free. Three genomes run your body. The truth of the three genomes creates new possibilities. Things you think are impossible become possible. Things you think true are revealed as false. I am about to walk you through an example. You will see just how powerful the distinction between one and three genomes is at the practical application layer. It's going to blow your mind. It will assault your deep beliefs about what is true and what is possible.

KEY IDEA: You can **train** digestion of carbs into your body.

CARB TRAINING

A practical application of the three genomes is what I call **carb training**. The widely accepted beliefs about carb digestion are based upon the idea of the one human genome. Our beliefs stemming from this idea dictate our actions.

THE BELIEF: We have issues with many foods because our DNA lacks the enzymes we need to digest them.

THE ACTION: We avoid lots of carbs.

We avoid carbs because we believe our DNA prevents us from digesting them. This drives baby talk. It drives the practice of avoiding all kinds of foods. For example, "dairy is bad. You don't have the enzymes to digest it." And it's all incorrect. The premise is false. Seeing the real truth changes everything. You have three genomes. As your beliefs change your actions change.

THE BELIEF: The genes needed to digest carbs can be acquired via the bacterial genome.

THE ACTION: Train digestion of carbs into the body to handle lactose, glutens and others.

All along the real truth was the genes needed to digest most carbs are not in the human genome to begin with. You don't need human genes to digest them.

You can simply acquire the genes needed to digest them!

All we need to do is selectively acquire key bacteria. These bacteria possess the genes to make the enzymes needed to digest carbs. The result? You can train the body to digest most any kind of carb, even carbs you can not currently handle.

You can even **acquire the ability to digest lactose and glutens!**

Let's do that now. In the process what you stand to gain is an **ability.**

ITS NOT THE FOODS. IT'S THE BUGS

What causes darkness? Is it lack of light? Or does darkness *eliminate* light? You probably answered lack of light causes darkness. This is true. To say darkness eliminates light **conflates** the effect with the cause. This is exactly what has happened in the modern era of nutrition. Gluten intolerance? Dairy intolerance? Bloating and gas? Foods cause those problems because we don't have the genes to digest them right? That's the predominate belief. It stems from thinking the human genome runs everything. Since you don't have the genes to digest carbs you need to eliminate them.

And yet what if this is simply a case of conflation?

What if I told you the cause is not the foods?

You can acquire the ability to handle glutens by acquiring bididobacteria. The same goes for lactose. You are about to gain the ability to digest lactose! In the process you will see everything you believed about lactose intolerance was never true. But wait, why would you want to digest lactose? The baby talk says "dairy is bad!" What you will see later is dairy foods have a lot of functional power. For example dairy is helpful to suppress ACE enzyme activity. Why would you want to do that? For starters, some of these new super viruses, like the SARS-COV 2, utilize the ACE receptor to enter the human body. Dairy can be used to impair ACE enzyme receptors, knock out hunger, speed up fat loss, and even help slow aging. As you can see, the three genomes is no small distinction. Its key to an immune centric approach to health and it changes just about everything. An immune centric approach to health changes your entire approach to your body. More than a different lens, its simply what's really true.

THE NEW ERA OF CARB TRAINING

The prevailing theory today is lactose digestion is controlled by human heredity. The *Theory of Lactase Persistence* says the genes to digest lactose fell out of the human genome hundreds of years ago. The result is dairy is to be avoided. The problem is the theory is both correct and **totally meaningless.** Digestion of lactose is **not** solely the function of the human genome.

There is a growing body of science literature that supports acquiring the ability to digest carbs**, even lactose and glutens!**

THE NEW RESEARCH

A 2017 study summarizing the root cause of gluten intolerance stated "...the root cause of (non celiac gluten intolerance) is a particular dysbiotic (unhealty gut bacteria) profile characterized by decreased Butyrate producing Firmicutes and/or *Bifidobacteria*, leading to low levels of intestinal Butyrate. "

Let me translate.

Low bifidobacteria=> low Butyrate=> gluten intolerance.

Another 2017 study in the Annual Review of Genetics demonstrated that humans with higher Bifidobacteria have a bacterial genotype that "***sidesteps*** *the theory of lactase persistence*. This was a finding consistent across human population groups." Let me translate. The word "sidesteps" means the theory of lactase persistence **does not apply** to humans with high bifidobacteria. You want more proof?

Several studies have shown that protocols to increase lactose fermenting bacteria in the gut alleviate symptoms of lactose intolerance. Here are just a few.

- A 2008 study in the *Journal of Applied Microbiology* showed lactose intolerant subjects for two weeks with bifidobacteria was shown to ameliorate symptoms of lactose intolerance.

- A 2017 study giving human subjects specialized milk fractions increased lactose fermenting species and alleviated symptoms of lactose intolerance.

- A 1997 study showed that small doses of lactose growing over time increase the ability of lactose intolerant subjects to handle dairy. The reason was simply that the lactose provided food for bifidobacteria.

FACT: The bacterial genome contains the genes to digest lactose.

BABIES USE BIFIDO

Our first dose of bacteria comes from mothers milk. It is only because of Bifidobacteria in mothers milk we can digest milk as babies. It's easy to prove**.** Sterilize mothers milk before you give it to a baby. You kill the bacteria the baby needs to digest the milk. I don't suggest you do this. It just illustrates the point. The sugars in milk are a primary food supply for Bifidobacteria. Passed on in mothers milk is a strain of bacteria called Bifidobacteria infantis, This bacteria prefers milk carbohydrates as the main source of energy. The genes of this bacteria make an enzyme specific for long chain milk sugars**, i.e. *lactose.***

Generally speaking Bifidobacteria populations decline with age. Over time you lost the bacteria you got from mom. You then lost the ability to digest dairy. So here is the good news. You can **grow back** the populations of bifidobacteria that digest milk! In the process you gain greater energy, immunity, longevity, and it's a lot easier to stay lean.

I used to break out horribly whenever I had any milk product. Today, I have no issues at all. I grew back the bacteria populations that digest dairy. And now I have a powerful tool. It allows me to knock out hunger on cue, offset weight gain, and gives me many others abilities. To train lactose digestion into the body we feed bifidobacteria. I have done it and have trained thousands to do it. You also have already begun doing it. You took the first step in Chapter 1 with Human Milk Oligosaccharides. This brings us to a bit of a paradox.

THE HORMETIC PARADOX.
At first the solution sounds like a paradox.

KEY IDEA: The foods that give you problems feed the bacteria that solve the problems.

It sounds counter intuitive, but it's how things work. The key is once again is fermentation. Here is the overview. This is not to be done if you have colitis or a medical condition. We will cover that in another chapter.

TO-DO: TRAINING LACTOSE DIGESTION 101

1. Begin with small amounts of Human Milk Oligosaccharides.
2. Add in small amounts of phenol powder.
3. Slowly increase amounts as bloating and gas decrease. Take at least 2-3 weeks on this phase.
4. Next, slowly add in small amounts of organic dairy items like cheese or yogurt and slowly scale over a period of weeks. Begin with amounts that can fit between thumb and forefinger.

Think of how much ground we covered here in one small chapter. By seeing the three genomes is how your body really works, major ideas and practices were vaporized! Your mind probably still resists the new information. It's to be expected. The final foundational piece will help a lot. We are going to reset what you know about food as energy.

TO-DO: THE INTEGRATED INTERVAL

Replicating daily exertion with no time.

The body rapidly adapts to daily exertion. It gets very strong very fast. The same is true in reverse when daily exertion is subtracted. The body withers quickly. There is no middle ground. Daily exertion historically was things like getting water, pushing a plow, hunting or making a fire. Daily exertion is **not** the same thing as our modern contrivances for working out. For thirteen years, I have worked out very little, but daily exertion is part of what I do every day. And it literally takes no time. **It has kept me young.** At 55, I can break into a full sprint with no warm up, walk on my hands for over a minute on a moments notice, put my palms on the ground anytime, anywhere. And it's all from daily exertion, meaning, things you don't need to go to a gym for, things you can do at home or from anywhere.

Over the next few series of to-do's, we will give you the power to add daily exertion back into your life. It will be easy. It's called **The Integrated Interval.** If you got nothing else out of this book, the Integrated Interval will radically and powerfully change your life.

THE POWER OF A MINUTE

Contained within sixty seconds is the power to totally exhaust your body for an entire day. Just ask anyone who has ever run an all out 400 meters. We use the idea of the power contained in a minute but spread out into twenty second intervals across your day.

THE TO DO:

Pick an exercise. It can be your favorite. Lunges, push ups, pull ups, stretching hamstrings, glute stretch, etc. Follow this schedule.

Right now: Do that exercise for 20 seconds. GO!

How do you feel? Great right? That's it for today. This was the first movement of a new life.

For 3 days: Repeat once per day.
Days 4-7: Do twice per day
Days 8-14: Do 3x per day.

Past the fourteen day mark integrate the Integrated Interval at least two times per day, every day.

These small pulses of exertion, integrated into your day, with no warmup, just twenty seconds and back to what you were doing, have the power to radically change your life. The power to effect your health, your immunity, and your rate of aging, are all contained in these small bursts of daily exertion.

At first this may be very hard. Your body will adapt and get strong very fast. Before long you will be Peak Human in this one movement. When I first began doing the integrated interval, I chose pull ups. I'm embarrassed to say I could only do a few. Within a few weeks I was doing fifteen to twenty with ease, anytime, with no warm up. The body adapts rapidly when we do something every day. Its what humans have done for thousands of years. Build daily exertion back into your life with the Integrated Interval. It will change your life in a way "working out" never could.

Chapter 7

New Foundations: Energy Harvest

The majority of thinking today about food is binary and linear. It's the game of calories in, calories out. In this way of thinking food is just units of energy - calories, grams, glycemic index. You just need to count the units.

Ironically, the idea that food is simply units of energy does not represent how food really works. Counting calories and grams can be an effective approach short term, but generally speaking it's not sustainable. More importantly, it's not what is really true about the effect of food on your body. While the scope of this book is far beyond diet, food is always a foundational tool. We need a new foundation to understand what is most true about food, and how it works inside your body.

ENERGY HARVEST

First of all it may surprise you that there isn't a formally recognized definition of the calorie in the International System of Units. I first wrote about this nearly thirteen years ago. It holds true today. All our working ideas and definitions of the calorie are not formally codified by any working scientific body. Look it up yourself. But beyond simple definitions, the core idea here is this

Caloric intake is not the same thing as **energy harvest.**

UNDERSTANDING ENERGY HARVEST

Energy harvest means the energy you **net** from digestion. It's like gross income vs net income. Calories are like gross income. Energy harvest is like net income. All of the newer food innovations in things like protein bars rely on manipulating energy harvest. Read the label. You will see things like "net carbs." Words like "net carbs" mean calories-in does not equal net calories.

Energy harvest is a real thing.

- Animal studies have shown that net calories from carbs can be reduced by altering ratios of bacteria types. This also **triggers and maintains** the active set of genes common to lean people. In other words, by using foods to alter gut bacteria composition, you can map Peak Human physiology on to your body.

- Cheeses and dairy products have been shown to decrease net calories absorbed from fats. They produce "calcium soaps" in the gut. These calcium soaps inhibit fat absorption.

- Selectively targeting production of Bifidobacteria in the gut helps the body **suppress fat storage** by production of FAIF, the protein you learned about in Chapter 1.

- The addition of phenols from things like berries before a meal has been shown to impair key enzymes needed to absorb sugar.

KEY IDEA: The energy you **harvest** from food is quite **variable.**

New scientific models have emerged in recent years reflecting how different foods have unique and functional metabolic properties. Many of these properties work *independent of calories.* For example, a recent paper outlining the Carbohydrate-Insulin Model of Obesity, noted regarding animals "....dietary composition has been clearly demonstrated to affect metabolism and body composition, **independently of calorie intake."** But what about humans?

2,000 calories of potato chips has a radically different effect on the body versus 2,000 calories of salmon. We all get this. The calories are equal. Both are loaded with fat. The effects are totally different. One will get you lean. The other will destroy your health.

Several factors influence how much energy you harvest from food. You can control most of them. My first body hack in 2007 was achieved purely via altering *energy harvest.* You can and will do the same. You can create *meaningful reductions* in the energy harvested from food.

KEY IDEA: You can learn to manipulate the calories harvested from food.

HOW BACTERIA MANAGE ABSORPTION

Experiments have shown animals with gut bacteria pass *87 percent more calories* in their poop than animals without gut bacteria. In the science these are called "germ free" animals. Germ free animals have to eat thirty percent more calories just to *maintain* weight!

These experiments **clearly debunk the idea** that calories in equals calories absorbed.

One mechanism impacting net calories is carbohydrate metabolism. The net energy from carbs varies dramatically depending on your gut bacteria. You just learned our human genome lacks many enzymes necessary to handle more complex types of carbs. In recent years numerous science papers have established that key **enterotype's** of gut bacteria correlate with weight gain, obesity and cancer. Others correlate to being lean and healthy.

SHORT CHAIN FATS FROM BACTERIA EFFECT NET CALORIES

One driver of net calories are the fats produced by bacteria in the gut. These fats, called short chain fatty acids, radically impact caloric absorption. One of them is called **acetate.** Acetate helps you make cholesterol. It also stores fats in the liver. Acetate is also the final form of alcohol your body burns off. Acetate is why high alcohol intake correlates to fatty liver.

KEY IDEA: Acetate correlates to higher net calories.

If your gut bacteria makes lots of acetate, you will net more calories. Acetate levels can fluctuate dramatically. It just depends on the bacteria in your gut. The bacteria in your gut will fluctuate wildly based on what you eat!

THREE FACTS OF ENERGY HARVEST

- Net calories can and do vary from total calories.
- Unique foods possess unique properties to alter net calories.
- Net calories *can* be manipulated.

THE NEW ERA OF FOOD AS FUNCTION

Carbs. Grams. Calories. Macro's. These are units of measure. They represent the idea that food is just energy. If food is simply energy, you don't need anything more than units of energy to understand how food works. This kind of thinking is everywhere; in books, social media, podcasts,. And it is simply **not** what is really true about food. How food works is not characterized merely as units of measure.

THE OLD: Food is just units of measure.

THE NEW: Food is signal, function, and gene activation.

The old framework of food has been outgrown by revelations of how food really works.

You **cannot** step into peak human physiology via the old way of thinking! Peak human physiology is precisely about feeding key bacteria, stimulating key signal pathways, manipulating genes and timing inputs to diurnal rhythm, all in the right order of operations. Thinking of food and using it only as units of measure **can not accomplish this**. The key to mapping Peak Human physiology to your body is using food for function.

KEY IDEA: Foods are unique whole entities. The effects are unique to the whole.

Foods can have unique effects on gene activation, cellular signaling and the three genomes. The effects seen are often unique to the whole. Let's look at the example of orange juice. You will see how the effects are unique to the whole and not the parts.

ORANGE JUICE AND HESPERATIN

Orange juice contains a flavonoid called hesperetin. Hesperetin raises blood levels of key phenols (the color pigments in orange juice). These phenols lower inflammation, reduce DNA damage, improve cholesterol and many other beneficial things like helping to improve memory. Not only that, hesperatin may be one of the most powerful natural defenses in existence to fight highly virulent viruses like H1N1 and Covid 19. It seems to suppress numerous mechanisms needed for these types of viruses to proliferate.

Experiments comparing hesperetin to whole orange juice have shown administering hesperetin alone does **not** raise blood serum levels of phenols the way whole orange juice does.

The effects are unique to the whole.

The benefits of hesperatin are only seen with orange juice, not hesparatin alone. This is a theme you will see repeated over and over. Unique foods take the separate parts, the unique fibers, sugars, proteins and fats and combine them into distinct functional entities. The effects on things like genes and cell signals are *unique to the whole.*

In the new paradigm orange juice contains color pigments. The pigments are called citrus flavonoids and carotenoids. They accumulate in the blood to activate genes and influence signal pathways. New research has shown chronic consumption of orange juice does the following.

- Protects against cognitive decline and aids cognitive function.
- Prevents DNA damage.
- Lowers total cholesterol and LDL.
- Reduces oxidative stress, particularly in the lining of your blood vessels, which as we age becomes a pivotal element accelerating inflammation.
- Reduces inflammation.
- Protects against weight gain and metabolic syndrome.

That last point is particularly interesting. Far from contributing to weight gain, regular consumption of orange juice actually protects against it. So what's going on here? Orange juice is a carb and carbs are sugar and they make us fat right?

This is the old way of thinking.

It's not really true that orange juice **is** a carb. Orange juice ***contains*** carbohydrate, but orange juice also contains many other things, like carotenoids and flavonoids. We now know inflammation and free radical stress profoundly influence body fat accumulation. Orange juice protects against both. It loads the blood with protective signal mediators. Orange juice as a whole lowers oxidative stress and activates genes that reduce inflammation. This has nothing to do with macro's. Instead **these are functional properties of the whole!**

The example of orange juice demonstrates what is really true. Food is not simply energy and units of measure.

Hesperatin from orange juice and viral spread.
As it turns out, orange juice - fresh, whole, organic - may just be an essential component of an immune centric diet. When it comes to impairing the spread of a virus like Covid 19.

- Hesperatin may inhibit PLpro, an necessary enzyme for coronavirus replication.
- Hesperatin may inhibit the S spike docking mechanism of coronavirus
- Hesperatin may inhibit RDRP, the enzyme needed for RNA to be copied to replicate the virus.

What is the best way to get Hesperatin into the body? It's via the whole, not the parts. When treated as a distinct whole entity, orange juice has properties for health and weight unique to the whole. This is true of many foods. This way of thinking gets us out of reductionism - the calories/macro's/ingredients way of thinking.

HEALING GUT ISSUES WITH ORANGE JUICE

The Objective: Healing issues with gut inflammation and a worn gut lining.

THE WHAT: Orange juice
THE WHEN: Mornings.
THE HOW: Combined with a minimum four hour fast upon waking.

If you have chronic gut inflammatory issues orange juice just may be your best friend. (But orange juice is a carb and carbs are bad.) When chronic oxidative stress takes hold in the gut, the tissues lining the gut become inflamed. In this state the gut lining must heal **before fibers can work.**

The worn gut lining presents a tricky problem. The short chain fatty acid Butyrate is the primary way the gut lining is maintained. The problem, however, is this; when the gut lining is worn down, key transporters needed for Butyrate **will not work.** In this case, a combination of fasting and orange juice may help the inflamed gut.

Research into inflammatory bowel disease shows ascorbic acid in the gut is reduced by up to 73% from oxidative stress. Fasting helps the gut make nitrogen. This feeds Akkermansia to restore and heal the gut lining. Orange juice lines the inflamed gut with ascorbate to reduce oxidative stress. **Make sure to strain the pulp out first.**

Later, you can and will demonstrate to yourself how foods have unique properties with hands on practical experiments.

YOUR THINKING WILL CHANGE

Thinking of food as units of measure creates a rigid mindset. Things become binary. We tend to think in terms of baby talk. Everything has to fit into a good/bad mindset. You may have reacted at first to orange juice exactly in this way. But to hack Peak Human biology we need to take into account many other things.

- Diurnal rhythm,

- What you ate last,
- What you will eat next,
- How different foods work together,
- The sequence of meals.

Once you take these things into account the old binary thinking shatters. Tracking units of energy and avoiding major classes of foods becomes so 10 years ago. Let's finish by updating our understanding of carbs.

The Old: Fruits and Fibers are carbs.
The New: Fruits and Fibers are **functional fermenters.**

Language conditions the way we think about things. If we want to stimulate new thinking and new directions we have to change the words we use. The words "carbs" and "fiber" are very *outdated words*. They do not accurately describe the things we now know we are dealing with. Want proof?

We use the word "carb" to describe fibers - things like beans, potatoes, green beans, lentils. We lump them all in as carbs. Subsequently we just avoid them. But when we look into this thing we call "fiber" there is something very compelling. There are dozens of different kinds of fibers! There are the resistant starches, the arabinoxolans, cellulose, hemi-cellulose, pectins, inulins, and many others. Each exerts unique effects. Each is a unique food source for different types of bacteria in the gut, which themselves exert unique global effects on the body.

The same can be said of different fruits. The color pigments in dark fruits act as food for very specific bacteria. Banana starch, a high glycemic carb in the old paradigm, can be a potent food source for bifidobacteria when consumed semi-green. The same is true of fructose. Fructose bound to whole foods works very different from fructose in isolation. Fructose contained in fruit is bound to many types of natural fibers and phenols in a matrix that works as a whole.

Overlooked in the baby talk of carbs are bad and "food is units of energy" is **fermentation.**

Fermentation is when bacteria in our gut feed on fibers and proliferate. One key to Peak Human physiology is *leveraging fermentation.* Here is the key.

KEY IDEA: Fermentation makes bacteria!!!

Let me say this again. It is vital you get this. *Gut fermentation produces gut bacteria.* In fact, it is estimated that for every 100 grams of carbs fermented in the gut a whopping *30 grams of bacteria is produced!*

KEY IDEA: 30 grams of bacteria are produced for every 100 grams of fiber fermented!

Using **what, when and how,** you can use specific fruits and fibers to steer the types of bacteria populating your gut. Doing so can rapidly map Peak Human physiology onto your body.

Ironically, this is accomplished with **"carbs!"**

For example, inulin fibers found in banana's and asparagus, when given to obese people selectively feed a strain of the bifidobacteria family called *b. adolescentis,* which promotes getting lean. The "what" are bananas and asparagus. When and how we use them is the other part of the equation.

The only thing in your way are words.

The words you use program your mind. It's time to step into what is really true. Fermentation is real. Learning to harness fermentation is a real power. You can use it to map peak human physiology onto your body. Using the language of real health- what, when and how - we can selectively feed the body specific fibers to ferment **overnight** the same bacteria found in the leanest, healthiest and longest lived humans.

This chapter was about de-programming your mind from the old way of thinking. Let's take break from big words for a few chapters. It's time to define the problem.

TO-DO: FERMENTING BACTERIA 101

Using key substrate to target signal pathways and bacteria cross talk.

YOU NEED:

Semi-green banana's, grapefruit, asparagus, onions, avocado, raspberries, vinegar and olive oil.

THE OBJECTIVE

Using a key sequence of foods, you will drive b-vitamin production sky high in a single day. You also activate key signal pathways while you sleep to slow aging. This is just for one day.

THE TO DO:

Breakfast : Banana's and grapefruit.
Lunch: Banana's and grapefruit.
Dinner: Bowl mixed with raw asparagus, onions, avocado, raspberries, vinegar and olive oil. Use no more than 1/2 avocado.

THE WHAT: Prebiotic foods.
THE WHEN: In the above sequence.
THE HOW: Bananas should be semi-green. You have to test your tolerability first. Start with less green. Over time you can work up to more green.

The amounts will surprise you. Roughly two bananas and whole grapefruit per meal. For dinner, asparagus and onion are most effective raw. If you don't like asparagus substitute raw green beans. If you don't like anything in the bowl mix, then just repeat lunch. Caution, have some cough syrup standing by. You may not sleep from all the b-vitamin production.

WHAT IT DOES:

Later on you will learn about a master regulator of aging called AMPK. Grapefruit naturally stimulates AMPK. Semi-green banana feeds bifidobacteria. These two foods are very synergistic. We are pre-amplifying all the beneficial signals that extend life during sleep. The foods for dinner all either feed bifido or further amplify signals to slow aging. It is the sequence of these things together that you will literally feel.

PART 3:

The Problems We Need To Solve

Chapter 8

The Problem of Time

Until very recently, time was the single biggest problem everyone faces. Pre-pandemic, the problem of time looked like this for most people...

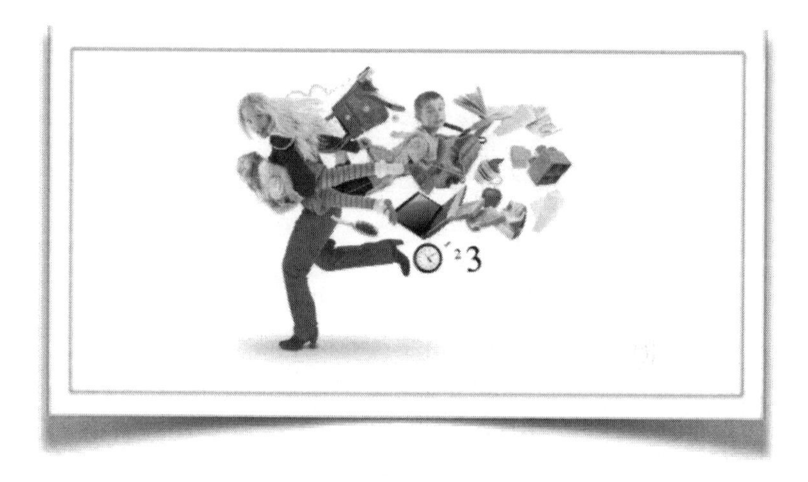

AND THIS

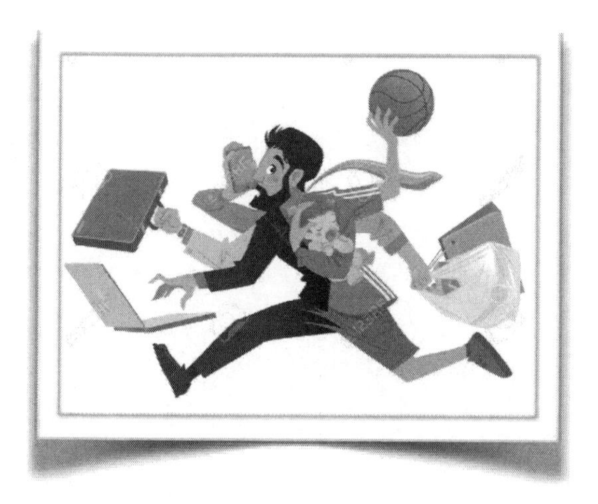

Get it?

It is likely your life was characterized at times by the image above. And then, suddenly, we were all homebound. We had too much time on our hands.

So what is does our new reality look like now?

Most likely our lives will have a mix of both. We will have seasons where we have no time, and seasons where we have too much time, spent mostly at home.

In Chapter 1 I posed the question, why does the simply solution, which is to stay healthy elude the vast majority of people over time? The answer is truth. We are not dealing with what's really true.

Think about something, if what you do isn't based on what's really true will you be satisfied? If you are not dealing with what really happens over time will you get what you want? Over and over in this book you will be confronted with real truth.

For example, These images represent the real world most people live in. Priorities and time management not withstanding, things get overwhelming. Often. We all know it. The modern era of fitness sells a fantasy. The fantasy is we can always make time. Stop listening to lies. Here is the real truth.

Time frequently goes to zero, and for long periods.

If you honestly inventory your own life history you can readily see this is the real truth. And now we have a new reality. It is one where we will have seasons of no time, and seasons of too much time.

GETTING REAL ABOUT TIME

To understand **what really happens** over the long term requires a perspective that encompasses the realities you will face across decades. This requires hyper honesty. The transitions from carefree and single, to roles and responsibilities, aging and injuries, drive very real seasons of life. These seasons exert very real pressure on any system or to-do list you may subscribe to. A foundation built on fitness fantasy always collapses under the weight of life's real pressures.

The foundation of staying younger, longer, is poured with the truth of what happens over time. I have seen how the decades play out. Here is what is fake.

FITNESS FANTASY - THE BLUE PILL

- You can solve the problem of time with priorities and time management.
- You will get in shape and stay there.
- You can always make time.
- If you get in your best shape you solved the problem.

None of this is true. It never was. You want real truth?

THE RED PILL

- You **will** have long seasons of being "off track."
- Getting in top shape means absolutely **nothing** long term.
- Your primary role creates probabilities that overpower priorities.
- Getting in shape can and does drive long term weight gain.

This is what is really true. And it's the first time anyone has ever laid out what is really true.

We are going to define the problem of time everyone in the real world faces. Just by defining the problem your entire approach to your health and body will change. Allow me to introduce to you the **Graph of Doom**.

THE GRAPH OF DOOM

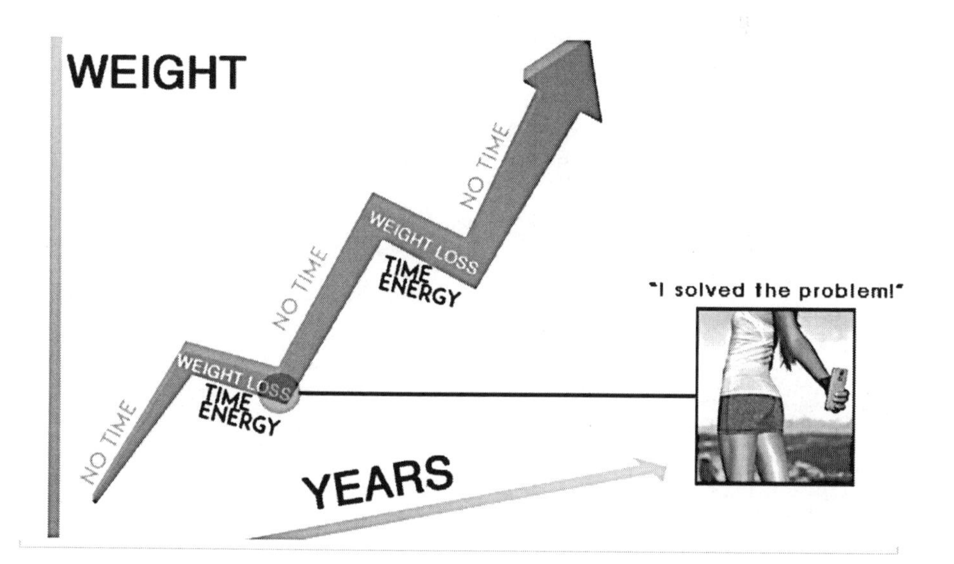

One of the central problems of modern life experienced by the vast majority are long periods where the time and energy needed for exercise and diet are not available. Over and over what we see are "seasons" of dieting, seasons of getting in shape, seasons of getting on track. And while **we do need to devote time intensive periods to taking care of our bodies**, the reality is there are also long periods of inactivity, and we *all know this is true.* This is what really happens over time for the majority of the bell curve. This even happens to some who consider themselves outliers if you simply observe them long enough. The downward dips in the Graph are seasons of getting in shape or losing weight. The peaks are seasons being "off track."

Notice something - many times you "get back on track" and get in shape. And yet the slope of the curve remains slanted **upward.** It's only when you widen your view to several decades the pattern is clear. It's groundhog day. The process repeats over and over. You get off track. You get back on track. You take selfies, do a social media victory lap, you think you solved the problem. These periods where you think you solved the problem can even last many years. And yet the Graph still tilts up. This is not some cutesy graph I came up with, this is the true life reality that actually happens to most people.

KEY IDEA: Seasons of being in shape are not solving the problem.

Lets summarize the major ideas behind the Graph of Doom.

- You spend long seasons being in shape.

- Over time there are seasons being "off track."

- Weight and appearance are the measure of success.

- Seasons of being lean and looking good are actually **part of the upward long term trend of weight gain.**

Interestingly, being single tends to correlate to being in shape, and family and relationships to seasons being "off track."

How do we know the Graph is true? First, the Graph is supported by the science. But it's also *self evident.* Millions of people moving into their thirties to forties to fifties and sixties, routinely learn it's true **the hard way**. The Graph is something most experience over three or four decades. Work, family, kids and pressures eventually drive seasons of being "off track"

PROBABILITIES ARE WHAT ACTUALLY DRIVE OUTCOMES

I am about to show you that long periods where time and energy are not available for diet and exercise are simply unavoidable for the vast majority of people in the modern habitat. **These "life seasons" are more the result of probability than priorities.** I want to say up front you don't have to agree with me to obtain the intended benefit.

There are two camps of people when I bring this up. The first camp consists of ordinary people. These are the mom's, accountants, business owners, cops, attorneys, commercial real estate brokers, etc. The ordinary people almost always agree. They universally nod their heads. They get it. They live it. Despite their best efforts these "off seasons" just tend to happen. If this is you, you are already breathing easier. The truth sets us free. I know your pain. It's what got me here.

Others tend to disagree with the argument of "off seasons." At his peak our friend Simon was one of these people. These people believe the problem is one of priorities and psychology. Once again, you don't have to agree with me if this is you. We are all seeking the optimal strategy. Let's make that our common ground - improving upon what we do. I will offer, however, that unless you have been consistently fit for over twenty years that, like Simon, you may well be in a ten or fifteen year cycle that is playing out. I have seen it many times, even with people who have appeared on magazine covers.

If you have ever found yourself saying the magic words, "I just have to get back into ***it***", the rest of this chapter will feel like a breath of fresh air. "***It***" are the, seasons of "I just haven't had the time", where all the weight gain happens.

A 2017 science paper from a team of Australian researchers quantified the barriers to adoption of the healthy lifestyle. The top reason people fail to adopt a healthy lifestyle are **time constraints.** More importantly, the study quantified exactly how much time is needed every day to maintain the "healthy lifestyle."

THE HIDDEN COST OF HEALTHY

One reason I'm not selling you on a lifestyle is you probably can't afford it. Before you buy into something you should know the cost right? The empirical research into the time needed for the healthy lifestyle is, well, shocking. Here it is.

2.3 HOURS PER DAY!

2.3 hours a day is the all in cost for the "healthy lifestyle." If the research is correct, time is not just **a** problem. Time is **the** problem.

2.3 hours a day at first sounds extreme. You may only spend thirty to forty minutes a day exercising. But let's dig a bit deeper. This is the *all in cost* . Ladies, how much time do you spend showering and doing your hair after a sweaty yoga or barre class? It all adds up. "Healthy" has hidden costs when it comes to time.

Here is a simple exercise to help identify your all in cost of the healthy lifestyle.

CALCULATE THE HIDDEN COST OF HEALTHY.

Do this exercise twice. First pencil in your estimate of each activity. Then over the next week time yourself and see what the actual time is.

Getting your clothes and gear together.________
Driving to the gym, or class or wherever you go.
____
Getting into and out of the place you workout out.________
Actually working out, whatever it is you do. ________
Showering after a workout.________
Getting yourself together after working out.________
Shopping for the food you need.________
Preparing the food you need.________
Shopping for supplements_______
Cleaning up after your meal. ________
Meal prepping. ________
Extra sleep needed from working out ______
Trips to the doctor ________
Time socializing around workouts ________

TOTAL COST OF HEALTHY IN TIME __________

If the research data is accurate how is 2.3 hours a day sustainable? Many experts say the answer is to set priorities and manage your time. That solution has a very big elephant in the room. The experts don't have your job. Remember, we can't solve a problem until we can replicate the conditions of the problem. The real world involves roles and responsibilities that compete for your time.

ROLE DYNAMICS AND LEFTOVER MINUTES

The science of **Role Dynamics Theory** says everyone has a primary role. Your primary role is your main thing: mom, VP of Sales, Instagram model, Dad, CEO, Computer Programmer. The concept is simple; your time is primarily allocated by your primary role.

One reason off seasons are inevitable is that most people use what I call *leftover minutes* vs primary minutes. Primary minutes are minutes that go into your primary role. Imagine two people. Person A has a primary role in some profession where you have to look good. Person B does not. Person A must allocate his or her primary minutes to looking good. Person B has to allocate *leftover minutes* looking good. Person A simply has fantastically better odds of looking good.

One of the underlying problems why a lot of advice does not translate, and why this debate creates such division, has to do with advice born out of primary minutes. Most of the advice givers achieve their result from primary minutes. Most of the advice takers have to use leftover minutes to get the same result. In fact this entire book was born out of my experiences with what happens trying to get the same result with leftover minutes.

Your primary role puts *unique pressures* and constraints on where your primary minutes go. Your primary role is like a deck of cards. It sets the odds and creates probabilities for how your time will be used.

What's left outside your primary minutes are ***leftover minutes.***

Everything else, socializing, shopping, showering, time with the spouse, doing your hair, deciding what to wear, washing your car, picking the kids up at school, and hundreds of other activities compete for leftover minutes with the items you listed above under the "Healthy Lifestyle." Here is a quick exercise to identify where your leftover minutes go.

MY PRIMARY ROLE IS _______________

Now list where your leftover minutes go

WHERE MY LEFTOVER MINUTES GO:

1.
2.
3.
4.
5.

If the time cost of the healthy lifestyle is 2.3 hours the answer to **who can sustain 2.3 hours a day** comes down almost entirely to your role.

FACT: If you listed a primary role that involves being fit you have a massive probability advantage.

If your primary role is devoted to being fit you are like a black jack dealer with a deck of face cards. Out of the 1,440 minutes in a day you have on average 500 minutes you can devote to being fit. You have better odds. If your primary role is being fit, getting real about the difference in the odds stemming from roles will give you an advantage with your clients.

Imagine a black jack expert sells you a strategy. The expert always seems to win. You assume his strategy will work for you as well. When you try the experts strategy, sometimes you win, sometimes you lose. Over time you lose more than you win. The expert says you are doing something wrong with the strategy. But there is an elephant in the room. The expert uses a different deck of cards than you. His deck is all face cards. Your deck has all the cards. One day you challenge the expert to play from the same deck as you. A funny thing happens. The expert does no better than you the longer the game is played.

HOW THE DECK OF LEFTOVER MINUTES IS PLAYED

Here are some averages from the US. Bureau of Labor and Statistics. These are just basic categories. We could come up with many others, like answering email, messaging and on and on. Here is how an average day breaks out.

Sleeping: 420 minutes.
Commuting/driving/going places: 101 minutes
Eating: 67 minutes
Cleaning: 60 minutes
Primary Role: 500 minutes
Time w/Children: 104 minutes
Getting ready: 22 minutes

The total here is 1,274 minutes. Now on top of this add in 150 minutes for the "healthy lifestyle." Now the total minutes in an average day is **1,424 minutes!** This leaves sixteen discretionary minutes in a day! The problem, however, is this is **not** reality. The day in and day out of real life is far, far more challenging.

You are getting ready to go exercise. You get a text. Your son was bullied at school and got in a fight. You can either workout, or drop everything and deal with your child's issue. Your child wins, hands down, right?

Robert is 35, a devoted family man, former powerlifter and fitness devotee. Like most he has a real job. He is an analyst for a major corporation. He heard me on a podcast and asked me to help him learn some of the things you are learning here. Ironically, as I was adding some fine touches to this chapter Robert and I had this exchange. His Primary Role has abruptly taken his leftover minutes to zero.

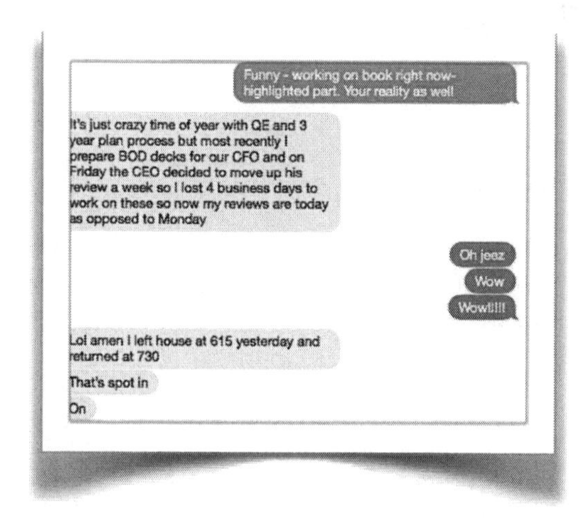

Robert's text is a good example of Role Dynamics and leftover minutes in real life. Time management can not solve this. Real life can easily overwhelm fitness fantasy about priorities. So here is the problem. Sustaining 2.3 hours a day from your leftover minutes has a **low probability of success long term.** In reality its not possible for the majority of the bell curve. But we need to go farther still to see the real root of the time problem.

LEFTOVER MINUTES GO TO ZERO

If 2.3 hours a day is not sustainable then what is the number that can be sustained? This brings us to the *real barrier of time.*

KEY IDEA: The real barrier of time is seasons when leftover minutes go to zero.

The storms of life are like a flash flood. They wipe your plans and priorities off the calendar. Unexpectedly pressures and events compound. They compete for leftover minutes. Inevitably leftover minutes are squeezed to zero. And for long periods. This is the barrier you must overcome. Everyone in the real world, the world of having a job, family, pressures, age, knows this is what's really true long term. We all have long periods of telling ourselves, " **I gotta get back on track. I need to get back into it."**

Over decades the real problem of time, *leftover minutes going to zero,* keeps resurfacing. The reason all the expert advice basically sums up to "You gotta make the time", is no one has a solution that works without time. The answer to the problem of time going to zero becomes, "don't let time go to zero."

But time does go to zero. Frequently. And for long periods, sometimes years. That's the problem.

THE WINNING STRATEGY

You need a winning strategy when leftover minutes go to **zero.** It has to work when you don't have time to eat right and exercise. It must do two things.

1. It must keep the body young.
2. It must prevent the weight gain that takes place when time goes to zero.

This is virgin territory.

This is a strategy to maintain weight when you can not eat right and exercise. When leftover minutes are zero you must be able to maintain. No strategy can or ever will work long term until you have this.

KEY IDEA: If the strategy doesn't solve the real problem of time it's not real.

It *can't* work. You will discover why in The Fat Loss Paradox.

I want to share my own experience of this problem and what I have seen after 40 plus years.

MY EXPERIENCE WITH THE MAIN PROBLEM OF TIME

The year is 1992. I'm 27. I'm single and work in telecom sales. I sit in my car, outside the gym at Beach and Adams in Huntington Beach. I'm downing my "metabolic optimizer". These were the ancestors of meal replacements and pre-workout drinks. Those things don't exist yet. There is no HITT training, no personal trainers, no pre-workout drinks Not many people were super fit in that era. Everyone was always asking what my secret was. My secret was working out 1-2 hours a day. That's always been everyones secret, plus or minus several physique enhancing substances.

An hour in, working my triceps, a bit of soreness gnaws at my elbows. I have always been very analytical. I start to mentally run the math. It's not very good. I can see how this kind of training is going to wear my body out prematurely.

Over the years, I have seen thousands of people who trained a lot when they were young wear their bodies out. Conversely, I have seen many people who never trained until the late forties or fifties get in incredible shape simply because the body is fresh. The body is not a set of tires with infinite tread. It has a shelf life. You can wear it out prematurely by how you use it.

KEY IDEA: Less beats more in the long run.

At only 27 I already had a lot of injuries. At age 16 my foot slipped on some chalk while clean and jerking 265 pounds overhead. I fell backwards with all the weight. At 19, my wrist slipped benching 335 pounds. The bar crashed into my collarbone. I began to mull the possibility of a long term net negative. All the time, effort and energy I was investing into my health had a high cost. Twenty percent of the effort yielded eighty percent of the health benefit. The remaining eighty percent of the effort made the difference in appearance. It was also driving eighty percent of the wear and tear. The more I thought about it the math sucked. I began to think about getting maximum results with minimal time and effort. There wasn't a word for it then, but I began hacking the body.

Bodies are a form of status. Standing out physically equates to a form of herd rank. People will do just about anything for more status. Where it concerns the body there is a huge caveat with doing more to the body to obtain more status.

You choose how fast to use up your body.

What if you had to buy one car for life? Assume money is no object. You can choose anything but you can only choose once. What would you choose? Most people would consider a number of factors: reliability, practicality, appearance, space, and yes, status.

WHAT YOU WOULD NOT DO

What you would not do is park your car for 6 months and then race it at the track for six months, and then repeat the cycle over and over. You would destroy the car. Fast. Letting a car sit for long periods is bad for the car. Racing a car all the time also wears the car out fast. Racing in particular has a very high toll on a car. Ironically, the vast majority of people do something just like this with their bodies over time.

You get off track. Just like the car you sit for six months. You decide to get back into it. You go hard, working out, doing the routines of physique stars and olympic athletes. It's just like taking your car to the track. Injury inevitably kicks in. Another cycle of sitting on the sidelines ensues. And then it's back on track. You go hard again.

If you could only have one car for life, you would never use the car in this way. Yet this is exactly what the vast majority is doing to their bodies.

KEY IDEA: High performance has a high cost.

The number of ex-athletes who can barely walk could fill stadiums. Pushing the body to extremes to get incremental benefits of appearance or performance has a high cost. It wears the body out prematurely.

Fast forward. The year is 2006. I'm forty now. Thirteen more years have passed. My ledger of wear and tear now records thousands of hours training: bench presses, clean and jerks, handstands, interval sprints years before HIIT was a word, lots of trips under 6% body fat, every diet you can think of, including fasting and time restricted feeding, Twenty years before those things became a thing. Despite all of this, a journey that started with Jack Lalanne in 1970, working out to Jack, his onesie, and his dog, has hit a dead end sign.

I'm fat.

Tens of thousands of hours invested*;* **return on investment zero.**

Ironically, only three years earlier at age 37, I was in top shape; 5% body fat and 212 pounds And I was the real deal. I never used steroids. I worked a regular job. Like most I was just a consumer in the pursuit of health.

On that day in 2006, I sat in my Newport Beach office, reflecting on my state, something amusing occurred to me. If put on a graph, my then current weight of 257 pounds would exactly match my companies growth curve over the last three years. Both had gone up a lot. I started telling myself, "Ok, I just have to get back on track.....I just gotta get back into it."

BACK ON TRACK: THE MODERN MANTRA OF HEALTH

The body mantra of the modern era is, **"I have to get back on track!"** *Everyone chants the mantra over time.* Millions are chanting it right now. Repetitive seasons of groundhog day for "getting back into it", are the new normal for the body.

Getting back on track is a ritual. It has all kinds of accompaniments - new clothes, before pictures, reprioritizing, after pics, the social media victory lap, advice giving on how you did it, learning big words, and then, sadly, the long term inevitability of competition for your time, the fat loss rebound effect, and many other things detailed in this book.

In 2006 the storm of building a company had taken a toll. Day after day of high stress pressures and putting out fires crushed my leftover minutes to zero. The decline of age was hitting. I didn't have the energy to workout in the evenings like I once did. Family and relationship pressures competed for my priorities and time. After thirty years of putting in the time everything I knew to do required time I simply did not have. The paradigm told me it was my fault, that I needed to make time and set priorities. I discovered the paradigm had no answers for the real problems we all face.

KEY IDEA: The current paradigm for the body has no answers for the real barriers time presents.

Ultimately why I got fat is why everyone gets fat: time constraints, age related decline, real life pressures, accumulated wear and tear. Let me leave you with one key idea regarding time.

KEY IDEA: You will never really solve anything until you get real about **the real problem of time.**

TO-DO: THE INTEGRATED INTERVAL

Bedtime Circulation and Mobility

Imagine a world where we take care of our teeth only by going to the dentist. In this world, the experts say things like your teeth should be a priority. You need to make time. So you do. Three times a week you go for a cleaning. As far as strategies go it kind of works. For a while. Inevitably the difficulty of seeing the dentist three times per week becomes impossible to maintain. You get off track. You have an off season with your teeth. During the off season your teeth decay. The reason the strategy didn't work was **time.** Taking an hour three times per week to see the dentist is too time intensive. The irony is this is exactly the same strategy most people have for their body. It's called working out. It takes about the same amount of time every week.

Your teeth illustrate a life necessity. You have a non-time intensive daily maintenance strategy for your teeth. Every day, without fail, you maintain your teeth. You may only spend two minutes total. Yet you never miss a day. Your body **needs** something similar. If you don't clean your teeth the decay is noticeable that day. Your body works the same way. You just don't feel don't feel the decay until its too late. What follows is a powerful life transformation. It only takes one minute. You do it at bedtime, just before you brush your teeth. It's toothbrush time for the body. **Do this starting tonight.**

THE WHAT: Two yoga flows.
THE WHEN: At bedtime just before brushing your teeth.
THE HOW: With three deep breaths, head inverted, and transition to the ancestral squat.

1. Start down dog. Take 3 deep breaths through your nose with head inverted.
2. Move to cobra position.
3. Move to Childs pose.
4. Come up to your feet and touch hands to ground, stretching hamstrings.
5. Repeat the flow again.

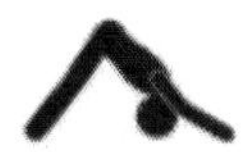 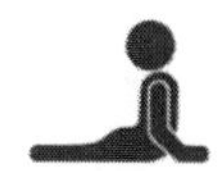 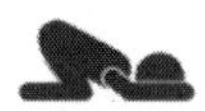 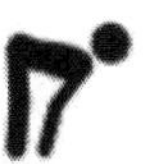

You will progress incrementally. If you can only touch your hands to your knees keep at it. Before long you will get your hands on the ground.

As a bonus, add in the ancestral squat after child's pose. It looks like this

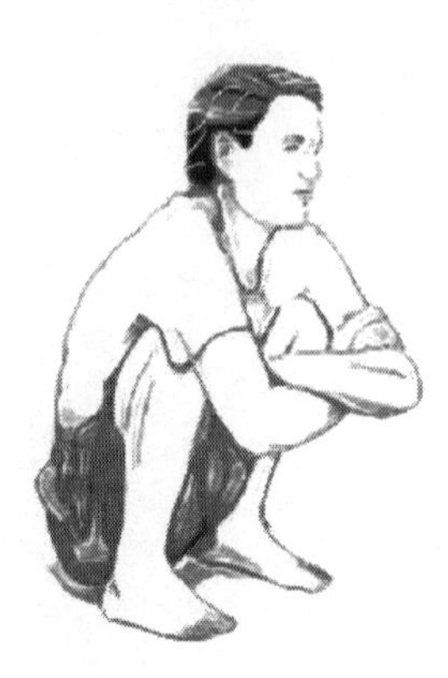

For thousands of years humans spent time every day in this position. It has numerous benefits. It helps prevent the hip, knee and ankle problems common with aging that destroy mobility. This position works them every day. It also helps with lower back issues and constipation. In general it helps your body stay young.

I do four total flows at bed time now days. It keeps me youthful and limber. I can touch my palms on the ground anytime, anywhere because of this simple bed time exercise.

Make this part of your nightly bed time routine **starting tonight!**

TONIGHTS TO-DO:
2 Yoga Flows at bedtime

Chapter 9

The Habitat Problem

Do you want to know the underlying cause of obesity and metabolic syndrome, above all others?

It's the refrigerator.

Metabolic disease can literally be traced to the advent of refrigerators and everything it takes to support them. Refrigerators require mechanized transportation and farming, electricity, local stores with abundant food, running water, and every other convenience the modern era brings. The presence of a refrigerator means more food can be stored than used at any given time. We live in a world where people are rushing to jam their refrigerators with as much food as possible. And when that happens? They buy more refrigerators and stuff them to the brim.

In an entire lifetime, carrying groceries to the refrigerator is likely the most energy the average person will ever expend to get food. If survival is the most powerful force in your body, the refrigerator embodies how the modern era has nerfed the forces tied to survival.

And yet now, facing a post pandemic world, it is exactly the force of survival the drives us to stuff multiple refrigerators with stores of food.

The forces of survival are always there. The modern era, exemplified by the refrigerator, keeps them nerfed long as there is abundant food.

THE META LIFESTYLE OF THE MODERN ERA

You live in a "meta lifestyle." It's the one afforded by modern industrialization. This is why I'm not selling you on some "healthy lifestyle." All "lifestyles" subordinate to the meta lifestyle. We all share it. It's the lifestyle of using transportation, refrigerators, electricity and lots of other things.

The net of the meta lifestyle, as far as your body is concerned, is to invert **energy balance**. Energy balance refers to the energy you take in versus what you expend. The meta lifestyle inverts energy balance when compared to history. Today it's much easier to store energy from food than expend it. It used to be the exact opposite. This is the core problem the modern meta lifestyle presents.

THE PROBLEM OF HABITAT INFUSION

As the 20th century progressed, a critical inflection point passed. **Life suddenly got easy.** Food became plentiful. Energy dense food became ubiquitous. The probabilities of energy balance **inverted.**

Once it was super hard for the average person to be fat.The *odds* were against you. For most of history food was scarce. Being overweight was a sign of wealth and health. Without servants life was hard. Most people who wanted clean clothes used a washboard. It looked and felt like a workout. An average person who wanted butter had to make it. That looked a lot like a workout too. The same was true for furniture. Making furniture also looked like a workout.

For all of history weight gain had constraints. Getting food required lots of labor. Often there was no food at all. We called those famines. When there was food it was generally low in energy. Pizza as we know it didn't really exist. Just about everything required hard labor. Once, there was no way to avoid expending lots of energy and food had **low energy density,** meaning everything was low cal.

This age presents the exact opposite problem. We have a problem of "too much." We have too much food, too much technology, too much abundant energy, and when confined to home, too much time on our hands. Opposing your efforts is a force of probability; it's easier to take in energy than expend it. This creates a probability that favors weight gain over the long term. This probability creates the main health problem of the meta lifestyle we all share. But it is only the first of many.

Why is there an unsettled debate regarding obesity and the overweight majority in modern societies? The answer seems intuitively obvious. Sugar and lack of exercise are what most people point to.

Upon closer examination the causes of metabolic disease and obesity are not so clear. Research suggests the problem has *multiple causes.* Many factors are attributed. It's hard to nail the cause down to any one thing: endocrine disruptors in the water, processed foods, EMF fields, fruits and vegetables depleted of flavor and nutrients, neurotransmitter depletion from constant information overload, sedentary lifestyles, and many other things seem to play a part. Our intuition seems challenged the closer we look. Still, no matter how much the science seems to negate a simple answer, our intuition can't get completely shaken. It whispers to us there is indeed a simple obvious answer.

There is, and at some level *we are all aware of it.*

I want to give you a new way to look at the problem. It will satisfy both our intuition and the science that says lots of things contribute to the problem.

I want to present to you the idea that obesity and metabolic disease is a **habitat problem.**

I first began to think of the overarching cause of metabolic disease as a habitat issue back in 2016. I was consulting with Quest Nutrition. One day I was having a conversation with the brilliant Carl Lenore, founder of Superhuman Radio. Carl is one of the most brilliant and innovative thinkers I know. He's always full of original and amazing ideas that never cease to astound me. Vitamin D was the hot topic of the day back then. During our conversation it struck me how numerous factors combined to have a distinct effect on our ancestors. The net of these things form a habitat. That habitat creates distinct probabilities. Likewise our modern habitat creates probabilities that favor aging and poor human health.

KEY IDEA: **Habitat infusion** is the foundation of the problem.

We are infused with our modern habitat. Our ancestors were also infused with theirs. Their feet touched the dirt.Their faces weathered in the sun.The microorganisms in the soil became one with their bodies. They got cold or hot and couldn't do much about it. People needed to depend on each other for survival. **All** of these factors, large and small, formed a distinct set of *stimuli:* low energy dense food, total darkness at night, daily temperature flux, shivering, high omega 3's in the diet, daily exposure to fresh air and sunshine, daily physical exertion, high levels of vitamin D, low to no EMF, and several other factors all worked together. In that habitat obesity and metabolic disease are highly improbable. It's extremely difficult to have metabolic disease, obesity or cancer in the ancestral habitat. The conditions are stacked against you.

Likewise, we are *infused* with our modern habitat.

Artificial light wreaking havoc with our body clock, emf fields contributing to disturbed insulin function, hormone disruptors in the water and cosmetics, deuterium rich water in our food promoting cancer, prescription drugs, carbon monoxide disrupting sleep, constant control of temperature, lack of hard chewing, neurotransmitter depletion from information addiction, mechanized transportation, energy dense food everywhere that takes little to no energy to obtain - these factors and many others collectively combine to form a *distinct habitat* that we are part of. Infusion with the modern habitat creates a distinct set of *conditions where* obesity and metabolic disease are **highly probable.**

An idea you see repeated many times in this book is the notion of **probabilities.** Probabilities tell us the likelihood of a thing.

KEY IDEA: Ecosystems drive probabilities.

We are always the product of our ecosystems. If you take two people of equal IQ, one went to Stanford, the other never went to college. The one who is the product of the Stanford ecosystem just has better odds. It doesn't mean both can not succeed, but it does mean one has much *better odds* than the other. Stanford and silicon valley are a unique ecosystem. It offers access to channels not available outside that ecosystem.The failure of the fitness paradigm to work on society at large can largely be explained as a problem of ecosystems. The fitness paradigm works great in its natural ecosystem. If you make your living in fitness it works. It only fails when applied **outside of that ecosystem.** As strategies go, it was never designed for the 9-5 world. It suffers from probabilistic constraints, as we detailed in the previous chapter. Within the fitness ecosystem, that paradigm has very good odds of working. If not, the odds are not so good.

The difficulty staying lean and healthy faced by most people in our modern habitat is the result of probability. The deck is stacked against you. It isn't any one thing. *It is the habitat itself.* Should the zombie apocalypse happen tomorrow, our intuition confirms no one would suffer from obesity. Everyone wants the simple solution for problems of weight, cancer and metabolic disease. Here it is. Here is the simple solution

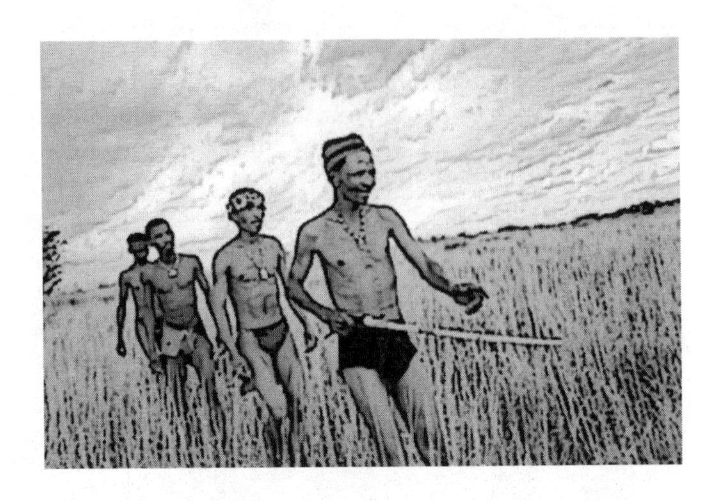

The simple solution. Works every time.

Just swap habitats. Become a hunter gatherer. It solves everything. Obesity will be impossible. The deck is stacked against you.

The simple solution, however, is not so simple. No one seems willing to relocate. The next chapter will complete the picture. You will learn *how humans really eat.* It explains why mimicking a hunter gatherers diet doesn't work long term either.

Still the point stands. Swap habitats and metabolic disease takes care of itself. Whatever the issue, thyroid, menopause, hormones, whatever, take away refrigerators, grocery stores, cars, power, running water, heated indoors, and suddenly **no one** has a weight problem. If you will spend fourteen hours a day finding food, merged with the natural habitat, chewing hard food, neither you, nor anyone you know, will count calories. No one will have a belly fat problem. Nor will you worry about looking jacked.

In my seminars I like to ask a funny question. It emphasizes the habitat problem. If civilization fell apart tomorrow, what would be your diet and workout strategy?

The answer, of course, is immediately obvious.

None.

If tomorrow the power grid goes down for good there will be no diet or fitness industry. Demand for gyms will be zero.

THE NATURE OF THE PROBLEM

You have well over thirty factors impinging upon you all at once. Each is between one to ten percent of the total problem. Here is a short list.

Energy dense food:
Modern food is very energy dense. Energy dense food induces over eating. Research establishes a critical threshold where super energy dense food breaks the bodies controls over satiety and hunger.

Abundant energy:
Today we have abundant electro-mechanical energy. It takes the place of *physical energy*. The chemical energy we once expended for food and transport has been replaced by energy from things like oil and gas.

Circadian Disruption:
Light pollution from cities, artificial light, and lack of darkness disrupt critical daily gene activation needed for the Genetic Rush Hour.

Flavor and Nutrient Depletion:
Modern "natural" foods are selectively bred. Flavor and nutrients in food are highly depleted from a century ago. Lack of flavor drives pleasure seeking from empty calories. Nutrient depletion drives over eating.

EMF Fields:
Electro magnetic fields and EM smog disrupt key cellular process and can even promote cancer.

Blocked Electron Flow:
Electrons are, in a sense, an essential nutrient. Lack of our feet making regular contact with the ground starves the body of electrons.

Quick Hack: Make contact with the ground for 15 minutes once per week.

Neurotransmitter depletion:
Over stimulation from smart phones and computers depletes the brain of key neurotransmitters. The "wired and tired" feeling drives stress and over eating.

Quick Hack: Once every 3 months take tyrosine for 2 weeks.

Deuterium Overload:
Modern water and food sources are saturated in deuterium ions which can promote cancer.

Endocrine Disruption;
Exo-estrogens and endocrine disruptors in water, cosmetics, plastics disrupt critical hormonal stasis.

These ten items are hardly an exhaustive list. Each represents a percentage of the problem. Now think about something, why can't we employ the same strategy in reverse?

TEN IMPROVEMENTS OF FIVE PERCENT.

Dozens of negative factors in the modern habitat drive reductions in health. The way we solve the problem is to do the same thing in reverse. Each chapter so far has given you a small to-do. Each to-do gives you a small improvement. Best of all, you can do them all at home. You don't need a gym. With these ten improvements of five percent you have something new and powerful. You have an immune centric approach to health you can do at home. Collectively, the things you learn here will exert a counter force. They will help you transcend the old time intensive strategy.

KEY IDEA: You fight incremental negatives with increment positives

TO-DO: HACKING THE ECOSYSTEM 101

Restoring what the modern ecosystem subtracts

RESTORING PERFECT DARKNESS

We live in an era of light pollution. Artificial light and EM overload from city lights, cell phones, screens and cell towers needs to be mitigated.

STEP 1: LIGHT PROOF YOUR SLEEP

You need to sleep in total darkness.

1. Cover blue lights from microwaves, washer dryer, stove, appliances.
2. Get an eye cover or black out drapes so your sleeping area rests in total darkness.
3. Change the settings on your phone to night mode when the sun goes down.
4. Hold your cell phone at arms length at night and limit its use. Experiments have shown it cell phone screen exposure at night can reduce melatonin secretion by up to 37%.
5. Do not look at laptop or phone screens thirty minutes prior to bed.

STEP 2: LOWER EM EXPOSURE DURING SLEEP

1. Disconnect Wi-Fi at night.
2. Put cell phones inside microwave. Your microwave is essentially a Faraday cage.
3. Make sure a television flat screen or computer system is not within five feet of your head, particularly behind an adjacent wall. Flat screen televisions emit a magnetic field even when off.

STEP 3:

1. If you are an early riser avoid artificial light before the natural break of dawn.
2. Make sure devices are in night mode when waking in darknes

Chapter 10

The Problem of How Humans Really Eat

The single most powerful force at work in your body is the need for survival.

It's very easy to prove. Here is a quick experiment to illustrate. Don't actually do this.

QUICK EXPERIMENT: Via force of will, hold your breath until you pass out.

Good luck. You won't be able to do it. Almost no one could. Your survival programming will kick in. Your will to oppose it breaks. Quite easily. But you get the idea. **The** most powerful mechanisms at work in your body are those related to *survival.* Toward the goal of survival, numerous **mechanisms** dedicated to keeping you alive, function in the background. Some regulate breathing, some regulate your heart beat, and some regulate *eating.* And that's the rub.

Mechanisms tied to survival are **far stronger** than any will attempting to oppose them. You just proved it. It looks like this.

Survival mechanisms > Will

You may have never considered this before, but the mechanisms in control of eating are tied to *survival.* Ironically, and for our purposes, the single largest factor aging the body is **eating.**

- Eating is the single biggest factor driving aging.
- It's the single biggest factor derailing health and immunity.
- It's the single biggest issue most people struggle with.

We have conquer the problem of eating to conquer the problem of immunity, health and aging. But to conquer the problem of eating we need to address *how humans really eat.*

Why does the simple solution, which is to simply stay healthy, elude the great mass of people? More truth. We have not been dealing with what's really true about how humans eat.

We have had seventy plus years of dieting and eating prescriptions to solve the problem of eating in the modern habitat. All of them have failed at large. I would like to suggest the reason why. The answer is actually very simple.

The mechanisms that control eating are survival mechanisms.

Panic buying from Covid-19 was driven by one thing - survival. Survival mechanisms are the most powerful driver of food intake and it's easy to see. Because eating is controlled by survival mechanisms humans are hard wired to eat a specific way. The way humans are hard wired to eat even has a scientific name. It's called Ad Libitum Eating. You are familiar with the short version of this word. It's called **Ad Lib.** To Ad Lib with food just means to eat **whatever.**

Eating whatever is the **default, hard wired, behavior** for human beings. Don't take my word for it! Look to science. Every scientific experiment ever conducted on eating is based on Ad Libitum eating. Every single experiment with food uses what's called a control group. The control group always eats Ad Libitum, meaning, the control group just eats whatever. Eating whatever is what all mammals, humans included, naturally do. Parents know this. If you let them, kids will eat whatever.

And that's the big problem: ***eating whatever.***

The modern era of nutrition, no matter the protocol or diet, is all about two lists. One is the list of foods you eat. The other list is the foods you don't eat. You have your own lists I am sure. The purpose of lists is precisely so you do **not** eat whatever. The purpose of the lists is to **avoid food. Our survival mechanism oppose avoiding food.**

Not eating *whatever* is the basis of every diet, every eating program, and every single solution you can think of. To put it plainly, every solution that exists today is saying "*do not eat the way survival has hard wired humans to eat!*" And what is the mechanism proposed to enforce not eating how survival has hard wired you to eat?

Will.

And yet, the new reality we live in is one where food can be scarce and we can be confined to home. Eating whatever is no longer taboo. In many cases its a *necessity.*

More importantly, its very easy to prove *will* can not overpower the survival mechanisms that control eating. Just as you did with breathing, you can readily prove your survival wiring for food overpowers your will. Just stop eating. Period. No food. Go as long as you can. Eventually, I guarantee, the survival mechanisms driving you to eat win out. You will eat. The mechanisms that drive survival are far stronger than your will opposing them not to eat. And if you think this is an extreme example, it is also **true by lesser degrees.**

When we attempt to oppose a survival mechanism with will, the will to oppose that mechanism will eventually break.

Survival mechanisms > will.

So we have a problem. If humans are hard wired to eat *whatever* for survival reasons, how can any protocol, which is ultimately enforced by **will,** and thus opposes your survival programming, be successful?

The answer is it can't. *Which explains why nothing has worked with the population at large.* But we need to dig in a bit into the actual mechanisms to understand the forces at work driving humans to eat whatever.

THE SURVIVAL MECHANISMS OF STARVATION

The one nutritional constant shared by all mammals, across all of history, is feast and famine. Humans also share in this one constant. Feast and famine runs across all generations, cultures and all of human history. And now feast and famine have appeared again, as they always have and always will. Mammals, you included, have some very powerful genetic programming and mechanisms in place to deal with both famine and feasting.

For example, after a period of starvation, here are just a few of the very powerful mechanisms that kick in to restore body weight.

STARVATION ADAPTIONS

Each of these by itself is a book. I am summarizing them in the most general way. The main point is to understand just how survival has hard wired your body to eat whatever, post starvation.

THE HUNGER HORMONE PROBLEM

Several hormones controlling food intake hyper activate from starvation. The most important is leptin. After starvation, circulating levels of leptin are lowered, together with the hunger hormone PYY. What drives lower leptin are shrunken fat cells and changes in gut bacteria. The result is you eat more. Simultaneously, after starvation sensitivity for the hormone **acylated ghrelin** skyrockets. The net is you eat more and it's harder to feel full. Taken together it looks like this.

Starvation => lowered circulating leptin + higher ghrelin sensitivity => eat more, harder to get full.

The effect on hunger hormones from starvation is like pulling the band on a slingshot. The more body weight you lose, the greater the tension in the band. Finally, when the band snaps back, it shoots *beyond* the original starting point. These post starvation overshoots of leptin, PYY and acylated ghrelin have a profound impact on long term food intake. They drive weight regain. The culprit? Shrinking fat cells.

THE FOOD PLEASURE PROBLEM

Food tastes better after starvation or fat loss. It's a fact. And it's a big problem. The perceived reward for food is amplified by food deprivation. It's also further amplified by reducing fat cells.

Increased food pleasure after starvation is a crucial survival mechanism. It insures you are hyper motivated to eat, which insures you will survive. Science has revealed a portion of the brain called the arcuate nucleus. This is the brain's pleasure center for food. If you have ever done a long hike and when you finally ate the food was mind boggling, this is the arcuate nucleus in action.

When you lose fat signals from the arcuate nucleus drive up pleasure from food. Hyper activation of the arcuate nucleus is like a points card. After starvation, food pleasure gets quadruple reward points. Since you are leaner, the perceived pain of eating more is minimized.

When a behavior has high reward and low, to no perceived pain, the behavior becomes very probable. In this case the likely behavior is eating more.

THE ENERGY GAP PROBLEM

Starvation, or losing body fat, has an inherent problem. The body now needs less energy. At the same time food intake goes up. You burn less. You eat more. This is called the **"energy gap."**

Reducing calories will reduce your resting metabolic rate. At the same time, decreased leptin from shrinking fat cells makes you eat more. The drive to eat more promotes eating Ad Libitum, or simply eating *whatever.*

The Energy Gap => Lower Metabolism + Eating More

Notably, the energy gap does not kick in until way after the starvation period. In today's language we call this the **maintenance phase.** Eating *whatever* puts back the weight lost via starvation (or dieting), which insures survival.

The energy gap explains why caloric reduction based fat loss always fails long term.

Just The Energy Gap alone will defeat over fifty percent of any and all attempts to permanently reduce body fat. Yet several additional mechanisms are also at work.

THE MICROBIOME PROBLEM:
New research has shown that fat loss, dieting, and weight loss, tend to recolonize the gut bacteria to promote weight regain!

While the reasons are very complex, essentially the process of oxidizing fat requires anti-oxidants, notably phenols. Depleted phenols starve the beneficial gut bacteria of the food sources they need. The bacteria that are left over drive cravings, storing fat, and increasing energy harvest. In short, post starvation, a shift in gut bacteria drives the efficient regain of the weight you lost.

MY CONFESSION
I have a confession. The section you just read was originally in the Fat Loss Paradox section of the book. The chapters were getting too big and the problem of How Humans Really Eat required some mechanistic underpinnings, so I moved them here. Here is my confession - wherever you see the word **"starvation"** above, it *originally* read **"fat loss"!**

"Starvation" is just word. So is "fat loss", or "diet", or "fasting." They all mean the exact same thing to your body - shrinking fat cells.

KEY IDEA: Dieting, fat loss, and fasting all have precisely the same effects as starvation. They all shrink fat cells.

FEASTING IS ESSENTIAL
New science has revealed the essential role that feasting has in promoting some extremely beneficial effects on the body. It only makes sense. Feasting after starvation is tied to survival. It is a simple thing to understand how feasting, post-starvation, promotes

survival. And it does. After starvation, feasting has extremely powerful, and very measurable effects on the body. Until recently, there was very little science to explain what was going on during feasting. In 2014, a study in the *Journal of Cellular Metabolism* showed periodic feasting to be the *missing link in body fat regulation.* Among other things, the study showed that:

* Feasting increases fat metabolism!

* Feasting increases metabolic activity and energy expenditure.

* Feasting may increase a "circulating catabolic factor." This is a molecule that prevents weight gain during overfeeding.

* Feasting induces hypophagia - a reduction in food intake and eating that can last up to several weeks.

As you can see, **survival** is at the core of some very powerful control mechanisms over eating behavior. But why are we concerned with starvation? The modern era has conquered famine in industrialized nations has it not?

You come into this world hard wired to eat a certain way. It's called Ad Libitum, or simply, eating whatever. No one had to train you to do it. Eating whatever is how humans naturally eat.

And along came the modern era. Food was plentiful. Work got easy. Everyone got fat. So we invented restricted eating. We used lots of cool labels - intermittent fasting, time restricted feeding, dieting, healthy choices, and on and on. And this spawned over seventy years of trying to change a thing that can not be changed. Survival has hard wired humans to eat up after starvation.

MECHANO-BIOLOGY: CONTROLLED FROM THE OUTSIDE-IN
There is an emerging scientific view that cells are controlled **from the "outside in."** This means signals from the outside effect the inner workings and inner state of the cell. These signals can be biochemical, or mechanical! In other words, cells can and are, quite literally programmed by *physical and mechanical forces.*

KEY IDEA: External physical and mechanical forces program cells.

Computers have software, hardware and firmware. The tissues of your body are very similar to hardware and firmware. In one sense your bodies tissues are programmable. The new science of **Mechano-biology** tells us how physical forces from the outside can reprogram cells. The physical and mechanical forces created when fat cells shrink control cellular programming for fat. As a result, the "programs" and mechanisms activated are a function survival. Whatever the label you want to use - dieting, weight loss, fasting or starvation - the result is the same.

Think about this. The mechanisms I listed above. They drive you to do what?

They drive you to **eat whatever.**

When do they kick in?

They kick in post fat loss.

What is their purpose?

Their purpose is to insure s**urvival.**

What triggers them?

They are triggered by shrinking fat cells - mechanobiology.

KEY IDEA: If it shrinks fat cells, your body only understands it as starvation.

We take for granted that shrinking fat cells is this something everyone wants. To most people who have ever lived this would seem insane. Across all of history, a prolonged duration of reducing body fat and shrinking fat cells was due to starvation!

HOW THE MODERN ERA MIMICS STARVATION AND FEASTING

You decide to get in shape. You diet, lose body fat, rock a few selfies. All those things have one thing in common. The measure of success is *getting fat cells to shrink.*

For a while you look great. After a time, however, the mechanisms we just inventoried are activated by mechanobiology. The act of shrinking fat cells activates programming tied to survival. After starvation, survival favors eating *whatever,* if food is plentiful. In this modern era plentiful food is always readily available. Your natural, hard wired eating behavior, to eat **Ad Libitum,** reasserts itself.

You label it with, "getting off track." Really this means you started **eating whatever.** Our modern labels trick the mind. We think the solution is to just get, "back on track." This means you stop eating whatever. The problem is your body doesn't care how you label shrinking fat cells. No matter the label, shrinking of fat cells across the whole body is a starvation signal. Likewise, the label, "getting off track", is the same thing as feasting after a famine experienced by our ancestors.

Because Ad Lib eating is a survival mechanism your will to oppose it will eventually break. Maybe some emotional life circumstance sped the process up, a divorce, a lost job, but that doesn't negate the fact that what's driving your eating are not modern contrivances, but **ancient programming tied to survival.** Getting in shape mimics starvation. Getting off track mimics feasting after starvation. Your body does not differentiate between the modern labels we use. The common denominator is shrinking fat cells.

KEY IDEA: The modern era of getting in shape unwittingly mimics famine and feasting.

SEVENTY YEARS IN THE WRONG DIRECTION

There is a powerful irony here. For several decades the solutions dedicated to solving the problem have unwittingly triggered powerful survival mechanisms that drive the problem. For over seventy years, since the very beginning of the modern era of diet, we have been trying, via force of will, to oppose what our bodies are naturally programmed to do after starvation. We have been trying to eliminate **eating whatever.**

It can't be done.

Eating whatever is not just how humans are naturally wired to eat, it is **how humans really eat.** We only need to observe them long enough. It's how all humans, across all history, have eaten. And now the world has changed. Immune centric health is now center stage. The possibility of food shortages and long periods at home has changed how we eat. Eating whatever, as a mechanism of survival, doesn't seem that far off.

In the pre-immune centric paradigm, most people were losing the long term war against eating whatever, despite winning a few battles.

So how do we overcome our survival programming which drives how humans really eat?

The answer is you can't.

Never could. For seventy years an approach was popular that tried to get us to do what survival has wired us not to do. New generation after new generation kept on trying. And for seventy years we were going in the wrong direction

A NEW HEADING - A NEW COURSE

Its a new world. Its time for a new course. We have new demands - immunity, uncertainty, and real health. I want to give you a new way to think about the problem of food. It's based not only how your body works, and is in line with the latest science, but meets the new realities fo working more from home. Its a course I have personally done for over thirteen years.

It's called **Offsetting.**

Offsetting is a component of the first power: Learning how to eat.

KEY IDEA: You can offset the intake of food via several mechanisms and tactics.

Let me show you what I mean. This is something you can actually **do right now.** Look at the chart below. It shows a graph of your blood sugar after eating a baked potato. The large and rapid spike in blood sugar promotes weight gain.

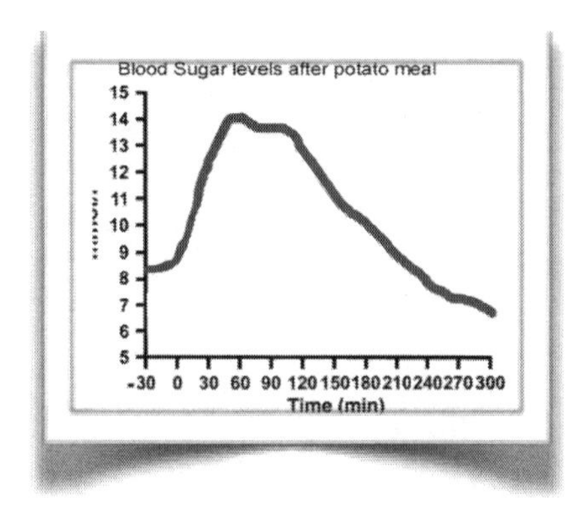

Now look at the next graph. There is **one small change.** We *add* calories! A whey protein shake was added with the baked potato. Now look at your blood sugar.

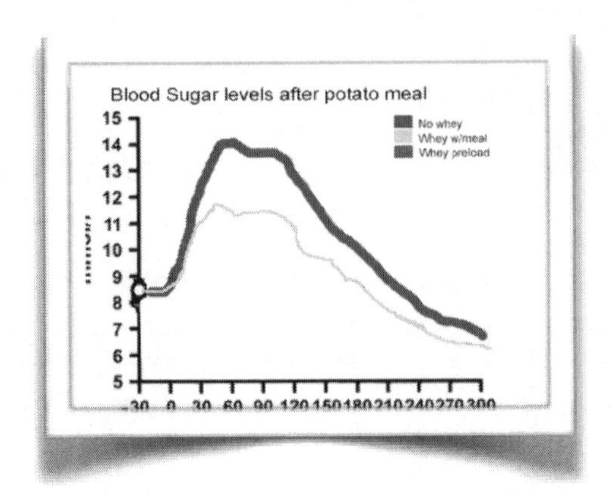

One small change yielded a twenty percent reduction in peak post meal blood sugar! Now let's factor in *"when."* Drink the shake thirty minutes **before** the potato. Now look.

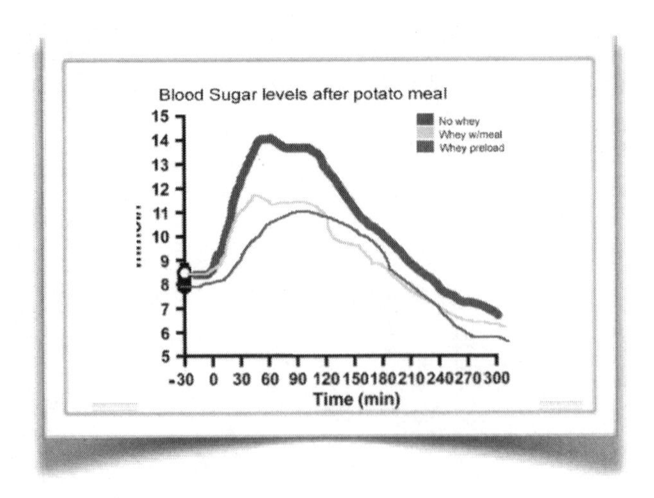

Factoring in *"when"* gave another ten percent reduction in blood glucose! More importantly, peak blood sugar is now delayed! It's been pushed back *a full hour!*

WHAT JUST HAPPENED
A weight gain meal is **becoming a fat loss meal.** We can continue.

- Next, *let the potato cool ten minutes.* Blood sugar will go even lower. It will also further delay the timing of peak blood sugar.

- Next, add cinnamon and olive oil to shake. This gives another few percentages of improvement.

- Next, add a small amount of butter to the baked potato. The small amount of fat slows digestion and also yields another small delay in peak blood sugar.

We could keep going. In Chapter 23, there are even more hacks. The main thing is it's easy! It does not require effort, only knowledge! With little effort, a baked potato can go from pro weight gain to a fat loss meal!

Are you getting the power here?

A NEW POWER FOR A NEW REALITY
This is not dieting. This is not about lists of foods to avoid. **This is a brand new ability.**

This is a *power.* Its a power essential in a world where you need real health but the future is uncertain. You need the power to eat whatever and maintain health by offsetting the pro weight gain effects of food. Offsetting involves leveraging science established, highly measurable and quantifiable know-how, to learn a powerful skill.

Offsetting can be done with virtually any food. We devote several chapters to this later. This is not what you know. This is offsetting.

THE OLD: Avoidance
THE NEW: Offsetting

Offsetting is far more than just a cool hack. Offsetting is an essential component of this new age.

You need the power to eat anything and stay healthy

The moment you get real about how humans really eat, and the realities of an uncertain future, how to offset food is like reading or driving a car. It's an essential life skill. I also want to be clear. I am not saying you should not try to eat healthy. That's ridiculous. **You should**. Before you finish this book the single healthiest eating protocol ever developed will be at your disposal. It will allow you to effortlessly hack into Peak Human physiology without meal prep and without fighting cravings.

PRE-LOAD HACKS TO OFFSET CARBS & BLOOD SUGAR

THE WHAT: Anything on this list
THE WHEN: 20-30 minutes prior to a meal.
THE HOW: See each individual item

In the new reality, where working from home is more common than ever, it is vital to be able to not just avoid foods, but to **offset them.** We begin with simple techniques for lowering blood sugar and carbs.

Whey protein
Whey has been clearly shown to lower your blood sugar significantly when you have carb heavy meals. It helps your body make insulin and pass sugars through the gut. Best thirty minutes prior as a preload meal. You can combine with other things like cinnamon and flax oil for additional effectiveness.

THE HOW: You can add cinnamon to whey to magnify its blood sugar lowering effects.

Berberine
Berberine is an amazing plant derivative that we can use in many ways. Berberine decreases the absorption of sugars in the intestines and is a potent tool offsetting carb intake.

THE HOW: You don't want to use this one often. Save it for very large meals or when you have meals very high in sugar or carbs

Berry phenols or berries
The color pigments in berries have been shown to impair the enzymes the body needs to digest carbs. Thirty minutes prior to a meal berries or berry powder can help improve blood sugar metabolism. Notice also that you actually ad calories.

THE HOW: Raspberries and blackberries together have a number of functional properties that are synergistic. About a cup prior to a meal is effective.

PART 3:

Young Fat & The Fat Loss Paradox

Chapter 11

The Fat Loss Paradox

THE END BEGINS

The modern era of weight loss and fitness can trace its roots back nearly seventy years. The underlying idea all this time has remained the same. It's the idea body fat is just stored energy and all you have to do is lose the fat. Said another way, the problem is solved if you get your fat cells to shrink. Upon this foundation every single program, every routine, every strategy, supplement and diet, you can think of has been based. Ironically, **none** of these things were based on what actually happens when fat cells shrink!

Why does the simple solution, which is to just stay healthy elude the vast majority? A big reason is not dealing with what is true about how fat cells work when you shrink them!

In the next three chapters you will learn what really happens when fat cells shrink. Body fat is going to leave the purview of weight loss and fitness. It will become a crucial part of a much bigger, more comprehensive umbrella. You are going to learn body fat is connected to **whole body immunity and aging.** How your body fat really works, and what happens when you lose it, is about to step into the 21st century.

These next three chapters have some big words and key concepts. Take your time. What you stand to gain is the most powerful shift of your lifetime regarding how you deal with fat. A lot of de-programming will take place.

Oh, you will still want to look good. You will still want to get and stay lean. The big picture, however, will expand in ways previously unimagined. Body fat will become a central mechanism you actively control in order to **control immunity and aging.** Along the way you will learn there is a paradox to fat loss. The **Fat Loss Paradox** is this:

The physical act of shrinking fat cells promotes weight gain.

ERIKA'S STORY

Erika was prettier than most. Her mixed ancestry made for an exotic appearance. Often people would tell her to look into modeling. She tended to put on weight easily. She never thought she could get thin enough to model. When the fitness boom of the late 90's came along she figured it was worth a try to get in shape. Perhaps she could get the lean look she had always coveted. It seemed pretty simple. She just had to set some priorities and goals, devote a bunch of time and energy for a few months, and then she could make a lasting transformation. And it worked!

For a while.

During her twenties Erika became a model. As the years went by and she passed into her thirties and forties, she began to notice something concerning. She began cycling her weight up and down repeatedly. With repeated weight cycling it became harder and harder for her to lose weight over time. By her mid forties she could not lose weight at all, or only with extreme difficulty. Summarized Erika's story is basically this.

Bunch of times getting in shape and losing weight. Things got worse.

Unfortunately, Erika's story is the reality most people will experience over time. What began for Erika in hopeful exuberance of a life transformation set off a cycle of weight loss and regain. It wasn't over in ninety days. It played out over *decades.*

Routinely, what I see is the vast majority of people who do fat loss transformations, when viewed over a twenty or thirty year period, **simply can't get lean anymore.** Recently, a new science paper looking at obesity made a very interesting comment.

"Lifestyle modifications including diet and exercise may help reverse obesity and improve chronic disease biomarkers but are **largely ineffective in achieving sustained weight loss and glycemic control"** - *Journal of Biochemical Pharmacology Jan 2019*

Let me translate. The study is saying, "we can create short term results, but long term those results won't bee sustained by most people. Ironically, do you want to know what the science says is the number one predictor of long term weight gain?

Fat loss.

Losing fat is the best predictor of future weight gain.

In the last chapter you learned of several survival mechanisms activated when fat cells shrink. Those mechanisms oppose the marketplace mythology that fat is just stored energy and all you have to do is lose it. **It's not true.**

For our purposes, however, the larger question is what does body fat have to do with slowing aging? The answer; everything.

What follows is a total reset about body fat. You will learn how **control of body fat is essential to control over immunity and aging.** You will discover body fat is an unacknowledged component of the immune system and the aging process.

The most critical mechanisms controlling body fat have never been recognized. No strategy has taken them into account. Until now, no system has existed to deal with them. They are at work every time you lose body fat. These unacknowledged mechanisms fall under **Mechanobiology,** how mechanical forces control cells. All along, they have been a ghost in the machine, silently steering the long term course of your body, short term success notwithstanding.

DAMAGE CONTROL: THE FAT LOSS DOMINO EFFECT
Shrinking fat cells trigger a row of biological dominos. A kind of "damage control program" is activated. "Program" refers to the idea fat cells get "reprogrammed" by fat loss. But it's not just fat cells.

When fat loss reprograms fat cells the process also reprograms collagen fibers. Amazingly, the collagen fibers in turn work to reprogram your fat. Collagen fibers do amazing things.

KEY IDEA: Collagen fibers control immune cell populations.

Collagen fibers can recruit more of the inflammatory macrophages! Collagen fibers also work like signal beacons. They can recruit key proteins, genes, and other things **into** your fat. The mix of things triggered by key collagen fibers can profoundly alter the "**configuration**" of your fat. You will see body fat is essentially a system. That system can have multiple configurations.

Perhaps the most stunning revelation regarding how fat cells really work is that shrinking of fat cells can trigger changes that lock in a cycle of weight regain!

Weight regain is exactly what the vast majority of people experience over the long haul when they shrink fat cells. The cycle can play out over many years. It can even play out over decades. Erika's story is a prime example. The old way of thinking was you just need to lose the fat. Ironically, all this time, *losing fat has been a **primary force** driving* long term weight gain.

NEW IDEAS: FAT LOSS IS AN INJURY

Injuries have both a short term and long term effect. Athletes are well of this. When properly treated, the long term effects of an injury can be completely negated. For example, you injure your knee; you get it scoped, go to physical therapy, strengthen the muscles around the knee, do ultrasound, and many other things. Properly treated the knee is good as new, sometimes even better than before.

Untreated injuries are a different story.

Even worse, are multiple untreated injuries to the same tissue. This is usually catastrophic long term. Athletes readily testify to the long term effects of untreated injuries. There are aches, chronic pain, and inflammatory related troubles. Worst of all, *things never work the same again.*

KEY IDEA: Losing body fat shrinks fat cells which creates ***injury at the cellular level.***

Millions of people around the world in their forties, fifties, and beyond, struggle to lose weight. Most say they have done many weight loss programs. It's always the same story. They had great success when they were younger. Now it's much more difficult. Weight gain snowballs into a progressive problem with age, despite seasons of getting lean. We tend to think the problem is simply getting older. But that line of thinking doesn't identify a mechanism where we can create meaningful changes. The reality of untreated injury will be revealed in the next Chapter as a powerful underlying mechanism. When untreated injuries accrue things simply don't work the same. This includes your body fat.

Today, entire industries devoted to weight loss and losing fat operate in total ignorance of the *micro cellular injury created by fat loss.* The underlying mechanisms have to do with the mechanical, genetic and biochemical consequences of shrinking fat cells. You will learn how this works and how to counter it. An entirely new paradigm of fat is going to run your thinking.

JOE ROGAN CALLS IT

Recently on the Joe Rogan Podcast, Joe was commenting on a fighter that missed making weight for a fight. I smiled as he said these words , "....it seems like after so many times dropping weight the body seems to develop a resistance to weight cutting." **Joe's intuition was spot on.** The long term result of repeated body transformations is the body resists transforming

A NEW FOUNDATION: IMMUNITY CONTROLS FAT LOSS

We are hypnotized to think fat loss solves everything. Our minds at first resist the notion it does not. This is where fitness ends. This is where a new paradigm begins. Weight gain is only one consequence triggered by fat loss. Newer revelations rest under the umbrella of immunity, aging and cancer.

THE OLD: Body fat is stored energy. You just have to lose it.

THE NEW: Body fat is a major control mechanism over whole body immunity.

I am going to show you why and how body fat is controlled by the **immune system.**

This new revelation will permanently shift your thinking.

The amount of your fat is important. Just as important is the **health** of your fat. The health of your body fat is controlled by immune mechanisms. Immunity is controlled by the Immunity Core: immune cells and signals and membranes. Think the Red team and the Blue team.The health of your fat effects aging, cancer and long term whole body health. And while **you must get and stay as lean as you can,** you must not compromise the health of your fat in doing so. This is especially true long term, where the real story plays out.

THE FOUR FOUNDATIONS

We begin with a few key concepts. You will need to these to understand how body fat really works. In the next chapter we will expand on all of these ideas.

First Key Idea: Fat loss and fat storage are governed by immune cells.

Body fat is really *a partnership.* Immune cells and fat cells work together as part of a system. Immune cells are the dominant partner in that system. If fat loss is a micro cellular injury, and injury is controlled by immunity, then *the immune system governs fat loss.* New science reveals immune signals control what the body does with fat; if fat cells store fat, burn fat, or create new cells to store more fat.

Second Key Idea: Fat loss alters immune cell populations

Losing fat *shifts* immune cell populations. These shifts effect inflammation signals. The results are a paradox. The short term results are usually beneficial, (But not always). Long term, however, is the real story. Losing fat promotes changes in **The Extra Cellular Matrix.** The Extra Cellular Matrix is the collagen filed exoskeleton surrounding your fat. Changes in the Extra Cellular Matrix promote *very important shifts in immune cells,* and thus effect whole body immunity. Simply put, fat loss changes the balance of the Red Team and Blue Team.

Third Key Idea: Fat and cancer are closely related.

The mechanisms controlling the growth of fat cells are nearly identical to the mechanisms controlling the growth of cancer cells! Both fat and cancer are have a nearly unlimited capacity to expand. This is not the case with other tissues. Muscles, organs, blood, and other tissues can not expand infinitely like fat or cancer. A powerful reason fat loss must come into a 21st century framework is the simple fact *body fat can feed cancer!* See Appendix A: Why Do Fit People Get Cancer?

Fourth Key Idea: Micro RNA'a - The Cellular Jump Drive

Think of a computer thumb drive or jump drive. Programs on the thumb drive can download onto other computers. Ironically, it turns out your body has something very similar. Small bits of instructions contained in your fat can be exported. Cell-like containers from your fat can envelope these instructions and circulate into the blood stream. The instructions can download into other cells. It's like a cell to cell thumb drive. These cellular jump drives are called **exosomes.** The instructions in exosomes are called micro RNA's. They *reprogram* cells elsewhere in the body. In a sense, they are basically viruses that our bodies produce internally. I don't mean they are viruses. I mean that the differences between exosomes and viruses come down to labels used and where they come from. This is how signals from your fat can drive immune and inflammation signals *across the whole body!*

Armed with these four concepts can make a radical shift in your understanding of body fat. Read them again if you need too. These concepts bring fat loss into a much more comprehensive and accurate picture.

This is the new picture.
Body fat => Immunity => Aging

From this chapter onward

- You will never again want to do any fat loss or weight loss or body transformation unless it solves the problems you learn about here.
- Your understanding of body fat will be forever changed.
- You will understand how body fat effects aging.
- You will learn to control the health of your fat. This encompasses not just how you look. It also includes aging better and mitigating risk of diseases and cancer.

Is your head hurting from all of this? Keep in mind what's at stake here - more time in a younger body. Now let's take a break. Here is a powerful application of the three genomes - **Intermittent Fat Browning.**

TO-DO:HACKING FAT 101

INTERMITTENT FAT BROWNING
How would you like to learn a hack you can use periodically to drop fat with no exercise and it positively works? I use this whenever I need to jump start or accelerate fat loss in the belly area. **It's a real thing.** It really works. It's based on the absolute cutting edge science of Mechanobiology. Cold induction into fat cells is one of the key ways we can steer whole body immunity. Cold induction helps **shift populations of immune cells.** You are about to learn and apply what is called fat browning. With this technique you can change your fat from the kind that stores energy to the kind that burns energy.

THE WHAT: Ice, menthol, and (optional) a doorway or pull up rack.
THE WHEN: Before bed and upon waking in the am before eating.
THE HOW: Apply menthol first. Then ice. Then abs for 5 minutes.

Rub menthol on your problem fat area. Now lay a t-shirt across the same area and ice it for ten to twenty minutes. You will feel a cool supercharged sensation from both the ice and menthol.

HOW IT WORKS:
Both ice and menthol trigger brown fat production in your fat. It works immediately. You are literally changing the signal state of your fat. **This is powerful Mechanobiology in real time.** Your fat will begin to switch over to a kind of fat that burns fat. Next, take five minutes and do a series of muscular contractions in your problem area. If you can, find a doorway or use a pull up rack in your doorway to streeeeeeetch the problem area as much as you possibly can. Now simply contract and squeeze. Repeat for thirty second intervals over five minutes. Muscular contractions take the place of insulin. Doing this helps fat cells utilize glucose to release fat.

A caution - ***DO NOT DO THIS PROTOCOL ON A REGULAR BASIS!***

Do it intermittently. Your fat **rapidly** adapts to cold induction. It will create the opposite effect if you do this too much. Do this *morning and night* for five nights. Then wait at least thirty days before doing again. If you do am cardio, do this after cardio. Then wait forty-five minutes to eat.

INTERESTING FYI

You have been spinning up the bacteria Akkermansia since Chapter 1. This works in conjunction with Akkermansia production. Akkermansia modulates cold induction and fat browning by helping fat to burn in the short term, and store more the longer cold persists. That's why you do this intermittently. It's also another reason you started on Akkermansia production in Chapter 1.

Chapter 12

The Fat Loss Paradox: Part 2

FAT LOSS AS A MICRO CELLULAR INJURY

After getting knocked out, many fighters want an immediate rematch. Usually this is a bad idea. Getting knocked cold is an injury. Until very recently, the effect of repeated head trauma was not completely understood. Too many fighters and football players have learned the hard way. The long term impact of repeated and untreated head trauma is things just don't work the same anymore. Something very similar pertains to body fat.

At first it may sound silly. How can losing body fat be an injury? And what does losing fat have to do with aging? To get a better understanding of how fat really works we lets see the physical structure of fat. Fat cells have a *very critical structural difference* from other cells. Fat cells are uniquely **vulnerable to damage.**

FAT CELLS ARE SUPER VULNERABLE
Fat cells are easy to damage. Look at the diagram below. Look where the nucleus is located for each cell

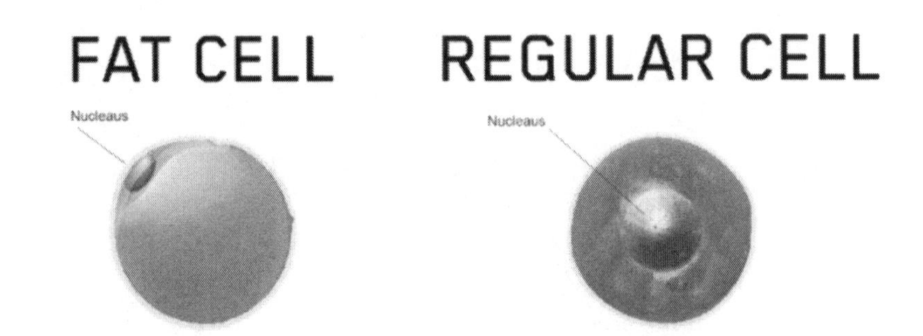

Imagine a glass Christmas tree ornament inside of a water balloon. As long as the ornament sits in the center it's protected. If the ornament moves to the side it becomes vulnerable to shattering. Fat cells are similar. Most cells have a nucleus in the center. It's surrounded by what amounts to a water balloon. Fat cells are different. The interior is taken up mostly by fat. The nucleus is pushed up against the cell wall. The result is fat cells are *very easy* rupture.

KEY IDEA: Fat cells are vulnerable.

It takes only a small amount of **mechanical stress** to damage a fat cell. For this reason, body fat has what amounts to an exo-skeleton. This exo-skeleton is the Extra Cellular Matrix. The Extra Cellular Matrix, or ECM for short, protects your fat.

HOW THE ECM WORKS

In the future skyscrapers may use AI in the building materials. This could allow them to dynamically adapt to structural stress. They could become stiffer when needed. The ECM surrounding your body fat works something like an AI building technology from the future. It is a super complex organ. In response to mechanical stress the ECM can become stiffer. A lot of back and forth "programming" takes place between the ECM and fat cells. Mechanical stress on the ECM can re-program your fat cells in several important ways. In return, fat cells can program the ECM to become stiffer over time.

Finally - we are getting to what is really true about how fat cells work when they shrink.

HOW LOSING FAT INJURES THE FAT CELL

The basis of fat loss is **fat cells shrink.** Fantastic right? Shrinking fat cells solve everything does it not? Think again. Let's see *what really happens* when fat cells shrink.

The Mechanobiology Of Weight Regain

You learned about Mechanobiology, how mechanical forces program cells from the outside/in. Lifting weights is a good example. The mechanical forces of lifting weights instructs muscle cells to grow. Fat loss also produces mechanical forces.

KEY IDEA: Mechanical forces from fat loss begin with a **misfit.**

The misfit is between the ECM and fat cells. The misfit, by its very nature, produces mechanical forces. The mechanical forces, in turn, re-program both the ECM and fat cells. More importantly, these mechanical forces actually *injure your fat mass!* Here is how it works.

The Shrunken Bricks Analogy

Think of a home with brick and mortar walls. Imagine one day the bricks shrink. The shrinking bricks cause a misfit. The mortar no longer fits to the bricks. The misfit causes a *transfer of mechanical forces.* The weight of the wall shifts. The weight goes from the bricks and mortar together, to just the mortar by itself. If this really happened the walls of the home would be severely damaged. The whole structure could even collapse. The reason would be due to ***sheering stress.*** The sheering stress is caused from a *transfer of mechanical forces.* Guess what, the *exact same thing* happens when you lose fat!

KEY IDEA: Mechanical sheering stress from fat loss injures both fat cell and ECM.

Mechanical sheering stress is not the only physical force to injure fat cells. There is another kind of mechanical stress injury from fat loss. This one is called a **Traction Stress Injury.**

TRACTION STRESS INJURY:
Traction Stress is what happens when you move an object by a single point. Moving an object by pulling on a single point can be very damaging. This is traction stress, or *pulling stress.*

Imagine you got in a fight. In the process your whole body is yanked around by your hair. At the same time your liver and heart are kicked out of place. You probably would be severely injured. Something very similar happens from fat loss.

Muscles move using special fibers. These fibers are called actin filaments. Fat also uses these same fibers. Fat, however, does not work like muscle. It does not move easily. Fat is anchored to the ECM by these filaments. When fat cells shrink the actin filaments are stretched or broken. In response they make **stress fibers.** The stress fibers work to *pull* your fat cells back and re-anchor them to the ECM.

Imagine a flash flood hits your home. Your entire house gets moved 30 feet off the foundation. A repair crew shows up and attaches a steel cable to your home. They reassure you they can pull the house back to the foundation. While they succeed, moving the entire house from a single point creates a lot of damage. Walls get cracked, the water heater gets knocked around. Something similar happens with fat cells. Pulling the fat cell back into position to fix the misfit ECM induces a lot of **traction stress,** or *pulling stress,* on the cell. Critical organs like the nucleus get kicked out of place. It's like your liver being kicked out of place, only at the cellular level. Moving the inner cellular machinery out of place injures the cell. To repair the damage stress proteins, called **heat shock proteins,** are produced. Heat shock proteins fix cellular damage. They are also a mechanism driving inflammatory signals and they tend to stick around a long time. New science has shown that after you have lost the fat, lingering inflammatory signals from heat shock proteins can provoke weight regain! This is just one immune mechanism. We will introduce several more. You can now see the real truth. Fat loss induces mechanical stress that **injures both the fat cell and the ECM.**

INJURY REPAIR IS TOP PRIORITY

After fat loss your priority is to keep the fat off. Top priority for your fat mass, however, is repairing the micro-cellular injury. E.C.M. Mariman, a prominent researcher at Maastrich University in the Netherlands, has studied the effect of mechanical forces on the ECM extensively. His work has has shown the mechanical stress on the ECM from fat loss must be resolved to avoid further injury to fat mass as a whole. The result is fat cells refill. Biology wins. Your priorities lose.

KEY IDEA: Weight regain is **inherent** to the injury repair process caused by mechanical forces of fat loss.

If you get nothing else from this chapter get this; **injury is governed by the immune system.**

In several papers, Dr. Mariman has shown the body has two options to repair injury from shrinking fat cells. Option one is to refill your fat cells with fat. You are now familiar with several survival mechanisms activated by fat loss. They all work to refill fat. Option two is to reshape, or **remodel the ECM.**

ECM REPAIR OPTION ONE: FILL THE FAT

The bodies go-to strategy to relieve mechanical stress from fat loss is to refill fat cells. Refilling fat solves the problem; fat cells refill, mechanical stress is relieved, problem solved. In Chapter 10, How Humans Eat, we learned how after fat loss lowered levels of leptin. This make you eat more. The trigger was shrinking fat cells.

Shrinking fat cells => lower leptin=> eating more=> fat cells refill.

You can readily see how weight regain is literally built in to fat loss! This is only one mechanism. There are many more activated when fat cells shrink.

Other Weight Regain Mechanisms

Shrinking fat cells also trigger specific genes. Many of these genes don't activate until well into the maintenance phase. A 2009 study in the *Journal of Diabetes,* by Dr. Ismael Capel, MD, PhD, showed entirely different sets of genes activate in the fat loss phase vs the weight maintenance phase. During the fat loss phase genes beneficial to health activate. *The* maintenance phase, however, is a very different story. In the maintenance phase genes can activate **that promote weight gain.**

The FAB4 Paradox: Not So Fab

The most important gene post fat loss is called Fatty Acid Binding Protein 4, or FABP4. As a memory meme, let's just call it FAB4 (for any of you Beatles fans). FAB4 is activated by fat loss. It helps escort fats into the furnace where they get used as energy. Paradoxically, FAB4 triggers the Red Team which inflames your fat. A 2015 science paper in the *Journal of Clinical Medical Insights* demonstrated **the paradox of FAB4.** We need FAB4 to burn fat. Conversely FAB4 can drive weight regain. It can also drive insulin resistance, inflammation, cancer.

FACT: You need FAB4 to burn fat and it is also the doorway to all of the bodies inflammatory pathways.

Genetic differences in things like FAB4 also explain the outliers. Some outliers seem to sidestep issues with weight regain. Part of the reason has to do with variances of genes like FAB4. The outliers have different genes that activate in the maintenance phase.

ECM REPAIR OPTION 2: RESHAPE THE ECM

Reshaping the ECM takes a lot of energy. During fat loss the energy needed to reshape the ECM may not be available. It's easier for your body to just refill fat cells than to reshape the ECM. In the brick and mortar analogy, if we have to redo the mortar its major reconstruction. The same goes for the body. Reshaping the ECM after fat loss a major remodel.

The high cost of reshaping the ECM is well known with obesity. Push your hand against a steel mesh fence. Your hand quickly gets red and inflamed. Something similar happens in obesity. In obesity fat cells push against the ECM. This creates chronic inflammation. To compensate the ECM re-programs obese fat cells to make stiffer collagen fibers. The stiffer fibers load into the ECM to hold the expanding fat together. The problem, however, is the stiffer the ECM becomes the harder it is to lose fat. A stiffer ECM also drives many health complications. The stiffer collagen fibers work like signal beacons and drive more Red Team populations in your fat. It looks like this:

Stiffer ECM=> more Red Team=> altered immune status =>harder to lose weight=> health issues.

KEY IDEA: Collagen fibers in the ECM steer immunity by shifting macrophage populations

Let me translate that. The membrane that surrounds your fat exerts vast control over immunity. People with metabolic disease, i.e., body fat problems were/are susceptible to Covid-19. Why? Immunity. When the health of your body fat is compromised it drives whole body immunity the wrong direction via populations of macrophages. This effects whole body health.

A key type of stiff collagen seen in obesity is Collagen 6. Collagen 6 stiffens up the ECM. The prevailing idea today is collagen is only good. In reality, collagen 6 drives cancer and inflammation. Collagen 6 also drives what are called *crown like structures* in your fat. These are areas where swarms of the Red Team surround dead fat cells in the shape of a crown.

Why am I comparing obesity with fat loss? Doesn't fat loss cure or ameliorate obesity? Welcome to the new rabbit hole of how your fat really works. Several surprising studies have shown *reshaping the ECM from fat loss can induce* characteristics of the ECM found in obesity!

- A 2010 study in the *Journal of Cell and Molecular Life Sciences* first postulated that characteristics of the ECM seen in obesity could be **replicated by fat loss!**

- In 2015 a team of researchers at Harvard Medical School submitted a doctoral thesis demonstrating fat loss could replicate the characteristics of inflamed fat found in obesity. The researchers found the culprit to be **remodeling the ECM.** The act of fat cells shrinking *drove stiffer collagen fibers into the ECM*! The stiffer fibers resulted in inflamed fat.

The pioneering Harvard study in 2015 by Dr. Gabriel Martinez-Sabatinez found something else very surprising. Paraphrasing from the research.

"...**weight loss significantly increases stiff collagen fibers in the ECM,** which promotes long term metabolic problems despite losing weight"

A **new view** of what happens from fat loss is emerging. The problem seems to lie with *repeated* remodeling of the ECM. The direction, outward from weight gain, or inward from fat loss, may be less important than the frequency of **repeatedly reshaping** the ECM.

One cause of the problem is most likely enzymes. Enzymes break things down. Special enzymes are needed to allow the ECM to expand or contract. One of these is called MMP-11. To make it simple, lets just call this enzyme **the remodeling crew.** The remodeling crew is another paradox. The ECM requires these enzymes to break down so it can remodel, either from fat loss or weight gain. Paradoxically, too much of this enzyme can drive chronic inflammation, altered immunity and weight regain! The analogy is you have too many construction workers at your house during remodeling. Normal function around the house gets interrupted. Likewise, the remodeling crew seems to be connected to metabolic problems. A known driver of metabolic problems is repeated weight cycling. Repeated weight cycling involves the enzymes needed for repeated reshaping of the ECM.

The *Journal of Experimental Cell Research* in 2017 published a paper showing how blocking the remodeling crew during fat loss **reduced** the inflammation of fat cells caused when they shrink. Further, blocking the remodeling crew prevented weight regain. It also prevented chronic weight cycling! You can see quite readily how the enzymes needed to remodel the ECM from fat loss can drive weight regain.

The emerging view in newer science papers suggests stiffening of the ECM is not simply the result of medical conditions like obesity. The emerging view is the more you mess with the ECM the stiffer it gets! Progressive stiffening of the ECM from repeated fat loss may just be the reality of how fat really works long term. Repeated expansion or contraction of the ECM, whatever the cause, tends to cause stiffening over time. The evidence for this is compelling. Part of the reason may be due to similarities between fat cells and cancer cells. See Appendix A: Why Do Fit People Get Cancer.

THE FAT LOSS HEALTH DICHOTOMY

Fat loss is very health promoting. It confers many metabolic benefits and improves health. Make no mistake, **you absolutely must get and stay lean.** So what's the problem?

The problem seems to be repeated cycling of fat loss.

Until now we have never dealt with what is really true about fat. Weight regain is inherent to the injury caused by the mechanical forces induced by fat loss. The forces of Mechanobiology driving weight regain are how things really have always worked. In 2017, Harvard researcher, Dr. Hagit Shapiro, in the *Journal of Future Microbiology*, codified what I had been writing about for over a dozen years. The paper stated "...dietary approaches fail due to difficulties in long-term post dieting weight maintenance, caused by *rapid weight gain that initiates repeated cycles of weight loss and regain.*"

The evolving picture seems to be repeated cycles of getting lean have a *long term toll on the body.* The toll is most likely **cumulative.** Here is what this looks like.

THE ACCURATE PICTURE
Shrinking fat cells =>
Mechanobiology stress =>
Micro injury to fat tissues=>
Immune system kicks in=>
Inflammation =>
Weight regain=>
ECM stiffening=>
Altered immune cell macrophage populations=>
Long term consequences with immunity, aging and weight.

Knowledge of these mechanisms mandates a very serious rethink.

Yes, we need a new paradigm. Lets start with the most important question.

Is reducing fat the measure of fat loss success?

Now, lets complete the paradigm shift.

TO-DO: LEPTIN INTERVENTION

Hacking Weight Regain From Fat Loss

THE TO DO:

Big meals are very important. Big meals act as hormonal control points. They stimulate a host of hormonal domains: stomach distention, satiety, satiation and other mechanisms. One way we hack weight regain is to ***hack leptin during fat loss.*** Stimulating leptin levels all through the fat loss process can help offset weight regain.

HOW IT WORKS:

Science published in 2013 showed very large breakfasts during fat loss can offset weight regain. The reason has to do with driving leptin up as body fat is coming down. These meals differ from cheat meals in a couple of ways. One is the timing. The second is the volume of food and the composition.

THE WHAT: Massive meals at breakfast twice per week.
THE WHEN: During the middle and late stages of **active fat loss.**
THE HOW: See below.

Wednesday is a very large healthy breakfast. The key with this meal is the sheer size. It is often north of 1,000 calories but is mostly healthy food. Sunday breakfast is more geared for pleasure. It is designed to lower feedback from the arcuate nucleus post fat loss.

HEALTHY WEDNESDAY BREAKFAST:

The foods are only a suggestion. Add your favorites. **The key is meal size.** Men should be in the 1,000 calorie range and women in the 700 calorie range.

Foods:
Oatmeal, honey, sourdough toast, Ezekiel toast, berries, whey protein, egg whites, eggs, healthy cereals, yogurt, bananas, grapefruit. steak

Macros: 40% protein, 40% carbs 20% fat.

SUNDAY BREAKFAST:

Preload: 2 scoops of whey protein, with olive oil, honey and cinnamon

Vegan Preload: Nuts.

Main Breakfast Foods:
Pancakes, steak, eggs, toast, chorizo, potatoes, sausage, syrup, honey, ham, bacon, turkey bacon. These are suggestions. You have a lot of discretion.

Make sure to get at least 40% protein. Flavor and total calories are the most important things and fat content can be higher at this meal.

NOTES: These are very large meals, often north of 1,000 calories.

WHY THIS WORKS:

You drive leptin up as fat goes down.

Chapter 13

Old Fat vs Young Fat: How Fat Steers Immunity and Aging

You have learned how a number of very powerful mechanisms oppose permanent reductions in body fat. Seeing them all together all at once is very helpful. It looks like this.

FAT LOSS	ECM remodeling Gut biome adaptions Hunger hormone adaptions Energy gap problem Food reward problem Genetic adaptions

The hype said all you need to do is lose the weight. You bought the hype. You lost the weight. Unfortunately, what no one bothered to mention was **the array of powerful counter measures** that were activated by losing the weight, or worse, what to do about them.

The counter measures above are a function of survival. They are also driven by immunity. Fat loss injurers the cell and it needs repair. The mechanisms opposing fat loss are powerful and many. Given both the power and sheer number, it turns out maintaining fat once you lose it is a **very, very low probability.**

Last chapter you learned how repeated and chronic cycling of fat mass can drive changes in the ECM. Changes in the ECM can promote shifts in macrophage populations. With repeated remodeling of the ECM the Red Team increases. Fat dominated by the Red Team is **very** bad for the aging process. You now have a clear mechanism to understand how repeated weight cycling can and does severely **damage** the health of your fat.

These new ideas move how we deal with body fat into new territory. If body fat taps into immunology, aging and cancer prevention, *we have outgrown the old framework.* **It must end.**

A new immune centric framework is needed. It's a new set of practices and a new paradigm. The immune centric framework for what fat is and how to lose it mandates a rethink fat itself.

WHAT IS FAT REALLY?

It turns out fat is not simply fat. The idea fat is simply fat cells was never really true. It turns out fat is something more like **a mothership.** Fat is really a system for harboring many kinds of cells. First there are the macrophages, but there are also many other kinds of immune cells harbored in your fat. In addition, fat also harbors stem cells that can become not only new fat cells, but also many other kinds of cells. All of these things - fat cells, stem cells, immune cells, collagen fibers and the ECM - all work together.

KEY IDEA: Your fat is really a **system.** It can have multiple **configurations.**

What I mean by *configurations* is the specific mix of immune cells, genes, fat cells, collagen fibers and stem cell fates. This brings us to the main point.

As we age our fat takes on an ***aged configuration.*** The aged configuration of body fat has massive consequences for immunity, aging and whole body health.

HOW BODY FAT STEERS IMMUNITY AND AGING

OLD FAT

Several science papers in the field of immunology have defined a concept known as **"old fat."** What is old fat? For starters its fat with high populations of inflammatory immune cells, mainly the Red Team macrophages, but also T-cells, and other immune cells.

KEY IDEA: Old fat is immune compromised fat. It's dominated by the Red Team.

New science connects **old fat** to weakened immunity and accelerated aging. Old fat also drives the onset of age related disease states, *particularly cancer but also viruses.* As you get older, the analogy of old fat is that of Grand Central Station. Your fat mass becomes a central gathering point, not for trains, but inflammatory **signals.** Inflammatory signals emanate out from body fat. This has big consequences across the entire body. Signals from fat can even accelerate the aging process. Here is how it works.

FAT AND STRESS

Your fat cells contain fat droplets. It turns out fat droplets do more than merely store fat. Fat droplets serve an amazing array of **anti-aging functions.**

KEY IDEA: Fat droplets are a powerful anti-aging mechanism that has gone unrecognized until now.

New research has uncovered amazing and powerful new roles for fat droplets. Nuclear power plants all have containment cells for nuclear waste. The containment cells keep the dangerous waste from hurting the environment. It turns our body fat does something similar. A recent paper in the *Journal of Geroscience* showed how *fat droplets actually protect the body from cellular damage.* During high stress, other systems in the body get overloaded. Fat droplets pick up the slack. They protect the body from very damaging molecules. They store the damaged molecules until the body can eliminate them. Let's use the example of sleep deprivation to illustrate.

Sleep deprivation is super stressful. Without sleep, cellular housekeeping does not function well. Damaged protein and fat molecules build up. The damaged parts can accrue so fast the cells natural disposal pathways get overloaded. Fat droplets function as the emergency back up. Damaged proteins and fats get sequestered into fat droplets. The fat droplets contain any potential damage and protect the mitochondria. Eventually, housekeeping in your fat eliminates them. The ability of fat droplets to sequester and detoxify the body when under high stress is newly uncovered key driver of longevity. When your fat gets old and can no longer act as a backup system, you age faster.

KEY IDEA: Young fat slows aging. Old fat accelerates aging.

WHY GETTING ULTRA LEAN IS SO HARD

The ability of fat to act as a stress buffer for damaged cellular parts also explains why its so hard to get extremely lean. It turns out getting super lean has a very damaging aspect. New research in the *Journal of Autophagy* showed that during starvation, or massive fat loss, we actually store brand new fat!

During extreme fat loss (or starvation) toxic and damaging forms of carnitines are produced. Carnitines are fat transporters. These toxic carnitines can do severe damage to the mitochondria if not eliminated. Like the nuclear waste analogy, new fat droplets form to sequester the dangerous carnitines. The ability of fat to shield other cells from damage in this manner is a brand new and previously unaccounted for *anti-aging mechanism.* As long as your fat is young, it has this ability to sequester damaged cellular junk. This is one key reason young fat helps keep you young. Young fat is anti-aging fat.

As we age fat loses its ability to function normally. When this happens fat goes from being an anti-aging mechanism, to a pro-aging mechanism. Here is how it starts.

THE FAT MUSCLE CONNECTION
The picture of the old body is this.

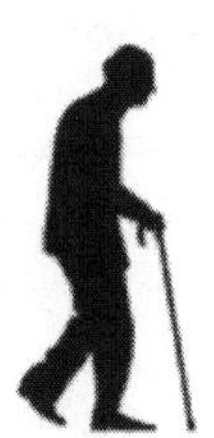

What stands out is limited mobility. Muscle has withered. Energy is gone. A majority of cells across the body are no longer dividing. One of the reasons our bodies get like this is due to a **signal feedback loop** taking place between fat and muscle.

Increased Fat Droplets In Muscle Tissue
We have all seen a nice thick juicy steak with loads of fat. If you are into health you may had grass fed steak. The grass fed steak is very lean and the flavor is rather gamey when compared to corn fed steak. Corn fed steak is simply not as healthy as the grass fed steak. One reason is all the fat contained in corn fed steak.

As we age our muscles become more like the corn fed steak. Fat deposits inside muscle increase. Muscle itself decreases. This kind of fat is called *intra-muscular fat.* As you might guess, muscle is really not the best place to store fat. There are big consequences when your muscles looks like corn fed steak. Intra-muscular fat droplets secrete key signal molecules that ***actually suppress*** **muscle growth.** It's easy to see with the steak analogy. Not only is the grass fed steak leaner, it *also has more muscle.*

KEY IDEA: Intra-muscular fat drives muscle wasting.

Fat and muscle share some common inflammatory signaling molecules. As intra-muscular fat increases, it creates a signal feedback loop between muscle and fat that weakens immunity and drives inflammation. Over time the signals magnify and get stronger. Age related muscle wasting driven by increasing intra-muscular fat is a prime driver of ***age related loss of mobility.*** The more intra-muscle fat, the more muscle renewal is suppressed. The result is we get weaker and less mobile as we get older. Want to hack this?

INTRA MUSCULAR FAT HACK:
THE WHAT: Molecular Hydrogen
THE WHEN: During The Amplified Fast (Ch 25)
THE HOW: With Omega 3's.

In 2015 I met a guy named Tyler LeBaron at a trade show. We had an exchange on the health benefits of hydrogen. I have met a lot of empty suits in this business; people with great credentials who don't stand up to scrutiny when pressed into fine details. Tyler is not one of them. He has vast knowledge of biochemistry. I was very impressed with him. Tyler convinced me of the functional utility of hydrogen, primarily in the form of hydrogen water, to enhance a number very desirable outcomes. One of the new outcomes of molecular hydrogen is it seemed to help patients recover faster during the pandemic. It's great for immunity. Another outcome is the ability of hydrogen to enhance a key molecule that suppresses intra-muscular fat. A simply way to hack the onset of age related intra-muscular fat may be molecular hydrogen water. Follow the protocols in Chapter 25 and 26 and add molecular hydrogen water on a regular basis.

The Body Fat Megaphone
As you learned in Chapter 2, body fat acts like a megaphone. It magnifies signals for whole body immunity. There is a giant science word for how immunity effects metabolism. Once again, it's really

two words stuck together. The first word derives from "immune" and the second word is "metabolism." When you put them together the word is ***immuno-metabolism***.

Immunometabolism is the study of how immunity effects metabolism, particularly in your fat cells, to control total body health.

Visceral Fat Sets In

Have you ever noticed the distended and bulging upper gut that is common with age? This is visceral fat. As the inflammatory signal loop between fat and muscle kicks in, our body fat *shifts locations.* Body fat moves from under the skin, to inside the body. This kind of fat, known as **visceral fat,** is particularly harmful to health. Visceral fat sits next to all of your major organs. It secretes lots of inflammatory signals. Inflammatory signals from visceral fat can jump to organs. When your fat gets to this stage, metabolism of fat, and the inability to properly store it, have massive negative consequences on the immune system as a whole.

VISCERAL FAT HACK: JELLO AT NIGHT

THE WHAT: No cal Jello to decrease visceral fat
THE WHEN: At bedtime
THE HOW: With the Pre Bed Module

Jello is loaded with glycine. Ingestion of glycine has been shown to reduce visceral fat by as much as 50 percent! Other benefits may be

- Boosts glutathione.
- Reduces oxidative stress
- Helps blood flow

Glycine via no cal jello at night is a nice way to end the day and long term may have an impact on visceral fat. We have used this hack for nearly a decade in VEEP. Anecdotal reports are it helps lose fat while sleeping.

THE SIGNAL CASCADE OF AGE

Remember fat is a system. It has multiple configurations. As fat infiltrates muscle and shifts to the internal body compartments, a comer in the aging process is turned. Our body fat takes on a configuration called the **SASP configuration.** SASP refers to secretions from fat. It stands for **Secretory Associated Phenotype.** Let's just call it SASP mode. In *SASP mode* body fat is secreting inflammatory signals on megaphone level. When your body fat goes into SASP mode, signals and hormones from your fat promote the activation of several sets of genes. These genes weaken immunity, drive *inflammation and rapid onset of the aging process.*

The **SASP** configuration essentially is like kindling. SASP mode ignites the fire of weakened immunity and aging. It accelerates the progression of senescent (non-dividing) cells in our body. Signals from fat then jump from organ to organ. The internal organs become inflamed. Then, the same signals infiltrate the blood. Once in the blood, signals generated by the SASP mode of body fat ignite system wide inflammation.

Stem Cells Mature Into Bad Guys
Fat renews itself from stem cells. When young and healthy, fat has a balanced mix of newly mature fat cells together with older fat cells. This is the healthy mix of fat cells. It gives your body flexibility to store fat or burn fat. As we age, the process of stem cells maturing to new fat cells short circuits. Stem cells stop becoming new fat cells. Body fat becomes imbalanced. There are too many old fat cells and not enough young ones. To make things worse stem cells change course.

Stem cells in your fat can actually mature into immune cells!

You wind up with an imbalance of Red Team macrophages! Think about that.

Your fat essentially becomes a giant factory producing inflammatory immune cells!

Loss of fat cell renewal, combined with increasing Red Team populations in your fat, work together to jump start SASP mode. SASP mode impairs whole body immunity. It also *accelerates the aging process.* These changes then effect whole body metabolism. Your fat neither stores fat nor burns it. Fat begins to get stored into places it should not go, like organs and muscles. I am leaving a lot of details out here on purpose to give you the main gist.

So what do we do about all of this?

How can we mitigate this, or better yet, reverse it? The answer boils down to three simple words.

Order of operations.

Doing the right things, in the right order and sequence, is how we solve the problem of the fat loss paradox and old fat. I am going to give you those things. But if you don't do them in the right order of operations, nothing will get solved. No matter how much science is behind the latest miracle pill, if you don't work in the right order and sequence, you are working *against* how your body works. Let's look at an example to understand how powerful the consequences can be for disregarding order of operations.

HOW SUPPLEMENTING NAD+ CAN ACCELERATE AGING

The latest fad as of this writing is using derivatives of b-vitamins to increase levels of NAD+. NAD+ is an enzyme. It's made from niacin. You need it to age well. Supplements that increase NAD+ promise to slow or even halt aging. That's a very big promise. Hypnotized by such powerful claims, consumers are gobbling up bottles of niacin derivatives. Done correctly, in the right order of operations, these things are fantastic tools to help slow aging. But a caution is well merited - when done *apart* from the proper order of operations, supplementing for NAD+ may actually **do the reverse and *accelerate aging***!

Supplement makers are quick to point out "NAD+ decreases with age." This sort of scientism based marketing makes you think taking a pill is all you need to do.

Not so fast.

NAD+: IT DOESN'T WORK LIKE THAT

When you have high populations of the Red Team, supplementing to increase NAD+ levels is the last thing you want to do. Why?

Inflammatory immune cells feed on NAD!

The Red Team needs NAD+ as a necessary enzyme to proliferate. It turns out the age related decline of NAD+ is driven by increases in the Red Team and other immune cells. The larger the Red Team populations the more NAD+ they gobble up. In fact, the **SASP mode** for body fat *feeds on NAD+!* The more NAD+ available, the more inflammatory immune cells your body can make and support. A person with age related inflammation could actually **speed up the aging process** by supplementing for NAD+!

This question is now being proposed in the very latest science articles. A June 2019 paper in the *Journal of Rejuvenation* research noted "The elimination of most senescent cells by senolysis *before initiating NAD+* therapies may be beneficial and ***increase safety".***

"Increase safety", is a code word. It means there is an order of operations. Before supplementing to increase NAD+ inflammation must first be reduced. Supplementing for NAD+ most likely *accelerates aging* if not done in the proper order of operations. Do you see why order of operations matters so much? Things go wrong in a specific order. We need to fix things in an exact order.

Without the proper order of operations you are just a sucker.

Without a master framework for the order of operations all things become equal. You have no way of qualifying anything. You don't know how to get the results you want. You stay stuck in one dimensional baby talk. Worse, you can actually do harm.

THE MASTER ORDER OF OPERATIONS FOR BODY FAT

Here is the new framework for how you handle body fat. It might seem strange at first, but remember, now that you understand body fat controls immunity to a large part, an immune centric approach to body fat isn't just a good idea - its mandatory.

From now on this is your master list of steps to take. This framework surpasses the seventy year old paradigm of fitness, dieting, and weight loss. Fat loss can finally come into the 21st century under the umbrella of whole body immunity, real health, and anti-aging.

1. Restore gut Lining.
2. Recolonize Gut.
3. Spin down inflammation.
4. Reduce body fat.
5. Offset mechanisms opposing fat loss.
6. Apply anti-aging protocols to obtain young fat.

The new umbrella for body fat is based on how fat has always really worked. It's based on what really happens when fat cells shrink.. This connects the gut, immunity, body fat, and aging. The reality is all of these things have always been connected.

Each of these steps has a **sub-order of operations**. For example, with the gut I started you on HMO's and Red phenols. This is the first step in an order.

LOSING BODY FAT MEANS FIRST SEAL THE GUT

KEY IDEA: The health of the gut mucous layer and the health of your body fat are one in the same!

Because immunity begins in the gut, and body fat and immunity are connected, fat loss actually begins in the gut lining.

BODY FAT: THE FIRST ORDER OF BUSINESS

The first order of business in the new paradigm of body fat **is not fat loss!** That alone is a major shift. Instead the first step is to seal and heal the gut lining. Without sealing the gut we can not address the health of your body fat. Fat loss and gut lining heath are connected. They must be addressed at the same time! Notice you also began to use cold induction in problem body fat areas. This is one of the ways we begin to flip macrophages from the Red to the Blue Team in your fat tissue. Let's detail the sub order for the first step.

BODY FAT STEP ONE:

1. Seal and heal the gut.
2. Flip gut macrophage state to anti-inflammatory.

Notice we haven't done any of the old things you normally do - count calories, hit the treadmill, diet strictly.

This is what I meant by the new **to-do.** *It's not the same stuff.*

You started restoring the gut lining in Chapter 1, with apple skins. We will continue adding on to this as you go through the book and you will have the power to maintain a healthy gut lining all your life.

Give yourself a massive pat on the back. These last three chapters asked much more of you. You have conquered them. I hope you re-read them many times over the coming years and spread them to everyone you know. We all want health, youth and vitality. The old paradigm of fat loss was never based on how the body really works and can only bring disappointment to the vast majority. You can be part of fixing the problem.

TO-DO: PRE-FAT LOSS PREP

We have seen how the old marketplace of strategies for body fat was an outdated paradigm and set of practices. An immune centric approach to body fat requires some prep is needed ***before*** *actually shrinking fat cells if you want to mitigate the downside..*

KEY IDEA: You need 4 weeks of prep before dropping fat.

If we want to keep fat off, there is a lot to be done before losing it. The good news is the list of to-do's is easy and non-time intensive. Before this book was published, I spent several years perfecting the techniques in my seminars.

THE WHAT: Preparing the liver for fat loss
THE WHEN: At bedtime
THE HOW: With 1000mg **Rutin**

RUTIN:
Rutin is a color pigment in plants. It does some amazing things. For one it is a potent anti-viral. It even helps prevent the H5N1 version of the flue. It also helps burn brown fat. **It restores NAD+ in the liver naturally.** Rutin also decreases carb absorption in the gut. It also stimulates insulin function. It further prevents glycation and is a powerful anti-oxidant. You just learned how we do not want to supplement directly for NAD+ with niacin derivatives unless inflammation is cleared. Rutin helps us get around this problem by restoring NAD+ naturally.

HOW IT WORKS:
Its normal to burn a bit of fat while you sleep. To do this your liver requires some raw materials, NAD+ being one of those. At the same time rutin helps turn white fat to brown so it is synergistic with the fat browning exercise you just learned. Rutin at bed for the next four weeks helps prep the body to lose fat, aid the liver and helps fat to generate more mitochondria. FYI, the to-do's so far have all been connected. They are actually part of prepping the body to drop fat and keep it off.

PART 4:

The Young Body

Chapter 14

Young Maintenance

HOUSEKEEPING: THE TRASH SWITCH

NASA is up in arms about the junk debris floating in space. Someday space travel may be impossible if we don't clean up the floating junk in orbit. The potential disruption of space travel from aggregating space junk illustrates a powerful truth of both life and biology.

KEY IDEA: Without housekeeping normal functioning stops.

If you take the idea of floating debris and apply it at the cellular level the same truth applies. As junk piles up normal function stops. As we age, junk from damaged fats and proteins accumulate in the cell. With age the natural mechanisms to remove debris decline. Eventually, accumulating cellular trash interferes with normal operation of the cell. When this happens, cells no longer become viable. The result is **you age much much faster.**

Genetic experiments show blocking housekeeping functions in cells induces *advanced aging.* Conversely, experiments stimulating housekeeping have been shown to slow aging. A game changing discovery is the same factors controlling housekeeping within cells also wield a lot of control over aging.

KEY IDEA: Old cells are dirty. Clean cells are young.

One of the simplest ways to dramatically age slower is to **take out the cellular trash** on a regular basis. The fantastic news is you can turn on cellular trash removal at will!

The Old To-Do: Workout three times a week.
The New To-Do: Take out the cellular trash 2 times week.

We will just call this process cellular housekeeping or taking out the trash. Once in a while, we will use the science name for this process. Auto-Phagic (pronounced fage-ik) clearance, or simply **Autophagy.**

In many ways cells are like factories. They assemble complex machinery. They don't always get it right. Luckily they have some pretty advanced quality control and housekeeping functions. Mis-assembled items have a couple of different ways to get recycled. Autophagy or housekeeping is the primary way junk is cleared. You also just learned how fat droplets can assist in this task when autophagy gets overwhelmed.

In mid 2016 when I began this book, autophagy was actually the first chapter I wrote. If you think you know this topic, be patient. Like body fat, you are about to re-think a number of things.

DUALITY AND AUTOPHAGY:
Like all the bodies systems, housekeeping is governed by **duality.** Mostly housekeeping is beneficial. It's at the top of the new to-do list. There are, however, cases where it is not a good. If you have any form of cancer onset, inducing housekeeping may not be a good thing. You would want to consult a doctor first.

WHAT MATTERS MOST: PEXOPHAGY

When guests are coming over we clean up what matters most first. Usually it's the bathroom. Our approach to autophagy is the same. There are different types and forms of autophagy. There is one that seems to matter most. It pertains to specialized machines within your cells. These specialized machines are called **peroxisomes.** Think peroxide. Peroxisomes are small organs within cells. They burn off really long chain omega fatty acids. They also maintain free radical balance within the cell. Peroxisomes are also central to immunity.

Housekeeping has a rightful home during sleep. It occurs naturally every night. The problem with age is sleep declines. Housekeeping declines with it. When sleep and the natural cycle of housekeeping decline we age faster. If we restore sleep correctly, we **really don't need to focus too much on general housekeeping.** In fact it may do more harm than good in many cases. If sleep is corrected, a little extra housekeeping is good, but too much may not be. It's simply balance once again.

Recently, fasting on a regular basis has gained popularity. One reason is fasting induces autophagy. Too much autophagy, however, is not good. I found that out for myself back in 2011. I had my body in autophagy a lot. It made me chronically sore and achy. I can tell you it doesn't work long term. You actually wind up **more inflamed** over the long haul. After many years of trial and error targeting autophagy and tons of research, I found where the real bang for the buck lies in terms of housekeeping.

KEY IDEA: Targeting peroxisomes for housekeeping is where the bang for the buck results lie.

When we want to single out peroxisomes for housekeeping the big word for this is **pexophagy.**

THE MITOCHONDRIA: NOT THE BE ALL AFTER ALL

Until very recently, the tiny power plants in your cells, the mitochondria, have had the majority of focus for anti-aging therapies and strategies. Much newer research suggests that idea needs a major re-think. See Appendix A: Rethinking Mitochondrial Aging Therapies.

A number of solutions in the marketplace focus on anti-oxidants within the mitochondria as a means of slowing the aging process. The problem, however, is this approach could *just as easily harm the mitochondria.* While small amounts of antioxidants in the mitochondria are essential for Peak Human physiology, indiscriminate anti-oxidants aimed at the mitochondria apart from *what, when and how* can very easily become pro-oxidative. Newer revelations have uncovered what may be a much better idea. The mitochondria are really best thought of as **partners with the peroxisomes**. Some scientists have used the phrase ***"co-organs"*** to describe how closely the two cellular organs work together. The analogy is that of two pedals on a bike. What you do to the one effects the other. They are so intertwined they may best be conceptualized as two parts of *a single thing*.

KEY IDEA: The Mitochondria and Peroxisomes may two halves of a whole.

VIRAL ENTRY AND PEROXISOMES

Peroxisomes work in conjunction with mitochondria to keep viruses from spreading to other cells. When a viral RNA penetrates a cell, both peroxisomes and the mitochondria are stimulated to activate immune defense protein called a MAV. MAV's initiate a whole cascade of defenses that help keep the viral RNA from spreading to other cells. In essence, peroxisomes are central to cellular immunity and co-equals with the mitochondria in that regard.

New science suggests the best way to get what we want in terms of aging slower is ***not*** by targeting the mitochondria directly! Instead, activation of the peroxisomes along with targeting them for housekeeping may be the ideal path to keeping cells young and with peak immune function.

A TOTALLY DIFFERENT APPROACH

Instead of trying to drown the mitochondria in antioxidants a newer focus is to find ***natural ways*** to help peroxisomes do their thing. This may be the safest, easiest and most effective mechanism to optimal immunity and better aging.

Why Peroxisomes Matter So Much

The peroxisomes wield vast control over both immunity and aging. At low levels, free radicals output by peroxisomes helps us stay young. Dr Vladamir Toritenko is one of the world's top peroxisome researchers. He happens to reside at Concordia college here in Irvine. He has written several highly respected papers on peroxisomes and aging. Dr. Toritenko posits, " At low levels, peroxisomal free radicals **activate an anti-aging program** in the cell; at concentrations beyond a specific threshold, a **pro-aging course** is triggered."

THE ANTI-AGING PROGRAM

Dr. Toritenko makes the case for a key threshold of free radical output into the cell. This output of free radicals is controlled by peroxisomes. Below the key threshold, peroxisomes turn on what amounts to an *anti-aging program.* When working optimally peroxisomes function as anti-aging factories! The peroxisome anti-aging program requires the anti-oxidant catalase. The difference between the anti-aging program and the pro-aging program is the *permeability* of the peroxisome membrane.

As we age the peroxisome membrane becomes less permeable. The anti-oxidant catalase can no longer pass the peroxisome membrane easily. The delicate balance of catalase and free radical output into the cell by peroxisomes is disrupted. Increasing numbers of free radicals spill into your cells. When this happens, the pro-aging program described by Dr. Toritenko activates. The peroxisomes go from being anti-aging factories to *pro-aging factories*! They spill "old age" into our cells minute by minute. We become susceptible to compromised immunity, aging, inflammation, and cancer. The pro-aging program drives an increasing feedback loop for aging. **The older you get, the faster you get older.** The cause is hydrogen peroxide, the same stuff you put on cuts! When hydrogen peroxide is imbalanced via aging of the peroxisomes *it drives aging in general.* If this goes on long enough, instructions to kill the cell are activated.

The good news is really good news. The peroxisome aging program is **switchable.** The answer is *pexophagy.*

KEY IDEA: Decline of peroxisomes can be slowed by pexophagy.

Pexophagy is unique among all tissues for housekeeping. It has vast benefits for aging above and beyond normal autophagy. Pexophagy seems to turn off the aging program and *turn back on the anti-aging program!* This keeps cellular immunity at peak levels and helps you to stay young.

Pexophagy: The What, When and How

THE WHAT: Pexophagy
THE WHEN: During **the Amplified Fast**
THE HOW: With Omega 3's and **small molecule activators and/or/ molecular hydrogen.** See Ch 25-26

One of the most powerful tools available to target pexophagy are omega 3 fats. They have very unique effects on peroxisomes *not shared by any other kind of fat.* Making Omega's work to target peroxisomes, however, needs an order of operations.

In the New Solutions section, you will apply both The Amplified Fast, and the 2 Day Immune Core Pattern, as a base foundation. On top of this base you can do a number of things. One of those is to target pexophagy on a weekly basis. It's easy and powerful.

Let's take a brief look at small molecule activators. These are substances that exert powerful pro housekeeping effects in a number of ways. These are things like pterostilbene, berberine and apigenin. Before you run out and buy all those things, remember, you need **the order of operations** more than you need the products themselves.

Pterostilbene:
Pterostilbene is a phenolic compound found in things like blueberries. It is similar to resveratrol in its structure and function except it is much stronger. Like resveratrol, Pterostilbene acts on some of the master regulators of youth like autophagy, but it has a much greater bioavailability and bioactivity than resveratrol. The health benefits of Pterostilbene are numerous and vast. Pterostilbene has powerful anti-viral action. in mice has been shown to increase oxygen consumption and fat metabolism. Pterostilbene is particularly potent in killing many types of cancer cells, particularly skin cancers and oral cancers. One mechanisms pterostilbene works by is via autophagy and activation of peroxisomes.

Berberine:
Berberine has been called legal Metformin by some, in reference to the host of similar health promoting effects Berberine shares with the diabetic drug metformin. Like Pterostilbene, Berberine activates the master controllers of youth. Berberine has been shown to increase fat metabolism, protect against fibrosis of the ECM that you learned about in Chapter 12, inhibit cancer cell proliferation and induces housekeeping. Berberine is of particular interest for its effects on metabolism. Berberine decreases insulin resistance and improves risk factors associated with Metabolic Syndrome.

Apigenin
Apigenin is a plant flavonoid found in things like grapefruit. I have used it for a number of years. It has shown a remarkable spectrum of health benefits ranging from helping to ameliorate Parkinson's and Alzheimer's disease, to improving rheumatoid arthritis, autoimmune disorders, and various types of cancers. It is particularly effective at inducing housekeeping in cancer cells which in most cases results in the death of the cell, in particular breast and cervical cancers. A caution is warranted however in advanced stages of cancer where sometimes autophagy can actually protect cancer cells. You should not automatically begin using Apigenin if you are currently under a cancer treatment program.

Butyrate:
We have a whole chapter devoted to Butyrate later in the book, but concerning housekeeping what you need to know is the bacteria metabolite Butyrate can induce housekeeping and cell death in certain tissues. In other tissues, like the colon, Butyrate is the primary life giving fuel. It feeds cells in the colon what they need to thrive while enabling the gut to heal and seal. Where Butyrate becomes extremely fascinating for our purposes is when combined with fasting it magnifies the beneficial effects of both.

You don't have to wait until the New Solutions Section. To get you started here are three simple steps you can do to begin switching on pexophagy.

TO-DO: PEXOPHAGY FOR STARTERS
Sleep is the original intermittent fast. It's the natural ecosystem of housekeeping. In the order of operations for housekeeping, sleep is where we want to start. Using nutrients it is possible to *steer peroxisomes.* The key to pexophagy is ***proliferation + clearance.*** By flooding cells with key fats we can force peroxisomes to proliferate. Then, by very strategic changes in feeding, we can force

peroxisomes into pexophagy! This has the net effect of making new peroxisomes while clearing out old ones.

An easy first step to activate housekeeping ***(the what)*** is at bedtime ***(the when)*** with Berberine followed by Omega 3 & small molecules upon waking ***(the how).***

1. Have the cold black beans lunch meal you learned in the Language of Real Health chapter. If you are vegan instead of chicken you can substitute garbanzo beans or fish if pescatarian.

2. At Bedtime, take 1000mg Berberine.

3. Upon waking take Berberine again. I highly suggest Amped Keto with it or at the back of Chapter 25 is the breakdown of small molecules you can do separately.

4. Take 1 teaspoon Omega 3 oil and fast until hungry.

Cold black beans at lunch loads the gut with resistant starch. You will produce Butyrate *while you sleep* that night. Butyrate magnifies the benefits of fasting during sleep. Berberine at bedtime helps activate housekeeping while sleeping. Upon waking, the small molecules in Amped Keto, or taken individually, contribute to autophagy. Omega 3 oil in a fasted state triggers peroxisomes to proliferate. Here is the net:

Improved autophagy during sleep => amplified housekeeping and proliferation after sleep => age slower.

This first step toward activating housekeeping is very powerful. If you got only this one thing out of this entire book, you would have a potent weapon against aging. Before we are done it will be improved upon significantly starting in the next chapter. You will learn how to manipulate peroxisomes by timing of select nutrient types. This has nothing to do with lifestyle. This is a powerful skill.

DECLINING IMMUNITY AND AGING AS A PROBLEM OF LOST DATA

New science over the last decade has revealed a critical role played by **data** in both immunity and aging. Data means information. There is information stored in DNA. The quality, or readability, of that information can drive aging. The net of these new revelations are three key concepts.

- As we age data in our DNA **shuts off.** The word is "silenced", meaning, it can no longer be read. The information is still there but it can't be accessed.
- If we can keep the data in DNA accessible, meaning **readable,** it helps our immune system work better and you you age slower.
- The process of copying data can be *regulated and improved.* There are simple, non-time intensive things you can do to help keep the data in your DNA readable.

What is really true about your body is that *information and instructions, in effect,* ***data,*** is essential. Without the instructions, i.e., the data, your immunity, health and aging are compromised. On a daily basis, critical segments of data need to be read for our bodies immune system work properly and age better.

KEY IDEA: As we age segments of our DNA turn off.

Science papers are rife with phrases like, "reversing gene silencing", in reference to the problem of aging and loss of data. A major area of cancer prevention research is devoted to finding ways to keep the data within DNA readable.

With age, more and more data in DNA is, in effect, lost. As you learned previously It's like a file on your computer that won't open. Losing data makes us age faster and more cancer prone. Research into gene silencing shows that if we can just keep our DNA **readable** *not only do we age better but our immunity to viral infection and other diseases is much stronger.* The good news is we can!

There are active to-do's you can take to make the data in your DNA readable. There are three primary ways we can make the data in your DNA more *available*. One of them is the via micro RNA's and exosomes you first learned about in Chapter 11. Another is to make it easier to copy DNA. This is known as DNA methylation. Finally, at the foundational level, for DNA to be copied it must first be readable.

HDAC INHIBITION, IMMUNITY AND AGING

The science word for keeping data in DNA readable is **HDAC**

Inhibition. Tell that to a friend today. "I'm doing HDAC inhibition." Saying "HDAC Inhibition" is another giant pain, so I will mix in the term **"making copies."** It means the same thing.

HDAC inhibition is one of the most powerful and promising areas of research in immunology, anti-aging and cancer prevention. For example, the drug Trichostatin A, is a powerful HDAC inhibitor. It seems to be able to flip the Red Team to the Blue Team by enhancing housekeeping. It's powerful stuff.

Making copies has a natural ecosystem in the Genetic Rush Hour. This is when many of the most important genes that need to be copied must be "readable." Making copies is also very complex and has biological duality, meaning it can work both ways. For this reason, the best practice centers on making copies around sleep cycles. Our sleep chapter will dial this in for you.

TOWARD A SET OF BEST PRACTICES FOR MAKING COPIES

Two keys to helping the body make copies are **diet and sleep.** Leveraging diet and sleep so the body can naturally make copies is a safe practice working with diurnal rhythm to keep natural immunity at peak function and to age slower.

Several foods can potentiate HDAC inhibition. Mustard and onions are two examples. Eating these at dinner helps the body set up for the Genetic Rush Hour to make copies. It's not a panacea. It's merely an incremental improvement. We will stack a number of these together starting with Butyrate, the most potent HDAC inhibitor we can leverage. Butyrate is known as a "class 3 HDAC inhibitor." Let's put a few of your previous to-do's together now to target HDAC inhibition.

TO-DO:
HDAC TARGETING DURING THE GENETIC RUSH HOUR

THE WHAT: Targeting HDAC inhibition during sleep
THE WHEN: At dinner and bedtime
THE HOW: Combine Signal Amplification 101 from Chapter 5 together with exogenous ketones

HOW IT WORKS:
If you were to do the Signal Amplification exercise from Chapter 5 at dinner time you would likely wake in the middle of the night from hunger. There is a hack for that. Exogenous ketones knock out hunger signaling. You can sleep and have an additive bonus. Ketones are a natural HDAC inhibitor! Butyrate is also a natural HDAC inhibitor. Combining ketones at bedtime with functional fermentation from the specific foods of the Signal Amplification exercise potentiates HDAC inhibition during sleep, where it naturally belongs. The best part is this is an all natural approach. It's based on how your body really works in the perfect diurnal timing.

WHAT YOU NEED:
Sodium Butyrate and magnesium Butyrate.

Chapter 15

Young Signaling: AMPK & The Sirtuins

AMPK: THE MASTER REGULATOR OF YOUTH

The lioness is on her 19th hunt for food. The previous 18 have failed. If she doesn't catch something soon, the possibility of death is very real. The need for survival has activated her bodies most powerful mechanisms. Although starving, an odd thing has been happening within her cells. Her bodies main source of energy, ATP, has been replenishing, yet it's **not** being used. It's being saved. There will be a last ditch, all-out effort. It will make the difference between living and dying.

Her body is not adding muscle. Adding muscle is growth. Growth requires energy. She has none to spare. Instead, everything is going into the furnace, so to speak. The housekeeping function inside her cells is recycling every last bit of trash to replenish ATP. It's a strange irony, she is slowly starving to death but cells have taken on a state of near immortality. Aging, for now, is on hold.

It's near dawn. Mist rises from the Serengeti. She has been locked on her pray for nearly 30 minutes, watching. She waits patiently, conserving energy. The wind is in her favor. Her prey has been blissfully grazing, wandering closer, and closer. She readies herself. With no warning, she bounds from the grass in a paroxysm of power. She goes from zero to all out sprint in just a couple of seconds. Her prey is fast. The built up ATP in her muscles is finally released. Everything goes into this last ditch effort. And with an extra push her claws catch the hind quarter of her prey. The rest happens quickly.

She feasts. She eats over 40 pounds of meat at this one sitting. Satiated, she sleeps, even though it's broad daylight. Abundant energy is once again available. While sleeping, her muscles begin to renew at a fantastic pace. At the cellular level, it's back to business as usual. Cells divide and grow. Repair begins. Tissues replenish. Stem cells move forward and mature. The business of living, and aging, can now resume.

THE NEW CULTURAL SCIENCE OF 2020

Before the 1960's, DNA was a word spoken by a handful of obscure scientists. Today it's a word used by everyone. The same thing happened with cholesterol, HDL's and LDL's. Once these words were used only in science papers. Now they are also commonplace.

Today we live in a knowledge acceleration society. The acquisition of knowledge is accelerating exponentially. I want to introduce you to some new science words that will be used by everyone in only a few years. I have been using these words for over ten years. Only a handful of people even knew of them or what they mean. In five years they will be as common as "DNA" and "cholesterol" Are today. You got here earlier than the crowd.

Here are the new new cultural science words of the next decade.

- AMPK
- SIRTUINS
- NAD
- CD38

These words will be commonplace in the near future because they powerfully influence immunity and aging. It's not if, it's just when. They are too important to remain unaware of. And that is why everyone will know about them. Our lioness just demonstrated the first word, AMPK.

AMPK: THE MASTER REGULATOR OF YOUTH

Ask yourself when was the last time you were

1. Really hungry
2. There was no food in sight
3. The only way you were going to eat was by expending a lot of energy to physically get food?

The answer is likely never.

Never in your life have you checked all three boxes. Life and death survival over food has been conquered in the modern world. Yet, for most of human history, the opposite was true. Most humans who have ever lived had to expend massive energy on a regular basis just to eat. Starvation was normal. It turns out that there are three conditions that **prolong life when they occur all at once.**

1. Being really hungry or starving
2. Time of day is around dawn.
3. Simultaneously expending a lot of energy.

These conditions together activate an ancient molecular switch. This switch is designed to insure survival. We share it with the lioness. In fact all mammals have this switch in common. It's called AMPK. In my inner circle of super science hack colleagues we all call it "AMP - K", like "amped."

AMPK stands for a long name I won't bore you with. In simplest terms AMPK is a protein. It's an energy sensor inside cells. It senses when energy levels within cells are low. AMPK activates a cascade of signals. It's called **the AMPK signal pathway.** It's part of your bodies inventory of survival programs. When AMPK is activated, a cascade of biological events take place. These events change how cells derive their energy. In the process our bodies switch from a state of aging to one of ***life extension.***

Harvard researcher, Kris Berkewitz, has stated that AMPK is, "**capable of defining the rate of aging."** AMPK is for all intents and purposes, like the "ON" toggle on your phone. AMPK turns on youth and turns off aging.

KEY IDEA: When AMPK is activated, aging is slowed.

Normally, AMPK is activated before dawn. This is one reason you age slower at different parts of the day. By its very nature, AMPK activates housekeeping. The body also seems to be afforded protection from numerous disease states when AMPK is activated, including cognitive decline, many types of cancer, metabolic disease, strokes, CVD disease, and many others.

The Game Changing Discovery: *Signals* that control growth and aging can be switched on and off.

The reason has to do with **energy and growth.** The lioness illustrates something critical to understanding AMPK. Eating and aging go together.

KEY IDEA: Wherever we see eating we see aging.

Wherever there is no eating, or food intake is reduced by at least 1/3, aging seems to slow. This is why caloric restriction as a means of aging slower has gained traction. Some of the reasons aging slows when food is restricted are...

- Suppression of the ACE enzyme. (Think ACE inhibitors.)
- Activation of housekeeping.
- Restriction of the amino acid methionine.
- Reduced free radical damage from oxidizing food for energy.

Above and beyond these reasons is a bigger reason lack of food slows aging.

Signals.

THE SIGNAL PATHWAY PARADIGM OF AGING

Aging was once thought to be basically the result of wear and tear. In 2009 I read a very fascinating paper by Dr. Eric Greer and Dr Ann Burnet published in the "Journal of Cell Science", called "Signal Networks in Aging." The paper showed how a few key signal pathways could in theory moderate the rate of aging.

The net of these discoveries was to connect energy production and growth, driven by cellular *signals, to aging.*

KEY IDEA: Cellular signals drive aging.

In Appendix A: What Are Genes Really, you will learn a fascinating idea. It's the idea that cells are essentially computers. The idea that cells are computers lends itself to the notion cells are programmable. And this is exactly what many breakthrough papers in science today deal with - **cellular reprogramming.**

As it turns out, cells are routinely programmed. There are even some scientists who espouse the idea that aging is in one sense a reversible cellular program. For our purposes, perhaps the single most important idea with respect to cellular programming is when cells make decisions to live or die. This is called "Senescence". As we get older, more and more cells decide to shut down. When this happens en mass, you age very fast.

KEY IDEA: We do not age at the same rate across life.

We have a "window of youth." Our window of youth is the period where our *rate of aging* is relatively slow. As we age a critical threshold is passed. Once past this threshold the bodies rate of aging begins to speed up. Our goal with this book, is to push out the "window of youth."

THE THREE WAVES OF AGING

New types of measures promise to tell us our real biological age. The best known of these "biological clocks" is measuring DNA markers for what is known as methylation. The newest and perhaps most promising of these types of biological clock measures has to do with proteins in the blood. Called the "Proteome Clock", a recent publication in the Journal of Science Nature, showed that groups of protein in the blood predict our real biological age with a very high degree of accuracy. Most shocking, by measuring blood proteins the paper demonstrated that **aging happens in three distinct "waves".**

The first major wave of aging is in the early thirties, roughly around 34. At this stage, key shifts in the Extra Cellular Matrix flood the blood with very distinct markers of aging and disease. The next major wave of aging happens at age 60, and the final one takes place roughly around age 78. If you are in your mid fifties and reading this book, your timing is perfect. You are just in time to push the next big wave back.

While we can not stop aging, perhaps we can effect a few key cellular processes that help our cells remain in the "window of youth" longer. There is a big science word that means "programmed cell death". Let's just call it ***"cellular death row".***

The main thing to understand is that **cellular death row** works like a computer program. Cells have energy sensors. AMPK is one of those. When the total peak power output of a cell falls below a certain level, it activates a program for death row. Cellular power output and long life go together. Our goal is to keep the program for cellular death row from becoming activated as long we can. But is this possible?

Yes. Absolutely.

It all begins with controlling signal pathways.

THE AGE ACCELERATOR: IIS

Scientists studying the bodies signal pathways have discovered an amazing thing. The bodies **rate of aging** seems to correlate with **signals for growth!** The most important of these signal pathways concerns insulin. When we eat signals controlling growth are activated. Our lioness gorged herself. An immediate cascade of signals put her body to sleep. The energy from food provided the raw material for repairing and growing her muscles.

The most important of the signal pathways for growth is called **the IIS pathway.** This pathway is activated by food. The IIS pathway is most powerfully activated when the body makes insulin. Bodybuilders have known this for years. To get maximum muscle growth it's common to inject insulin. New research has shown something very interesting.

KEY IDEA: The more signal inputs down the IIS pathway the faster we age.

Conversely, fewer signal inputs down the IIS pathway can actually **slow the rate of aging.** Our lioness was starving. The IIS pathway was shut down. Instead, the AMPK signal pathway was activated. The result was to table aging until later. The energy needed for growth required her to have food.

Growth of tissue drives aging, Once you understand this it will change your focus.

5X INCREASE IN LIFESPAN

The IIS pathway is the most powerful pro-aging pathway. Scientists have recently shown that by combining inhibition of the IIS pathway with that of another key growth pathway, the mTor pathway, yielded a 5x increase in lifespan in worms. While this has yet to translate to humans, the patterns you will implement in Chapter 25 and 26 are designed with this idea in mind. You will balance bursts of growth with regular inhibition of the pro-aging pathways IIS and mTor. You will also sensitize insulin so you need to make less. At the end of Chapter 17, there is an exercise you can do for controlled bursts of muscle growth to balance off the inhibition of growth pathways and keep muscle young.

The current fitness paradigm is about growth. Because growth drives signals down the IIS pathway, it drives aging. In fact, studies using growth hormone have shown GH shortens lifespan. This is one reason I don't work out a ton. It's also why I don't take testosterone or growth hormone, even though I am now in my mid-fifties. Once you understand how they affect aging, it changes **how and when you use them**. It's like a race car with nitrous. You want to save it for the finish. I believe the proper home of those things is later in life, like the late sixties or early seventies.

THE IMMORTAL PARTNERSHIP: AMPK AND SIRT1

You are seeing many important aspects of our biology, once thought to be solo acts, are really duets. Fat is best thought of as a partnership between fat cells and immune cells. The mitochondria are best thought of as co-organs in partnership with peroxisomes. The same is true of AMPK. AMPK, it turns out, does not work alone.

KEY IDEA: AMPK is essentially a partnership.

When the AMPK signal pathway is activated it turns up an entire family of proteins involved with housekeeping, free radical balance, and many other longevity based mechanisms. These genes are called the **Silent Information Regulator Proteins**, or the Sirtuin genes. Basically, they turn things on an off. They are HDAC inhibitors! Together with AMPK, the Sirtuins regulate youth. The Sirtuin most involved in longevity is called Sirtuin 1, or **SIRT1.**

KEY IDEA: AMPK and the SIRT genes activate one another.

AMPK and the SIRT genes are part of a cycle. Each effects the other. All your life this cycle of youth, driven by AMPK and SIRT1, has been peddling on its own, naturally, when you sleep. With age, these two twin pedals stop turning on their own. You begin to age faster. Both AMPK and SIRT1 work together with HIF-1, which you learned about in the first chapter. These three mechanisms are all part of your survival programming. They are each survival mechanisms.

A BRIEF HISTORY OF AMPK TARGETING

I began implementing a series of protocols centered around activation of AMPK and SIRT1 in 2010. By 2013, I showed Quest Nutrition a couple of PDF's centered around some cutting edge things I was doing. One of them was on the gut biome. That PDF got circulated internally. The other got overlooked. It was entitled **"SIRT Training."** It showed a protocol for training once a week, centering around activation of AMPK and SIRT1. The result was my body looked much younger than it should. By 2015, I was introducing targeted AMPK activation to the fitness world on cutting edge podcasts. In 2017, I rolled out Amped Keto, the world's first product to amplify fasting via AMPK.

You can see it here.

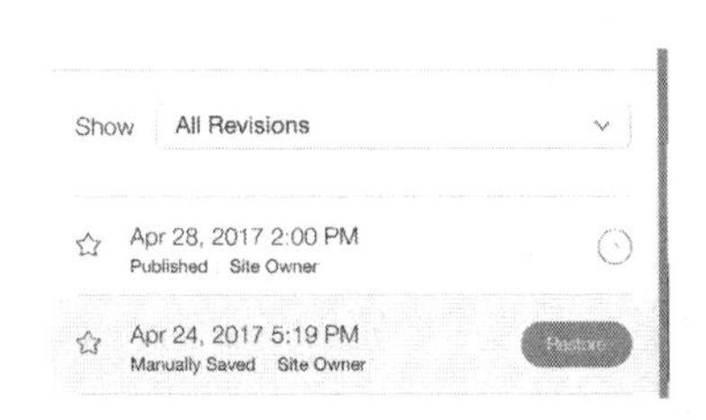

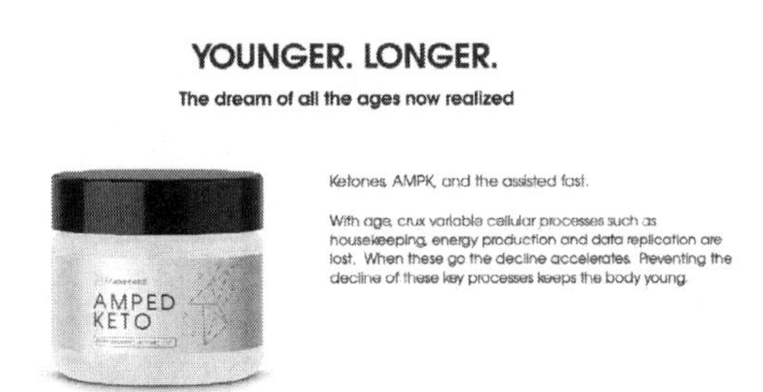

In that same year, I rolled out my Body Hack Seminar. Body Hack teaches people how to hack AMPK and the SIRT genes. Many of the to-do's in this book I piloted in Body Hack.

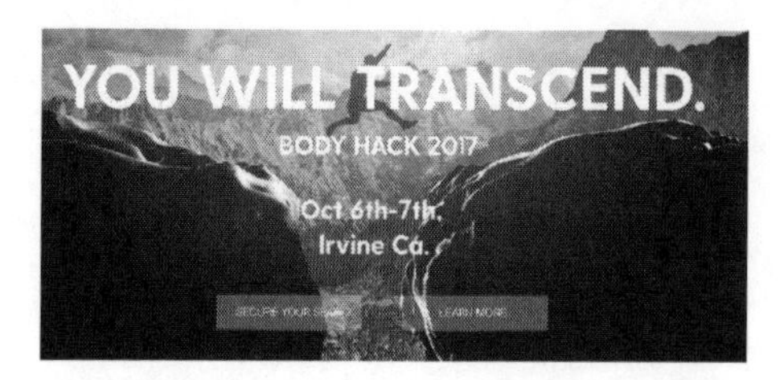

DAY 1

Switch on Youth.

The Amplified Fast: 8 am - 10.
You will show up fasted. We will immediately amplify the youth pathway signals. Topics include Ketones and their proper ecosystem.

I mention this history with AMPK and SIRT1 so you know over 10 years of research and implementation go into what you are about to read. That's 10 years of trial and error, not just on myself, but in my nutrition system and in my seminars as well. I think the result brings you the most comprehensive and effective techniques for AMPK activation.

SIGNAL PATHWAY BEST PRACTICES

If aging can be defined by key signals in the body and we can actively stimulate the right signals we can slow aging right?

Not so fast.

We can stimulate signal pathways to take control of aging. That's fantastic. You will learn how. But it comes with a caveat. **Influence of signal pathways has duality.** It can be both good and bad. Too much can be as bad as too little. I mentioned in Chapter 14 I learned this in 2012. I was doing too much stimulation of autophagy. I was sore all the time. I found out the hard way **less is more.**

Signal pathways are powerful. They exert life altering power of things like aging, muscle growth, immunity, and health. They all occur in a natural set of circumstances. For control over signal pathways like AMPK, SIRT, autophagy, it is important to establish a foundation of best practices. These will keep you from over doing it.

BEST PRACTICES FOR SIGNAL PATHWAYS

- Where, when, and how does the signal pathway naturally occur? Sleep for example.

- Maximize and amplify **the natural occurrence** of signals.

- Add small amounts of additional signal strength using what, when and how.

- Do **not** overdo it.

AMPK & SIRT1: THE LANGUAGE OF REAL HEALTH

Learning to control AMPK & SIRT1 to control aging, like everything else, really comes down to the proper order of operations and best practices.

AMPK and SIRT1 have a natural habitat in the Genetic Rush hour. When we are young, they activate in the middle of the night when sleeping. What you saw with our lion, is that along with sleep, there is a set of circumstances where AMPK and SIRT1 naturally activate. In short, AMPK & SIRT1 have a proper ecosystem. Until now, the proper ecosystem for activation of AMPK & SIRT1 has been totally ignored.

The natural and proper ecosystem of AMPK and SIRT1:

1. Around dawn
2. In a fasted state
3. Ideally under exercise and cold.

That's a problem. Those 3 conditions simply eliminate most people. Most people are not willing to get up early and exercise in a starved state while cold. We invented modern society precisely so we would not have to do those things! Luckily, we can **hack the process.** This is where 10 years of doing this comes in to play. Let's look at AMPK and SIRT1 activation from the Language of Real Health

THE WHAT: AMPK & SIRT1 activation.
THE WHEN: During sleep and during the amplified fast.
THE HOW: With roots and fiber precursors. **Clear HIF-1 first**

The first thing to understand about AMPK targeting, is **order of operations.**

KEY IDEA: Eliminating sleep hypoxia and excess HIF-1 comes first.

In your 20's AMPK activation keeps you young. In your 60's AMPK activation can create problems. The reason? Hypoxia. AMPK can work differently if hypoxia is present. **HIF-1 can activate AMPK.**

This is why HIF-1 came first in Chapter 1. This means you should be doing the Seattle protocol and the HIF-1 clearing protocols from Chapter 2 first. Do those for 3 weeks before beginning to target AMPK.

ROOT AND FIBER PRECURSORS

A unique aspect of how we are approaching AMPK activation is the importance of roots and fibers. Butyrate and bacteria are precursors to activation of AMPK. Roots and fibers are precursors to Butyrate and bacteria.

KEY IDEA: We can **amplify AMPK activation via** Butyrate production while we sleep.

Roots and fibers have a place in the cycle of famine and feast. When starving, the last thing humans would typically eat were roots. Apart from taste preference, the reason roots are last on the list to eat is energy yield. They have little energy and take lots of energy to digest. Survival favors eating game because there is more energy. Roots are the food of last resort. Ironically, however, balance rules. Roots can drive bacteria in the gut that activate AMPK and SIRT1 all by themselves. This helps replenish ATP for that last ditch effort to get game. For thousands of years humans ate roots as a last resort preceding feasting on game. The basis of The Amplified Fast replicates this ancestral pattern.

Using fibers and roots **we can pre-amplify AMPK and SIRT1 activation.**

TO-DO:
AMPK/SIRT 1 SUPERCHARGING WITH BAICALIN

THE WHAT: Baicalin
THE WHEN: 1x per month. Morning of The Amplified Fast. Tuesdays & Thursdays.
THE HOW: Combine Signal Amplification 101 from Chapter 5

WHAT IT IS:

There are a number things that activate AMPK and SIRT1. Some work better than others. Quite possibly, the most widely therapeutic of all may be Baicalin. Baicalin is a flavonoid derivative of Chinese Skullcap. Below are research headlines regarding everything Baicalin does. It almost seems like an ad for pixie dust except these are all findings in science papers.

One of the most amazing attributes of Baicalin is it impairs the enzyme Furin. The Covid-19 virus, once it penetrates into a human cell, requires the enzyme Furin to go into replication. Baicalin may impede or interfere with Furin in this respect. Other things Baicalin does...

- Protects against pulmonary hypertension
- Improves and prevents PCOS
- Suppresses gut inflammation
- Inhibits influenza virus
- Inhibits proliferation of many kinds of cancer cells
- Enhances bone cell development
- Alleviates age related macular degeneration
- Alleviates insulin resistance in the liver
- Helps with vitiligo

Baicalin has long been a favorite of mine to amplify AMPK and SIRT1 because of its broad potential to improve many kinds of health issues.

CAUTION

One study notes the potential for liver issues with Baicalin because it lowers urate. Conversely, several other papers show Baicalin improves liver health. To err on the side of caution I personally use it once per month during the Amplified Fast. Do your own research. Ask a well a doctor familiar with Baicalin and decide for yourself.

Chapter 16

Young Energy: NAD & CD38

100 years ago Pellagra was common in Europe. In the US it became a serious epidemic. The cure for Pellagra traces back to Dr. Joseph Goldberger. Dr. Goldberger's story typifies the American Dream. One of 6 kids born to a family from Hungary, his family immigrated to the US and settled in Manhattan. He went to City College of New York, decided to pursue medicine, transferred to Bellevue Hospital Medical College and eventually got his MD. He was intellectually curious. In private practice he became restless. This led him to a number of positions in public health. He began to publish research. Eventually the US Surgeon General himself, asked Dr. Goldberger to investigate the Pellagra epidemic in the southern US. Dr. Goldberger traced the culprit to a lack of animal foods in the diet. (Relax plant based people. I'm just giving you history.). Dr. Goldberger's solution was simple and powerful. He took patients with Pellagra off corn based diets. Instead he put them on milk, eggs and meat. Pellagra was cured! Later, a researcher named Conrad Elvehjem traced the culprit to the b-vitamin niacin. In the body niacin is converted to the co-enzyme NAD+.

NAD: MOTOR OIL FOR THE ENGINE OF LIFE

Our goal is to give you a new to-do list. The purpose of the new list is give you immune centric heath to keep your body young. On that list is increasing a key molecule called NAD+.

Simply put this molecule, NAD+, regulates immunity.

It regulates immunity via, you guessed it, macrophages, the Red and Blue Team. Macrophage populations require this molecule to proliferate. The signals created in the synthesis of this molecule for macrophages exert vast control over immunity. When I said learning to steer macrophages would become equal to diet and exercise in the first chapter I wasn't kidding.

ITS LIKE MOTOR OIL- THE ENGINE WON'T RUN WITHOUT IT

The simple metaphor of motor oil helps us understand what NAD is and why we need it. Without motor oil, a gas engine can not operate. The oil makes **the reactions possible** that allow the engine to work. Motor oil by itself, doesn't make the car go, but the car won't go without it. As long as the motor oil is clean and full, the engine experiences minimal wear and tear. When the motor oil gets dirty, or it gets low, then the engine wears out much, much faster.

Your body works very much like this.

KEY IDEA: NAD+ is like motor oil. It makes the reactions possible that keep the body young.

Inside and surrounding your cells are a pair of molecules that, in a sense, are **the motor oil of your body.** These two molecules are named NAD and NADP. They are needed for virtually all the major reactions your cells require for immunity and to stay alive and young. These two molecules have many derivatives and forms. I won't go into them, except to say it all begins to look like acronym soup when you inventory all of them - NAD+, NAADP, NADPH, NAMPT - it just keeps going.

The Main One - The Oxidized Form:
When you see NAD with a plus sign next to it - like this NAD+ - this refers to the oxidized form of NAD. NAD+ is an enzyme and enzymes fuel reactions but are not directly a source of fuel like ATP or ketones. Just as we use the term DNA everyday, the label NAD+ works just fine. We don't need to go into the big word science names, other than to say the "N" in NAD+ stands for nicotinamide, which we all know as niacin.

WHERE WE GET IT

NAD+ is made naturally a few different ways in our body. One way is during sleep. When tryptophan is metabolized NAD+ is made. NAD+ is also restored during fasting via activation of the AMPK and SIRT1 pathway. NAD+ is also made from niacin in the diet.

WHAT NAD DOES

NAD does 3 things principally.

REDOX AND NAD+
First, NAD+ keeps you from rusting. NAD and NADP are electron carriers. They are a primary reservoir of molecules to offset **oxidation.** Just like the oil reservoir of a gas powered car, each of your trillions of cells has a reservoir of NAD to keep each cell from rusting.

KEY IDEA: As we age, your reservoir of NAD+ dwindles.

When the bodies reservoirs of NAD+ dwindle, it effects immunity and you will age faster as a result.

YOUNG ENERGY AND NAD+
Next, you need NAD+ to make energy. It's needed for virtually all of

the reactions that drive energy production in our bodies. In fact, you couldn't make use of blood sugar without a form of NAD+.

NAD+ is vital for the energy production of the cell. At all stages our cells need it to make the cells primary fuel source, Previously, you learned about **cellular death row -** how the total energy output of a cell controls the decision to live or die for the cell. As we age, NAD+ declines. The cells ability to make energy declines with it! Loss of NAD+ is linked to cellular death row.

KEY IDEA: Healthy young bodies have lots of NAD+. Old immune compromised bodies have low levels of NAD+.

When NAD+ declines across the body, it effects the total power out of cells across the entire body. In turn this effects macrophage immune function and **you age much faster.** More and more cells will get sentenced to death row.

YOUNG SIGNALING AND NAD+

Finally, and perhaps most importantly, we need NAD to **carry signals.** NAD and its derivatives act as carriers for many signals both for the immune system and to stay young.

NAD+: WHY WE NEED IT FOR IMMUNITY AND YOUTH

The SIRT1 gene needs NAD+ to activate. It's also needed by the mitochondria. They decline without it. Here are just a few of the things NAD+ does to our immune system working and to keep us young.

- NAD+ acts as a "immune switch". When you cells have a ready supply of it, macrophages use it to maintain normal immune function. Without a ready supply of NAD+ macrophages drive compromised immune function.

- NAD+ is needed for many functions that help keep you young, like making copies and housekeeping.

- When NAD+ declines with age a key protein needed to repair DNA declines as well. When this happens DNA damage increases.

- NAD+ is a key control point over the bodies 24 hour circadian clocks, and helps regulate sleep which effects immunity.

- Declining NAD+ levels in macrophages throw gas on the fire of inflammaging.

- Declining NAD+ levels in the cell nucleus help promote "pseudo-hypoxia", where the hypoxia protein HIF-1 accumulates, interfering with DNA repair.

- Declining NAD+ levels may be a major factor in Alzheimer's onset.

KEY IDEA: NAD+ is directly involved with Immunity, aging and cell senescence.

WHY NAD+ IS DECLINING AND WHAT TO DO ABOUT IT

There are several different ways we can restore NAD+ levels. Most of them are actually very easy, even free to inexpensive. What is most important, however, is to understand the big picture. The big picture is what solves the bigger problem of keeping the body young.

In 2018, on an appearance on Superhuman Radio, I broke down for the bio-hacking community the number one way to restore NAD+. The audience was stunned to hear the answer.

Sleep.

Sleep is how the body naturally restores NAD+.

FACT: The primary way all mammals restore NAD+ is during sleep via the salvage of niacin.

Under normal circumstances, getting sound sleep is simply the best and most powerful way to restore NAD+. In fact, you will notice in the list below, of how to restore NAD+, the next most powerful method to restore NAD+ is **fasting.** Sleep accomplishes both. Sleep is fasting. Even better, it restores NAD+ in the right time of day. Notice I said "Under normal circumstances." As we age two key problems present themselves. First, is that sleep declines, and that part of the reason is a paradox. NAD+ exerts control over diurnal rhythms. Less NAD+ available translates to less sleep. Conversely, the less you sleep, the less NAD+ available. This is why restoring sleep is our first priority and the best way to restore NAD+.

This brings us to the second reason NAD+ declines, **inflammation.** As you learned in Chapter 14, inflammatory immune cells increase with age. In the process they consume NAD+

CD38 AND THE YOUNG BODY

In 2009, a paper in the *Journal of Cell Metabolism* identified the major culprit of NAD+ decline. It's a protein on the surface of immune cells, things like the Red Team. The protein is a sensor. The scientific name is CD38. "CD" stands for Cluster of Differentiation. The CD sensors are at the forefront of the latest research in the field of immunology. Some of them are critically involved in immunity. For example, one of the ways the Covid 19 virus gets into the body is via a CD receptor, CD 26.

By targeting and manipulating the CD sensors on immune cells powerful outcomes are possible. This brings us to CD38. It turns out targeting CD38 inhibition is something anyone can do, and it may hold the key to spinning down inflammation and staying young.

CD38 AND THE YOUNG BODY

As we age, levels of CD38 increase. CD38 increasing has a one to one correlation with NAD+ declining. There is a really good reason for this. **CD38+ requires NAD+ to proliferate.** CD38 also destroys the precursor to NAD, NMN, so generally speaking, CD38 wipes out the bodies reservoirs of NAD+.

KEY IDEA: CD38 increases drive decreases in NAD+.

In fact, decreases in NAD+ with aging perfectly match increases in CD38. It looks like this.

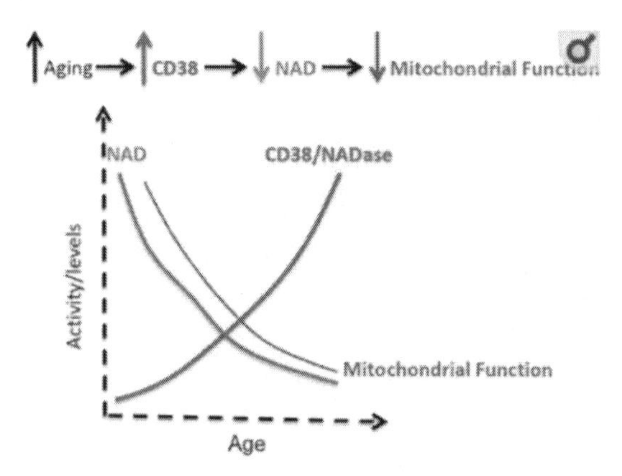

CD38/NADase increases during aging, and causes NAD decline and subsequent mitochondrial dysfunction.

Increases in CD38 are linked to mitochondria dysfunction, inflammaging, and insulin resistance. CD38 is particularly important in your fat tissue, CD38 drives fat storage. High levels in body fat of CD38 generally coincides with fat cell health going downward. As fat cell health goes downward, whole body immunity is compromised.

KEY IDEA: Lowering inflammation lowers CD38 levels.

LOWERING CD38 TO FOR IMMUNE HEALTH AND ANTI-AGING
Lowering CD38 has been shown to have a number of immune centric effects on the body. For example.

- CD38 Inhibition has been shown to **reverse age related NAD+ decline.**

- **CD38 inhibition improves immune function** by lowering the Red Team and increasing the Blue Team.

- Mice bred without CD38 showed significant protection against heart attack and cancer

- Higher CD38 levels have been shown to be essential for obesity onset.

As you can see, if we can lower CD38 we can increase NAD+. CD38 is a key player in the types of macrophages that dominate in your body. For this reason CD38 has a lot to do with inflammation and inflammaging.

THE DARK SIDE OF NAD+

If you do a search on NAD+, you will see nothing but links for supplements and life extension. You would think we have found the cure for everything. What you won't see anywhere is information about NAD+ and cancer. In Appendix A, you can read about how long term Keto diets could actually promote cancer. Once again, biological duality comes into play with NAD+.

Raising NAD+ can be a key element of keeping the body young- **if you don't already have later stage cancer.**

HIGH NAD+ FUELS CANCER CELLS

In late stage cancer, supplementing to increase NAD+ can actually make the problem worse. Cancer cells need to rely on glycolysis. NAD+ makes that reaction possible. In cancer cells, higher NAD+ levels actually fuel the cancer. Supplementing to increase NAD+ levels is not something you would want to do if you have late stage cancer. If you don't, then increasing NAD+ is a foundational tool for aging better. As you can begin to see, the Language of Real Health, the what, the when, and the how, dictates how you do anything and everything.

KEY IDEA: If you have cancer do not supplement for NAD+

METHODS TO INCREASE NAD+

There are several ways we can restore NAD+ in the body. Lets inventory the various ways we can restore NAD+. This will lead us into a correct order of operations.

1. Sleep
2. Fasting
3. Spin down inflammation
4. Increase bifidobacteria
5. Activate AMPK/SIRT1
6. Supplement directly with Nicotinamide Riboside, or Nicotinamide Mononucleotide
7. Supplement directly to inhibit CD38

If you believe the hype, the only way to restore NAD+, is via supplements. I am not against supplementing for NAD+. My Amped Keto does that. But I want you to do it in the most powerful way possible. Natural rhythms of NAD+ restoration and safety come first.

KEY IDEA: There are several ways to restore NAD+.

The future will rapidly bring many more ways to restore NAD+. One of the most promising new methods is the inhibition of an enzyme called ACMSD. ACMSD is involved in tryptophan metabolism. Inhibiting this enzyme has been shown to boost NAD+.

For now, we have lots of ways to restore NAD+.

Activation of the AMPK or SIRT1 pathway restores NAD+ You have already seen a number of AMPK activators listed so far. Using patterns in the 2 Day Core in section 6, will give you powerful natural ways to restore NAD+ via AMPK, restoring Butyrate, and using timing and food patterns. The natural home of NAD+ restoration is deep sleep. Paradoxically, NAD+ helps regulate sleep. Like many things, each effects the other. This brings us to the most important question regarding NAD+.

What is the proper order of operations to restore NAD?

THE ORDER OF OPERATIONS TO RESTORE NAD

The proper order of operations to restore NAD+ is this.

Restore the gut=>
Restore sleep=>
Reduce inflammation=>
Implement the 2 Day Immunity Core Pattern=>
Supplement for CD38 and NAD+

TO DO: REPLETE NAD+

This is a simple exercise you can do anytime to maximally restore NAD+ levels very fast. Rather than a single thing, this exercise combines several core modules.

THE WHAT: NAD+ repletion
THE WHEN: After doing the Inflammation Spin Down.
THE HOW: See below.

Dinner: Omelette with cheese and asparagus.

1. Oleamide
2. GABA
3. Melatonin
4. 300mg Nicotinamide Mononucleotide or Nicotinamide Riboside or plain old niacin.
5. Pterostilbene and curcumin.

Several things are happening with these simple steps. Oleamide, GABA and Melatonin insure a fantastic nights sleep. An omelette with cheese gives you abundant natural niacin from the diet. Asparagus helps bidobacteria production while sleeping which further stimulates b-vitamin synthesis. The NAD+ precursors Nicotinamide Mononucleotide or Nicotinamide Riboside also drive NAD+ production and help you sleep. Combining everything with curcumin helps prevent immune cells from cannabalizing NAD+.

Chapter 17

Young Muscle & Young Blood

Old muscle is at the center of the body becoming a prison.

As much as **one third** the muscle present in a young body is lost during aging.

One third!

Lost muscle is clearly one of the most dramatic distinctions between young bodies and old ones. But it isn't just muscle size. Key differences in old muscle have a dramatic effect on both immunity and aging. Young bodies have energetic, supple muscle. It is springy, pliable, and recovers well from exercise. Old bodies have slow muscle. It withers. It's easily injured. It limits our mobility and experience of life. To keep your body young we need to keep your muscles young.

So far we learned old muscle starts to store fat. Old muscles become like marbled corn fed beef. Fat droplets inside muscle suppress the renewal and growth of new muscle Worse, intra-muscular fat, drives the SASP feedback loop. Signals between your fat mass and muscle potentiate the senescent signal state of inflammaging.

One of our key strategies will be to give you non-time intensive ways to reduce intramuscular fat droplets and to increase signals that potentiate muscles to stay young.

WHY MUSCLE GETS OLD

The reasons why muscles get old are not simple. Increasing inflammation and decreased circulation play a part. At the top of the list, however, there is one master mechanism. Everything seems to converge on stem cells. These stem cells, called "satellite cells", are as starter dough is to sourdough bread. **Muscle cells don't divide.** They renew from stem cells. As long as your starter dough remains intact, you can make bread. As long as muscle satellite cells replenish you can renew muscle. With age your muscle "starter dough" diminishes. The satellite cells needed for muscle to renew **do not replenish.** The question is why? The answer, leads us into a new way to think about muscle. Just as body fat is actually an immune centric organ, so is muscle. Young muscle, and the ability of muscle to renew itself from satellite cells is really a function of immunity.

One of the primary causes behind loss of muscle satellite cells are , you guessed it, macrophages. Muscle growth and regeneration depends a lot on the immune system, particularly macrophages. In short, the macrophages in your bone marrow get old. When that happens, you get **old bone marrow.** Old bone marrow drives a reduction in muscle satellite cells.

KEY IDEA: Old macrophages in muscle are reversed. The Blue Team become the bad guys.

Remember in the first chapter I said the Red Team/Blue Team analogy holds in most cases? This is the one case it does not. It old muscle, the bone marrow gets an imbalance of too many of the **Blue Team!** We actually need to steer a bit more of the Red Team into old muscle.

AGED MUSCLE HACK:
Most of the hacks in this book are very advanced. This one is not. It's very simple. Many advanced readers will at first roll their eyes, but it is so universally applicable to average people, it needs to be here. It will not apply to people who consume lots of pre-workout drinks, for reasons that will soon be made clear.

An simple way to most people can help older muscle regenerate is to drive *small amounts* of the gas nitric oxide into the muscle. This is widely applicable to a vast majority of people over age 45.

THE WHAT: Nitric Oxide enhancing supplements: Beet root, arginine, agmatine sulfate, citruline
THE WHEN:Before a workout
THE HOW: With Folic Acid

Notice I said **small amounts.** If you do not regularly consume products that raise nitric oxide, then this is a good idea for you. If you are a regular user of pre-workout supplements and products that drive nitric oxide, this is **not a good idea** to increase the dose. Most people need to make more nitric oxide. Heavy users of pre-workout supplements need to make less. Too much nitric oxide production is just as bad as too little.

MUSCLE DAMAGE
As we age, damaged end products in muscle accumulate. Simultaneously, synthesis of new muscle declines. The imbalance starts small, with accumulated and untreated micro-injury to muscle. Over time the damage imbalances new muscle. You wind up with

muscle that doesn't respond to exercise. The muscle has lost its starter dough. Ironically, one of the primary ways **this happens is via working out.**

KEY IDEA: Working out creates micro injuries that can accumulate and create "old muscle."

When you want to know how to do something you go to the best in the world. The best in the world at adding muscle are high level bodybuilders. At the very highest level, the best of the best bodybuilders routinely do "body work." Body work is a form of highly invasive tissue massage to remove fused muscle fibers and muscle damage. It keeps muscles growing and young.

KEY IDEA: Once way to keep muscles young is to clear muscle damage.

Clearing muscle damage helps prevent the age imbalance of damage to new muscle.

AUTOPHAGY AND YOUNG MUSCLE

Another way to clear muscle damage is via housekeeping. Housekeeping helps muscles clear damaged end products. As you learned, housekeeping also declines with age. The decline of housekeeping and the increase of damaged end products in muscle creates muscle withering. At the extreme the word for this is **sarcopenia.** Sarcopenia is the muscle wasting we see with age.

Long before things get to the Sarcopenia stage, however, immune function is already beginning to wane and as a result muscle is already getting old. This is the time to take action. The single most effective method known to clear damaged end products from muscle is to initiate autophagy via exercise. In practice, however, this is not enough. Old muscle can not respond to exercise the way young muscle can. You need an edge. That edge is **signal amplification.**

TARGETED GROWTH WITH SIGNAL AMPLIFICATION

Returning to our lioness for a moment, when she finally had a successful hunt, she gorged. She then slept and rapidly restored muscle lost during starvation. Although this narrative is only a story, it illustrates something very real.

KEY IDEA: Starvation signals "amplify" signals for muscle growth.

Post starvation, our bodies are primed to add muscle. A few keys from the lioness story give us clues.

1. There is a period without food.
2. There is exercise during this period of no food.
3. There is a subsequent period of feasting and over eating.
4. There is plenty of sleep.

The lioness narrative lays out a simple, powerful, formula, based on leveraging survival mechanisms. Post starvation the body is primed to gain muscle. We can use modern science to expand this idea. The takeaway will be a formula to keep muscles young by **amplifying signal pathways.** The ingredients of the formula are not unique. The way the ingredients are sequenced, the recipe of what, when and how is what is unique and where the power lies.

Recently, a very well known figure in the keto space came to me for help with diet. Using a combination of very large meals of just the right foods in just the right sequence, we were able to mimic extreme starvation. Blood ketones measured well into starvation levels. The purpose was to prime muscle growth. The next phase involved over eating. My client was able to rapidly gain muscle with extreme muscle pumps. The key was supercharging AMPK signals prior to feasting. Signals for extreme starvation rapidly initiated housekeeping in muscle, clearing the way for more muscle "stater dough."

You can do the same thing at a much less extreme level. And it's easy

YOUNG MUSCLE HACK #1:
One of the ways we can keep the body young is to activate the SIRT genes. With age, loss of SIRT activation in muscle tissue promotes "old muscle." Activation of SIRT genes seems to preserve the starter dough of young muscle.

Here is a basic formula to regularly activate SIRT genes in muscle to then amplify growth signals. The pre-requisites for this are The 2 Day Core and The Inflammation Spin Down. The complete step through is at the end of the chapter.

- Pre amplify fasting using roots and fibers.
- Supercharge fasting signals with small molecules.
- Moderate exercise using the integrated interval during fasting. 1 minute per hour

- Post fasting giant meal intake.
- Muscle massage at night.
- Bedtime sleep aids.

This simple formula is about "when" and "how" to strategically target autophagy in muscles 2x per week or any time you need to.

KEY IDEA: The first step is to **amplify housekeeping signals** during exercise.

KEY IDEA: The next step is to **amplify growth signals.**

This is very easy to do and non time-intensive. If you will make this a part of your weekly routine, you can and will help your muscles stay young,. You can even help reverse "old muscle" to "young muscle."

MUSCLE LOSS, INFLAMMATION AND CIRCULATION

Numerous science publications link inflammatory signals and declining circulation with "old muscle." Young muscle, its seems, depends on "young blood." One example is a protein controlling muscle growth called ERK.

ERK AND MUSCLE SUPPRESSION

Simon's story gave us a framework to understand how with time, many people experience a reality of exercise.

KEY IDEA: Exercise works much better when you are young than old.

We have been led to believe that exercise is a neutral force, conferring its benefits at any age. The reality is very different. Exercise has a much more powerful effect on young bodies. Old bodies respond differently to exercise than young bodies. Simon found this out the hard way. One reason young bodies respond better is due to immunity and recovery. Old muscle recovers from exercise poorly because immunity is compromised as we age.

ERK 1/2 AND AGED MUSCLE

New science has uncovered a key mechanism behind the poor recovery of aged muscle. The key is a protein called **ERK.** In the science it's called ERK 1/2, which is a complete pain to read and pronounce, so let's just shorten it to ERK.

ERK sits on the cell surface of muscles. It's effectively a switch. It tells muscle stem cells to renew. It also controls activation of genes for muscle neurotransmitters. It works very differently in old vs young muscle. A 2016 study in the Journal of Molecular and Cellular Biology clearly showed muscle needs ERK to activate to stay young and healthy.

YOUNG MUSCLE: ERK activates post workout.
OLD MUSCLE: ERK tends to **not activate.**

ERK explains a key difference in exercise recovery between young and old muscle. To net it out, young muscles get sore but they recover, adapt and grow. **Old muscles just get chronically sore.** You can workout but they recover poorly. The lack of ERK activation in old muscle is at the core of why this happens.

The graph below shows the difference in ERK activation between young and old muscle after a workout. Old muscle are the squares on the chart. You can see at the peak, ERK activation is **half that of young muscle.**

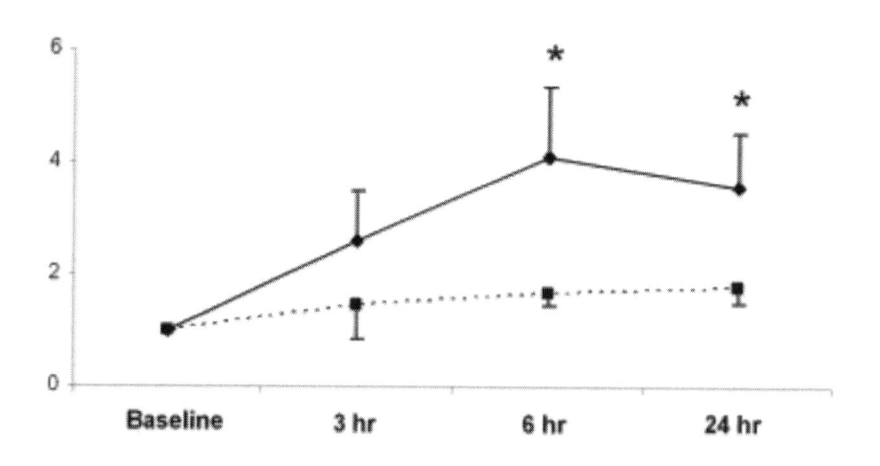

WHY ERK IN MUSCLE SLOWS WITH AGING

The reason ERK activation declines with age seems connected to aging blood and declining circulation. As we age and the blood tends to get clumpier and less viscous. The less viscous your blood the less ERK activates. It also seems tied to the decline of fluid volume in the body (Think ACE inhibitors. Old people are on them for a reason). It looks like this.

Old Blood => Poor circulation=> Old Muscle

Not surprisingly, mounds of new research support an old therapy to keep muscle young - massage.

YOUNG MUSCLE HACK #2: ERK TARGETING WITH MASSAGE
Emerging science demonstrates massage clearly helps muscles stay young. Research has shown just a single session of massage after exercise **increases muscle satellite stem cells**. In fact, a newer massage modality called **Cyclic Compression Loading** has actually been demonstrated to increase muscle size in humans apart from exercise!

KEY IDEA: Regular massage keeps muscles young.

As circulation declines with age, massage becomes an essential tool,

Massage mimics the circulation of "young blood." Once again, it's never just the "what." It's the "what, when and how" together. The goal of this hack is to combine massage with ERK targeting post exercise.

THE WHAT: Massage and ERK targeting.
THE WHEN: 1-4 hours post exercise and 24 hours after exercise
THE HOW: Dietary coconut oil post workout with massage.

A downstream derivative of coconut oil is palmitic acid. **Palmitic acid directly activates ERK.** Post exercise, coconut oil and massage together have a small but noticeable effect on recovery.

Caution. With all things balance rules. Too much coconut oil in the diet is bad in other ways. Use this hack a couple of times per week and limit the amount of coconut oil intake.

TO-DO: After your next workout, take coconut oil 1 hour post workout and massage the muscles exercised at the 2rd hour post workout. Repeat the following day. Your goal is to increase maximum ERK stimulation at the 6 hour mark post exercise.

CAUTION: ERK IN BRAIN NOT SO GOOD
A caution with stimulating ERK activation. With age we want more of it in muscle and less of it in the brain.

KEY IDEA: More ERK in muscle is good. More ERK in brain not good.

Once again, biological duality reigns supreme. Excess ERK activation in the brain as you age can promote Alzheimers. This is why we look to muscle massage to do the heavy lifting on aged muscle. Coconut oil seems to have a beneficial temporary effect on the brain. For this reason, limited use of coconut oil with massage helps both brain and muscle. You don't want excess ERK activation in the brain as you age which is partly why I caution against excess use of coconut oil.

INFLAMMATION AND CIRCULATION:
In Chapter 13 you learned of the inflammatory feedback loop between fat and muscle. As you age this loop suppresses muscle growth by driving fat into muscle. Expanding upon that idea, new science shows a relationship between total inflammatory markers circulating in the blood and loss of muscle stem cells. This brings us to the idea of inflammation and the blood itself. Part of the solution is **The Inflammation Spin Down** in the next section of the book. As promised in Chapter 1, you will learn to spin down inflammation on a regular basis. This will help you to have "young muscle" all the days of your life. The practice of invigorating the body with young blood goes back thousands of years. It's a history that is both gory and craven in many respects.

YOUNG BLOOD

Upon death in the gladiator ring, spectators would rush into the arena and drink the flowing blood of the dying gladiator! The horrific practice was done in the hope of receiving an infusion of invigorating life essence. Pliny the Elder, witness to the horror, wrote, "...These persons, forsooth, consider it a most effectual cure for their disease, to quaff the warm, breathing, blood from man himself, and, as they apply their mouth to the wound, to draw forth his very life."

Starting in 2005, science papers in the field of **Parabiosis** have demonstrated the rejuvenating power of young blood transfusions. Parabiosis is joining an old mammal to a young one via the blood. Experiments with Parabiosis have shown remarkable improvements regenerating liver, muscle, and stem cells. Recently, the practice of platelet rich plasma injections has grown in popularity. Platelet rich plasma injections derive from enriching blood factors. The enriched blood factors enhance renewal of stem cells.

Clearly there are attributes and factors in young blood that are different from old blood. The good news is we do not have to become a parasite society where the "haves" prey upon the "have not's" for their young blood. New science with young to old blood infusion has yielded remarkable insights into the specific components found in young blood that seem to be missing or declining in old blood.

The Map of Peak Human has a number of items all related to circulation. Simply by looking at statistics for circulatory related disease its a simple thing to understand your blood has a powerful effect on health and aging. But beyond tried and true facts, there are newer, more potent reasons for placing special emphasis on both circulation and the quality of your blood.

Let's briefly inventory the key factors of young blood. These are things within our influence to change via simple mechanisms.

YOUNG BLOOD VS OLD BLOOD: WHATS DIFFERENT

IMMUNE CELL CHANGES IN AGED BLOOD

It is estimated that every day you produce over 500 billion new blood cells! This thing we call "Blood" consists of different types of cells. There are two broad categories: immune cells and red blood cells. Ideally, immune cell populations in the blood are balanced.

KEY IDEA: "Old blood" has imbalanced populations of immune cells.

A team of researchers at University Hospital in Zurich, published a paper in 2016, connecting inflammation of the blood with aging and inflammaging. The team found that during aging, we don't make enough white blood cells. Beta and T cell populations also shrink.

With old blood, the immune system becomes overworked.

It's like age is an infection. The whole body gets inflamed. The way blood is produced shifts. The blood is flooded with blood cells that fail to replenish the bloods "starter dough" of stem cells.

KEY IDEA: With age blood made from stem cells increases.

This has the effect of depleting stem cells that make blood. One of the reasons *parabiosis seems to work is it helps to renew the immune system.*

KEY IDEA: Renewing the bloods stem cell system rejuvenates immunity.

We also have fewer red blood cells as we age. Our tissues become oxygen starved from blood that is fundamentally different from young blood. Summing up the changes in old blood

- Decline in key immune cells
- Decline of function in other immune cells
- Decline of red blood cell number and function
- Decline of stem cell renewal

As the blood itself becomes an inflammatory medium, tissues do not get properly oxygenated. Hypoxia of tissues and inflammation spread everywhere.

KEY IDEA: We need to increase the oxidative capacity of blood as we age.

BLOOD VISCOSITY AND AGE

The next problem of aged blood is blood viscosity is reduced with age. Worse, blood cells tend to clump together more as we age. This presents a massive problem for circulation. The smallest circulatory vessels of the body can only take one red blood cell at a time. But there is another problem. With age, the deformability of red blood cells declines due to a decline in flexibility of the red blood cell membrane.

The net result of these age related changes is that the smallest capillaries in your body don't get fed. We think of this as a lack of blood in the extremities. The result in terms of biology is hypoxia and accumulation of HIF-1. One key protein at work here is called **fibrinogen.**

Fibrinogen is one of the primary blood coagulation proteins. During injury, fibrinogen is converted to fibrin, which promotes clotting. Remember from Chapter 2 when I stated that with age, the immune system treats aging like it's one giant injury? Fibrinogen is a piece of evidence that this seems to be the case. With age, levels of fibrinogen increase in the blood making blood clumpier and less viscous, and less able to flow into the smallest capillaries. One of the ways we can drive an incremental hack of the aging process is by helping blood to flow better.

The drug Heparin has long been used as a blood thinner in aged populations. While effective, it has some considerations in terms of side effects. Recently, progress has been made in the area of Heparin Mimetics. These are substances, both natural and synthetic, that mimic the action of Heparin. We learned of Fucoidan and it's ability to steer interleukins in Chapter 4. It turns out Fucoidan is perhaps the most promising Heparin mimetic. It's a natural fiber polysaccharide made seaweed. It is an advanced and powerful goto for immune function. It is also a powerful anti-cancer agent, **increases muscle synthesis**, and is *an anti-coagulant.*

BLOOD CIRCULATION HACK:
THE WHAT: Fucoidan
THE WHEN: 8 hours after workout. After workouts
THE HOW: Together with Vitamin C

Young muscle and young blood are connected. The ability to add muscle depends on circulation. Using this protocol we attack on both fronts. Using Fucoidan as a post workout tool may help improve circulation and simultaneously improve muscle regeneration from workouts.

KEY IDEA: Fucoidan has the unique ability to effect macrophages in the gut.

Fucoidan helps to spin down Interluekin 6. Interleukin 6, it turns out, is not just gas on the fire of the SARS COV2 virus, it is also the primary signal molecule that **opens the gut up.**

VITAMIN C AND TET2
One of the key proteins that declines in old blood is a key enzyme called TET2. TET2 has been shown to rejuvenate aging brains when young blood is transferred to old bodies. The mechanism seems to be that TET2 restores the balance of red blood cells to aging blood. New research has shown that Vitamin C can help to restore TET2 levels.

PUTTING IT ALL TOGETHER:
This hack, combining Vitamin C with Fucoidan timed to max ERK12/ signaling after a workout, addresses both old muscle and old blood at the same time. ERK 1/2 activation peaks at the 6 hour mark post workout. This hack is designed to mimic a youthful profile of blood

and muscle at the precise time when you need it post workout. By addressing TET, ERK`1/2, and blood fibrins around working out, this is a master hack you can use on a regular basis to keep blood and muscle young.

TO-DO: MUSCLE GROWTH VIA AMPLIFED STARVATION SIGNALS

Our lioness slept after eating. She rapidly put on lost muscle. Why? Starvation. The most powerful mechanisms in the body, for anything, are survival mechanisms.

Muscle growth is supercharged post starvation in the presence of feasting.

Feasting after starvation has a number of documented effects I listed earlier. The reason is **signal amplification.** Signals for growth are primed by strong signals in the opposite direction. It's a survival defense. One way you can ameliorate age related muscle loss to amplifying starvation signals. In turn signals for muscle growth are primed. It's very easy. Let me give this to you in a new formula.

Amplify AMPK = > Amplify MTOR

MTOR is a signal pathway for growth. It is the bodies primary signal pathway to add muscle. The formula shows you can use starvation signals, AMPK and SIRT1, to amplify MTOR for muscle growth. I've done it many times. I routinely do this with people who come to me for help. It's all in the what, when and how.

This is a formula you can do once every six months. As you age this powerful formula massively cleans and then adds muscle. Amazingly, it's nothing more than food used to amplify signals.

This is an advanced hack. It puts together many things from the book. The modules here are presented and expounded on in the following chapters.

Reference Chapters:
Modules & The Amplified Fast - Ch 26
Daisy Cutter - Ch 21

THE WHAT: Stimulate muscle growth
THE WHEN: After 3-5 days of AMPK stimulation.
THE HOW: See below

BEDTIME HORMONE MODULE

1. Vitamin D
2. ZMA
3. Chelated minerals

INFLAMMATION SMALL MOLECULE MODULE

1. Fisetin +
2. Exogenous Ketones
3. Niacin
4. NAC
5. Vitamin D

- STEP ONE: 3-5 Days of the Amplified Fast. (Ch 25)
    - DAY ONE: Amplified fast + Small Molecules Module (ch 25) + Pre-bed Inflammation Module.
    - DAY TWO: Omega Fats Module + Small Molecules Module + Pre Bed Inflammation Module.
    - DAY THREE: Daisy Cutter Module by itself.
- STEP TWO: FEASTING: 3-5 Days: + Inflammation Small Molecules Module at bedtime+ Hormone Bedtime Module.
    - During feasting period **you must 2x your normal calories.** Eat mostly whole foods. You do not have to eat perfect. It's very difficult to eat a lot with whole foods. Lots of steaks are helpful. To get in adequate calories things like cereals, burritos, and rice help a lot.
    - Macro ratios during feasting are generally **40% protein, 40% carbs, 20% fat.**
    - Lift heavy weights. If you don't lift weights or can not, then use the Integrated Interval. Do 10 minutes a day of body weight movements. It must be strenuous: wall squats, push ups, pull ups, hand stands,

Chapter 18

Young Membranes

Some things matter more than others. At the top of the list are **membranes.** No discussion about real immunity can take place without discussing membranes and membrane linings.

WHAT ARE MEMBRANES?

A membrane is an **interface.** Membranes interface between stuff on the outside and stuff on the inside. Membranes are gatekeepers. They let some things in and keep others out. Dysfunction of membranes may be the single most unacknowledged part of the equation of immunity and aging with the power to radically improve the immune system and aging. I'm about to show you that you can't fix anything, or address anything about the body unless your first address membranes.

Membranes matter most.

Because of their status as gatekeepers, membranes are often first in line for things to go wrong with the body..

KEY IDEA: Membranes are the first point of contact for immunity

For example, when the gut membrane lining is compromised, LPS infiltrates fat mass. The result can be inflammation across the entire body.

The same is true of a handful of other membranes in your body. A prioritized list of these membranes would look like this.

The Membrane Plan of Attack

1. The gut lining membrane.
2. The gum line membrane.
3. The inner lining of your vasculature known as the endothelium membrane.
4. The phospholipid bi-layer membrane that makes up the cells of your body
5. The single layer membrane that envelopes the peroxisomes.
6. The 2 layer membrane system of the mitochondria, the tiny power plants in your cells.

The gut lining we have focused on elsewhere at length, so I won't go into it here. Let's look at the other membranes and why they are so important.

THE GUM LINING:
Until recently, the gum lining has been totally overlooked as a key factor controlling immune health and longevity. Pockets of bacteria and inflammation in the gum lining can have massive long term consequences. We learned how inflammatory signals from one part of the body can be "downloaded" into other areas of the body. This holds true for the gums where pathogenic bacteria can take hold.

- The gum lining has been linked with cardiovascular disease. Treatment of the gums has been shown decrease cardiovascular risk.

- Periodontitis in the gum lining is now linked to Alzheimers and arthritis.

- Women with gum disease have **2-3x higher likelihood of breast cancer.**

- Dental disease has been shown to correlate to obesity. It may even drive bacteria in the mouth that make you eat more!

The long neglected relationship between the gum lining with immunity, aging and disease is finally coming to light. New research has demonstrated pathogens and inflammatory signals in the gum lining can trigger system wide immune reactions. For example, if you have fusobacteria in the gut, you have a very good chance of getting cancer. The same is true of the gums. A 2013 meta review of the oral biome from Case Western University School of Periodontics, showed how fusobacterium of the oral cavity is proven to correlate with cancer of the colon!

In terms of priorities, the gum lining goes right at the top of the list.

You **can not treat the gum lining at home.** Treating gum lining bacteria involves scaling and *root planing* below the gumline. These services require professional dental help.

KEY IDEA: Deep cleaning of the mouth keeps the whole body young.

GUM LINING 101

Get a **deep cleaning** in the gums every 3 to 4 months.

If your goal, is to keep your body young a deep cleaning every 3-4 months **is essential.** Deep scaling and root planing of bacteria below the gumline is not possible apart from a professional dental visit.

TO DO: Put down the book right now and schedule your next deep cleaning.

THE VASCULATURE LINING - THE ENDOTHELIUM:
The term"vasculature" refers to your blood vessels. The inner lining of your blood vessels is called the **endothelium.** In today's pop sci nutrition world, the endothelium is perhaps the least talked about and least understood piece of immune centric health and aging.

Collectively, the lining of your blood vessels constitutes a giant membrane. It is every bit as important to aging and immunity as the gut lining. The cells of the endothelium have to do a critical job. They allow the raw materials of life into your cells, things like oxygen and glucose. Just like cells of the gut lining, the cells of the endothelium are unique and different from other cells in your body.

HACKING INFLAMMATION OF THE ENDOTHELIUM
When the lining of your inner vasculature becomes inflamed you are essentially screwed. For one thing you can get cancer. Cells lining the endothelium can "undock" and "transition" into what are called mesenchymal cells. This process, called the EMT transition, is how many diseases, including cancer, initiate. It's a flash point over whole body inflammation and aging. Accordingly, keeping the endothelium free from inflammation is centric to immunity and real health. Its a really, really big deal.

The Mediterranean diet has long been known for its vascular protective properties. Recently, new research has unveiled one of the key mechanisms. A 2019 study in the *European Journal of Nutrition* was able to show that a key phenol in olive oil, called Hydroxytosol, not only prevented inflammation of the vasculature, it even can prevent the EMT transition!

THE WHAT: Hydroxytyrosol
THE WHEN: During the Inflammation Spin Down - See Section 6
THE HOW: Combined with The Amplified Fast: See Section 6

CELL MEMBRANES AND AGING
One classic theory of aging says aging is really the oxidation of fats within cell membranes, combined with over production of free

radicals in the mitochondria. You have seen how aging is many things. In line with this more classical theory is a very important thing; cell membranes. Aging does very specific things to cell membranes. With age two major things happen to cell membranes.

KEY IDEA: With age cells membranes get stiff and less permeable.

Age is rigidity. Youth is suppleness. This is true at the macro body level and it holds at the cellular level. You have seen how membranes are really interfaces. They need to keep some things out and let other things in. The membranes making up the cells of your body must be permeable and flexible. When cells lose their suppleness and permeability you get old faster. The cell membrane is composed of what are called **phospholipids.** Phospholipids are specialized long chain fats. Lecithin is the one you are most familiar with. These fats for a two sided layer in our cell membranes. They can bind with things like choline to make cell membranes supple and permeable.

A research validated way to improve the suppleness and permeability of cell membranes is via supplementation with omega 3 fatty acids. Several studies have shown these fats are able to be incorporated into the cell membrane with the formation of "replacement" phospholipids. For example, a 2019 study published in the Journal Frontiers of Physiology showed that 12 weeks of supplementing with Omega 3's increased the phospholipid content in muscle cells by 57%! That sounds fantastic right? Now the bad news.

CENATENARIANS AND SERUM FATS

Newer research into very long lived humans shows sustained high levels of serum omega **3's shorten lifespan.** The reason is these long chain fats oxidize. Research with super long lived humans shows they are able to prevent oxidation of long chain fats in the blood. Generally speaking, continual dosing of Omega fats in the diet may drive up serum levels of these fats and oxidation along with them. Sustained oxidation of Omega fats in your blood most likely shortens life.

KEY IDEA: Sustained high levels of Omega fats in your blood may shorten lifespan.

So what can we do about this? How do we obtain the benefits of Omega fat supplementation for our cell membranes and mitigate the potential negative impact on lifespan? I believe the answer is, once again, **balance and order of operations.** The baby talk says Omega 3's are either good or bad. I believe the answer lies in when and how we use them.

The 2 Day Immunity Core Pattern (Chapter 25) is designed to solve this problem by taking everything into account. There are a few keys I will cover here.

1. The first key is you don't take Omega 3 fats every day.
2. In between days of having Omega 3 fats, we increase serum phenols
3. We have Omega 3's in small pulses timed several hours apart.

The 2 Day Immunity Core Pattern and The Amplified Fast are designed to give cell membranes the long chain fats they need to keep your body young. At the same time the issue of oxidation of these fats in the serum is built into how you do it. Here is one additional hack you can add to the 2 day core specific for cell membranes. The 2 Day Immunity Core Pattern is also designed to aid peroxisome membranes at the same time.

CELL MEMBRANE HACK:
THE WHAT: Lecithin
THE WHEN: Mornings on day two of the 2 Day Immunity Core Pattern
THE HOW: With 100mg of vitamin C. Do not overdose.

Supplementation with Lecithin has been shown to restore and augment cell membrane phospholipids. A small amount of vitamin C timed with ingestion may help prevent oxidation of fats.

PEROXISOME AND MITOCHONDRIAL MEMBRANES
In Chapter 16 we introduced the idea of Cellular Death Row. The total power output of a cell drives how fast you age. Mitochondria and the peroxisomes are the twin pedals cellular power output. They work together. When the membranes of either one, of these cellular organs start to go, your body as a whole is not far behind. Fortunately new science has revealed a surprising way to maintain the health of these membranes. One key I mentioned already is Pexohpagy. What I am about to show you is a way to help keep both organs young. This represents some of **the most advanced manipulation of nutrition ever presented** for functional outcomes. The key is driving production of the fat Oleate through both organs. In the process, we can do two things.

1. Target Pexohpagy
2. Target the membranes of the mitochondria and the peroxisomes.

THE MEMBRANE HACK: Mitochondria and Peroxisomes
THE WHAT: The Pexohpagy Module
THE WHEN: During the Inflammation Spin Down - Chapter 28
THE HOW: See below.

HOW THIS WORKS:
Stearic acid, the fat found in coconut oil, has been shown to promote health of the mitochondria membranes. It also converts to oleate (Omega 9) New research suggests one way to force pexohpagy on the peroxisomes is to feed oleate (omega 9) into the diet and then ***switch*** to glucose. After sustained feeding of oleate into the peroxisomes, as you do in the Pexophagy Module, a sudden rush of glucose into the cell forces peroxisomes into pexohpagy! The peroxisomes go into housekeeping. It looks like this.

Pre-amplify fasting with fibers => Proliferation with fats =>Pexophagy with glucose

In Chapter 25 and 26 you learn the steps of the 2 Day Core and The Inflammation Spin Down. This is a variant on both. The key is to substitute a day or two of Omega 3's with high Omega 9's. See Chapter 25 and 26 for the full step through of this hack.

PART 6:

The New Solution

Chapter 19

Sleep and Immunity

SLEEP: THE PRIMARY AGE ACCELERANT.

So far you have seen that we don't age at the same rate across our lives. The older we get, the faster we get older. Perhaps ***the*** primary cause, all factors considered, is disrupted sleep. With age, sleep becomes disrupted for a number of reasons. Disrupted sleep disrupts the most important mechanisms that keep you young.

- Housekeeping
- AMPK and SIRT1
- Data transfer
- Restoration of NAD+

In the first part of our lives, we age slower during sleep. All of the above processes more or less work optimally. As we age the script gets flipped. Sleep becomes the place where much of the age related damage is done. The causes are both many, and sum into a single thing. Disrupted sleep disrupts immunity and ages the body. In fact no real discussion about immunity can take place without addressing sleep. You are most likely to catch a virus after a poor nights sleep. The reasons as to why fill a rogues gallery of the usual suspects; apnea, hypoxia, inflammation, immune cell production, circulation, excess hif-1, disrupted expression of genes related to sleep clocks, and several others.

To make matters worse, we live in an era where lots of people are jumping on the fasting bandwagon. The reason for fasting is to get the benefits of the things I just listed. And yet **fasting disrupts sleep.**

HOW INTERMITTENT FASTING DISRUPTS SLEEP

Sleep is the original intermittent fast. Why do you think breakfast is called "break-fast."

Sleep is intermittent fasting.

As you first learned in Chapter 10, all of the benefits of fasting also occur during sleep with one key difference.

The same benefits derived from fasting are *much stronger* from sleeping.

Housekeeping, AMPK activation, data transfer and the restoration of NAD+, all of these things, naturally occur during sleep. At least they are supposed to. As we age sleep quality diminishes and so do all of these processes.

Millions of people around the world are unknowingly disrupting sleep with fasting. In an attempt to gain the life extending benefits of autophagy, AMPK activation and HDAC inhibition, during the day, millions of people are unknowingly disrupting these things during sleep. New research shows that fasting seems to disrupt our dream sleep or REM sleep.

FASTING DISRUPTS REM SLEEP

Simply put, fasting disrupts dreaming. This is no small thing. Lack of dreaming may have a far more profound impact than previously thought. Some researchers theorize lack of REM sleep may drive depression, poor immune function, weight gain and obesity. In 2017 Dr. Rubin Naiman, a professor of sleep at the University of Arizona Center for Integrative medicine, published a thought provoking paper in the *Annals of the New York Academy of Sciences.* Dr Naiman reviewed more than seventy books and scientific articles in his paper. He theorized that dreaming may modulate immunity and loss of REM sleep may be the culprit behind sleep deprivation. He postulates lack of dreaming can compromise whole body health, promote obesity, memory loss, and cardiovascular disease! While more research is needed to confirm Dr. Naimen's theory, the important take away is this...

Fasting at the expense of REM sleep is not ideal long term.

While fasting has numerous benefits, it also has several pitfalls we have to be aware of.

The Dark Side of Fasting:

- Disrupted sleep and loss of dreams.
- Increased hunger signaling
- Activation of the body's starvation defense mechanisms.

FIRST IN THE ORDER OF OPERATIONS

If you are routinely fasting and not sleeping **stop!** Restoring Peak Human sleep is the first order of operations.

Age related sleep disruption acts like a snowball down the hill to rapid aging. By restoring sleep we can can dramatically impact the body's ability to age better. While this is no simple thing, it is a solvable problem. You may have to treat it as a job for a while. Age related sleep disruption has several causes. These causes represent an accumulation of factors over time. The sooner you begin to address them the better.

To get an overview of the problem of sleep, let's look at some interesting research with ancestral populations.

THE ECOSYSTEM PROBLEM OF SLEEP

Research with African hunter gatherer tribes such as the Hazda, the San and the Tsimané have shown some surprising insights into ancestral sleep and the differences with modern sleep. Here are the highlights

- They sleep on average 6.4 hours with duration averaging 1.5 hours longer, i.e in bed 8 hours to get 6.4 hours of sleep.
- They go to sleep 3 hours after sunset on average. They wake just before sunrise.
- They begin sleeping when air temperature drops and wake when air temp is lowest.
- They sleep less in summer, about 55 minutes less.
- They do not have a word for insomnia. It’s prevalence is around 1% opposed to 10-30 percent in industrialized societies.

Here are some differences.

Ancestral Sleep	Modern Sleep
Sleep within 3 hours post sunset	Longer duration awake post sunset
Wake at sunrise	Post sunrise waking.
Relatively high o2. Low CO	Lower o2. Higher CO.
Low EM	High EM
Low stress.	High stress
Hard chewing	Soft chewing
Low comfort	High comfort
No insomnia	Prevalent Insomnia
Frequent waking. Rapid return to sleep.	Frequent waking. Difficulty returning to sleep
Temperature flux	Temperature controlled sleep

There are a few key take aways we can gather from ancestral sleep patterns. The first is they don't sleep more. They do sleep better. Paradoxically they have less comfort than we do. It's colder, the ground is hard, and they are not behind locked doors. Yet, they don't have trouble falling asleep or struggle with insomnia.

The second key difference is sleep and wake timing. They don't seem to have late risers. Everyone gets up early. Chronotype doesn't exist. Sleep and waking are much more attuned to rising before dawn and sleeping a few hours after sunset. Interestingly, these ancestral societies don't have perfect sleep. There is a lot of room for improvement. They don't sleep on comfortable beds. They wake several times during the night, but quickly return to a deep restorative sleep.

The Net of Light:
Research with workers in the Amazon with and without light reveals the net difference having artificial light seems to have upon sleep. Amazon workers without electricity sleep about thirty minutes more than ones who have electricity. Yet as we can see with the data on ancestral cultures, total time sleeping is only one of many factors.

We can boil the difference in sleep between ancestral cultures and our modern ecosystem down to two things.

1. They maximize periods of deep sleep
2. They minimize sleep disruption.

WAKING AND RISING

Available data suggests ancestral sleep is characterized not staying up too late and getting up around dawn. What's interesting is this is exactly what we do in modern societies when we are children. The most youthful and energetic period of life is when as children, we go to sleep a few hours after sunset and wake just before dawn.

This pre dawn waking sleep cycle is optimal for the Genetic Rush Hour and activation of the AMPK pathway and the SIRT genes. Exercise in a fasted state around this time (things like hunting or farming) creates maximum activation of AMPK, and in turn activates the SIRT youth genes, restores NAD+ and induces autophagy. And it makes sense. At dawn hunting and farming took place.

SLEEP HACK: THE ANCESTRAL SLEEP AND WAKE CYCLE

Give the ancestral waking schedule a try. Try going to bed by 9pm and getting up around 5 am. You can use the other sleep hacks in this chapter to help you fall asleep at an earlier hour. It may take a while to acclimate, If you are not currently doing it, many report that shifting to an early to bed early to rise pattern, has a marked effect on energy and productivity.

LOSS OF HARD CHEWING:

One of the most important and overlooked differences effecting ancestral sleep quality may be something totally overlooked - hard chewing.

Hard Chewing: The Missing Epigenetic Link to Sleep Apnea

The outside-in, mechanical force of hard chewing, directly stimulates genes in the face and skull to grow. In the absence of hard chewing the opposite is also true. Modern societies have removed hard chewing. Ancestral societies chew hard foods. Modern societies chew soft foods. The results are massive.

- Improved facial bone structure.
- Maintenance of throat airway size and volume.
- Improved oxygenation during sleep.
- Lean healthy bodies.

Loss of hard chewing has the opposite effect.

- Facial bone loss with aging.
- Shrinking of throat airway.
- Sleep apnea and sleep hypoxia.
- Obesity, metabolic disease and even cancer.

KEY IDEA: Chewing hard foods is Mechanobiology. It keeps the facial structure young.

To understand the power hard chewing has to drive epigenetic signals that control bone growth look at the man below. I took this photo at an invite only gathering in 2017 with Quest Nutrition. The top thought leaders in nutrition were invited to share and collaborate on their innovations. This is a 70 year old man who has regrown his facial bone structure by mimicking hard chewing. This is a real thing.

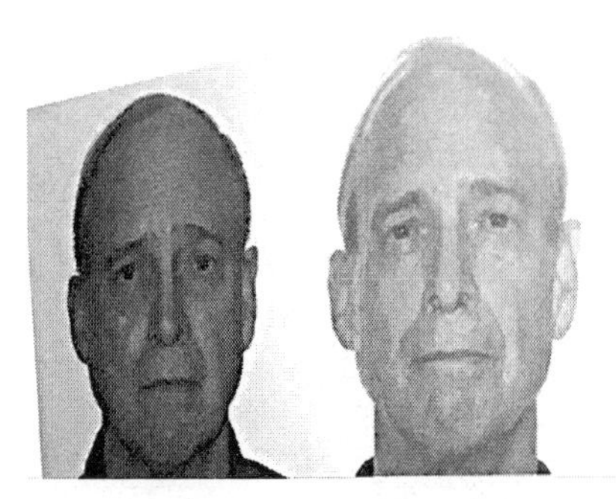

To get a better understanding of the impact soft chewing is having on our health, I spoke to Dr Gregory Clibon, DDS, a prominent dentist in Southern California and frequent lecturer at UCLA. Dr Clibon is passionate about sleep apnea and the impact of chewing soft foods on sleep, obesity, and human health.

I asked Dr. Clibon how chewing soft foods from infancy onward effects our health.

"Soft foods, such as baby food, is one of multiple factors that can have a detrimental affect on the development of the face, during our infantile growth years. This epigenetic altered development of our face affects the jaws, the palate, the space for the tongue, and the muscles used for chewing ...... This insufficient facial development leads to constrictions of our airway. These constrictions in our airway affect our ability to breath normally. Disordered breathing results in abnormalities in our sleeping behavior. Poor sleep or worse, sleep apnea, contribute to a multitude of health conditions. In children these conditions can include ADHD , asthma, allergies, mouth breathing, snoring, teeth grinding, and poor posture. Now as we progress into adulthood, these airway problems contribute to chronic fatigue, headaches, jaw joint pain, stress on the heart, poor memory, an increase in inflammation, a decrease in libido, and poor weight management."

Let me summarize.

Soft chewing =>
ADHD, snoring, sleep apnea =>
Chronic fatigue, headaches, weight problems, memory problems.

Just this one hack, returning hard chewing, can dramatically impact your life.

SLEEP HACK: IMPROVING THE AIRWAY BY HACKING THE FACE

One of the fastest ways to improve your quality of life and facial appearance is to spend 1 minute a day doing hard chewing. I do this routinely. You will notice the results very rapidly. Over time what you will see is the bones of your face take on a youthful look.

THE WHAT: Hard chewing.
THE WHEN: Use the Integrated Interval and do this in twenty second to one minute bursts.
THE HOW: Use raw green beans or a facial exercise appliance.

An easy way to do this is with raw green beans. Chewing them is fantastic exercise for the bones of the face. You can spit them out if you don't like green beans. Alternatively you can use a facial exercise appliance. If you choose to use one of those, Dr. Clibon cautions to use it on both sides of the jaw as well as the front. Overdoing exercise with pressure to the front of the jaw can imbalance the mandibular joint and create bite problems.

INFLAMMATION AND LOSS OF DIURNAL RHYTHM

As we age time keeping mechanisms within each cell that regulate diurnal rhythm becomes disrupted, which disrupts sleep. This is significant because all of protective mechanisms against aging and cancer occur during the Genetic Rush Hour within each cell.

AGE RELATED INFLAMMATION DISRUPTS SLEEP

One underlying mechanism identified in recent years is loss of NAD+. The core clock mechanism within cells needs NAD+ to function properly. Once again, it's easy to think we just need to supplement with B-vitamin derivatives and problem solved right? Yet In Chapter 13, we discovered loss of NAD+ is driven by increases in inflammation. Accordingly, **age related inflammatory issues** seem to be a major mechanism disrupting sleep cycles.

A 2016 Meta review of sleep and inflammation from the UCLA center for neuro immunology look at 72 different studies and found commonalities with key inflammatory markers and sleep disturbance. Most notable were C-reactive protein and interleukin 6.

Both of these inflammatory markers were found to correlate with poor sleep.

Inflammation and sleep disruption is easy to validate on a personal level. Aches and pains disrupt sleep. Disruption of sleep cycles from inflammatory related aches is pervasive with age. With age, waking with aches and stiffness becomes common. Sleep ceases to become restful and becomes a form of slow torture. The underlying cause, however, is not so simple. **One clear mechanism seems to be visceral fat.** The growth of fat in the internal body compartments correlates with obesity and sleep apnea. Further research with sleep apnea in children now correlates inflammation as a first cause preceding the onset of apnea during sleep.

POOR SLEEP DRIVES MORE POOR SLEEP

Research with inflammatory markers suggest a *feedback loop* is at work. The less you sleep, the more inflammation signals propagate. The more inflammation signals propagate, the less you sleep and the worse your immune system works.. For example, inflammation disrupts key cells in the brain needed to regulate sleep. When inflamed, these cells, (astrocytes) put several key inflammatory factors into circulation. These factors affect the core gene regulating diurnal rhythm, the CLOCK gene. Then in a feedback loop, disturbed sleep activates the immune system. This drives brain-inflammation.

KEY IDEA: The more inflamed you are, the less you sleep, and the less you sleep the more inflamed you become.

ADDING IT ALL UP:

Declining NAD+, increases in Interluekin 6, signals from visceral fat, apnea driven by inflammatory signals, and many other data points all lead to one big broadsword stroke.

KEY IDEA: We can't address immunity without addressing sleep and we can't address sleep without *addressing inflammation.*

See Section 6: The Inflammation Spin Down.

SLEEP HACK: OLEAMIDE

New research shows that the endocannaboid receptors have a very significant impact on sleep onset. In particular, a key receptor, ECB-1 seems to be activated by a special type of fat called Oleamide. I first introduced Oleamide to audiences in 2016 on Carl Lanore's Superhuman Radio, where I did a show on circadian rhythms and the suprachiasmatic nucleus. Oleamide is a fantastic tool that really works to augment sleep onset.

THE WHAT: Oleamide
THE WHEN: 30 minutes before bedtime.
THE HOW: With melatonin.

SLEEP HACK: ORAL APPLIANCE
THE WHAT: An oral jaw appliance
THE WHEN: During sleep.
THE HOW: Only from a trained dental professional

If you have applied the Seattle Protocol and you are still experiencing snoring during sleep, you must get an oral sleep appliance. This is **the single most important thing** you can do. Snoring during sleep is simply improper airway flow. Improper airway flow drives hypoxia during sleep. An oral appliance advances the jaw and opens up the airway. Improved airway flow during sleep will slow your rate of aging more than any pill or virtually anything else. I caution you to get one of these only from a trained dental technician. They must be custom fit to your jaw.

FEEDING PATTERS AND SLEEP IMPROVEMENT

New science is finally setting something of an ongoing question about what is the most powerful factor that effects sleep. For a while it seemed like cycles of light and dark were the big winner. More recently, research into food and metabolism has shown that diurnal cycles related to metabolism and food intake are the most powerful effectors of sleep cycles.

THE TIMEKEEPERS: WHO'S REALLY IN CHARGE OF SLEEP

The Brain's Master Clock: Controlled by light and dark cycles.
The Organ Clocks: Controlled by food and metabolism
The Winner: Food and metabolism

Metabolism and food intake are the most powerful input controls over sleep. And it's super easy to prove to yourself. At lunch, in broad daylight, eat between 3,000-5,000 calories of whatever you want. Watch what happens. You will go to sleep. It doesn't matter that it's mid day and light is everywhere. Conversely, do the Signal Amplification hack from end of Chapter 5, but do it at night. Odds are you will wake up in the middle of the night from hunger. Sleeping while starving is very difficult, even in total darkness.

KEY IDEA: Food patterns regulate sleep cycles more than any other factor.

The knowledge that food can control sleep onset and sleep cycles gives us a very powerful tool to aid Peak Human Sleep. New research with food pulses at night has shown different types of food inputs at night can help sleep. For example, a study in the *American Journal of Clinical Nutrition* has demonstrated that small, high glycemic index meals at night can help you fall asleep.

KEY IDEA: We can use timing, meal size and combinations of food *to help regulate sleep.*

Here is a food based sleep hack that improves upon that idea substantially.

SLEEP HACK: GRILLED CHEESE ON SOURDOUGH

If you have trouble falling asleep here is a dinner that will help you hack that problem. You can actually use this as part of the Amplified Fast as the dinner portion. Give it a try to get a feel for the power of food to induce and control sleep.

THE WHAT: Grilled cheese sandwich
THE WHEN: One or two hours before bed
THE HOW: On sourdough, with mustard on the inside and jalepenos.

What makes this work are the timing and the functional elements of the foods. Sourdough bread helps ferment good bacteria while you sleep. A bit of mustard and jalepenos on the inside help increase metabolism. If you don't like jalepenos you can leave off.

SLEEP HACKS FOR SPECIFIC PROBLEMS

TROUBLE SHUTTING BRAIN OFF TO FALL ASLEEP

THE WHAT: 1 Gram of GABA
THE WHEN: Twenty minutes before bedtime
THE HOW: Soak hands and/or feet in warm to hot water for two minutes

Does that last one sound sketchy? It's actually pure science. It's from a paper in the *Journal of Nature,* that showed dilation of blood vessels in the hands and feet, is the best physiological predictor for the rapid onset of sleep. Soaking the feet or hands before bed helps drive rapid sleep onset. Science aside, we all know that heat makes you drowsy, cold wakes you up.

There is also an internet myth about GABA that says it does not cross the blood brain barrier. I went back and examined all the original research. Totally not true. GABA can and does cross the blood brain barrier and is effective and sleep induction. Try this one. It's powerful.

SLEEP HACK: TROUBLE WITH DEEP SLEEP

An amazing science based technique, with numerous documented benefits for improving sleep, is slow breathing. The technique is simple, works immediately and you will notice the difference right away.

THE WHAT: Slow breathing.
THE WHEN: At bedtime.
THE HOW: See below.

Here is how you begin. Do this at bedtime.

Step 1: Get out your smartphone and set your stop watch.
Step 2: Click the "start" button and inhale through your nose for five seconds
Step 3: Exhale for five seconds
Step 4: Repeat for three minutes initially and work your way up to fifteen minutes

Slow breathing involves taking a maximum of six breaths per minute **through the nose with mouth closed**. Each inhale is five seconds. Each exhale is five seconds. Take three breaths every thirty seconds. Take six breaths per minute. Your goal is to work up to fifteen minutes prior to bedtime. When I really need to make sure I get a good nights sleep I do twelve minutes at six breaths and then wind down to two breaths per minute for the next two minutes and finish with six breaths for the last minute. Here are just a few of the scientifically validated benefits of this technique

- Improved sleep.
- Improved microcirculation.
- Enhanced arterial oxygenation.
- Improved cardiovascular function.
- Decreased blood pressure and hypertension.
- Improved heart rate variability.

TO-DO: PUTTING IT ALL TOGETHER TO SLEEP LIKE A BABY

THE WHAT: When you absolutely must have a great nights sleep.
THE WHEN: Starting at dinner.
THE HOW: See below.

STEP ONE: Grilled cheese at dinner or carb heavy meal.

STEP TWO: Integrated Interval Pre bed yoga flows.

STEP THREE: Soak feet and hands in hot water 2 min.

STEP FOUR: 6 breaths per minute exercise.

STEP FIVE: Supplement with:

- 10,000 i.u. vitamin D.
- 1 Gram GABA.
- 500 mg Oleamide.
- Melatonin.

STEP SIX: WiFi and lights protocol.

Chapter 20

The Immune Gut

The mechanistic origin of immunity in the body has a lot to do with your gut. Over the fourteen years since I began my journey studying and hacking the gut biome, a lot has changed. For the first eight years, things were pretty quiet. The techniques and IP I created for the gut biome stayed in the walled garden of my VEEP System. I was the only game in town. In 2014, the topic began to take hold in the public with a few early adopters, and by 2018 the gut biome had hit mainstream.

In the three and 1/2 years it took to get this book done, there was an explosion of venture capital flow into the microbiome. One entrepreneur after another was raising money for a microbiome project to develop drugs, tests, and prebiotics, based on the gut. Speaker after speaker was giving a keynote on the promise of new treatments and therapies based on the gut. Podcast after podcast talked about the need for "improving diversity." I knew from years of hard won experience that many of these things **were either not necessary or even incorrect.**

In this chapter, you are going to get the distillation of my many years and results with thousands of people, and stacks of studies going all the way back to Dr. Gordons very first one in 2006. In the process, much, if not most, of what you have heard about the microbiome will vaporize.

Why does the simple solution, which is to just stay healthy elude the vast majority? More truth. We have not been dealing with what's really true about the gut.

Some of the resets you are about to learn are.

- Why diversity of bacteria in the gut is meaningless as a practical objective
- Why you almost never need probiotics.
- Why poop testing is almost useless.
- Why you only need to focus on two bacteria.
- Why nearly all proposed therapies and treatments can never be nearly as effective as food.

If you thought our fat loss chapters were a reset, just wait. Let's begin by deconstructing the idea of bacteria diversity.

WHY DIVERSITY OF GUT BACTERIA IS MEANINGLESS IN PRACTICE

Today on podcasts and Youtube videos, nearly everyday, some well-meaning person preaches the idea of having a diverse range of bacteria in the gut. It's a nice idea. It comes from the word being used a lot in research publications. And it has no meaning in the real world.

KEY IDEA: Focusing on gut bacteria diversity has little practical value.

You do not need to focus on diversity to have a healthy gut. You just need to focus on 2 bacteria - Akkermansia and Bifidobacteria. We will dive into both at length here. If you have those two in abundance you will have peak immunity and keep your body young. By focusing on only those two, *you get diversity in the gut.*

KEY IDEA: You can have diversity of bacteria and have poor health.

You can have a diversity of bacteria in your gut, and if you don't have Akkermansia and Bifidobacteria, you won't have real immunity. They are the crux variable bacteria of the gut.

KEY IDEA: The main practical outcome of diversity is carb digestion

Where you obtain a practical outcome with diversity of gut bacteria is with digesting carbs. If you don't have diversity in the gut, you won't digest carbs well. If you have diversity of bacteria you can handle a wider range of carbs. This includes glutens and dairy. But once again, the way you get there is by focusing on Akkermansia and Bifidobacteria

WHY YOU ALMOST NEVER NEED PROBIOTICS

Food is far, far more powerful to effect radical, immediate change on the body than probiotics. And its super easy to prove. If you have doubts, do the Daisy Cutter at the end of the chapter. In three to five days you can easily prove it to yourself. Your poop won't have any odor. Your energy will be sky high when you come off it, and you will rapidly recolonize the gut in a way probiotics simply can not do.

The problem with probiotics I have seen time and again, is where they release in the gut. It is very difficult to precisely control. Over the last 4 years I have witnessed an explosion of SIBO. SIBO is when you have good bacteria in the wrong place in the gut. Most of the SIBO epidemic I attribute to probiotic usage. Time after time, I have seen people go on probiotics only to have major issues with SIBO after a couple of years. Only food delivers the precise mix of fibers that ferment the right bacteria in the right place.

That being said, there is a rightful place of probiotics. The rightful home of their administration are specific medical conditions under guidance of a skilled practitioner, who knows what they are doing. There are very specific instances where administration of a precise strain can alleviate specific medical symptoms. For example. with Giadin induced gut disbiosis, both Bifidobacteria Longham and Lactobacillus Casei can help rebuild the gut layer. This is a growing science, so again I stress **medical conditions** and a **skilled medical practitioner.**

WHY POOP TESTING IS NEARLY USELESS

A new trend that has emerged is testing fecal samples to determine your gut bacteria. As a practice, this has little value and it's fairly expensive. There are several reasons why.

The first reason poop testing is useless is gut bacteria are rapidly and totally modifiable. It is well established. Beginning in 2009, research demonstrating that gut communities could be totally recolonized in just a few days, began circulating. If you do the Daisy Cutter you will prove it quite easily. There is an even easier proof. Eat a bunch of junk food and watch how fast you have really bad gas. The bad gas is from fermentation. Fermentation makes bacteria. Bad gas is a sign you are making bad bacteria. The same is true in the opposite direction. This is why the gut is so powerful. It can be recolonized very fast. A direct outcome is the power to rewire cravings totally in about seven days.

Poop testing of the biome is based on the idea that your biome is a fixed proposition. It's not. The data you get back can easily be negated by diet patterns in just a couple of days. By the time you get the data, it's doesn't reflect the your gut.

The next reason poop testing isn't very useful is you don't have just one microbiome.

KEY IDEA: You have three primary microbiomes.

You have the fecal which represents the colon, then there is the luminal, which represents the contents of your intestines, and then you have the mucosal, which represents the thin film of the gut lining. Poop testing measures primarily the fecal. It doesn't really tell you the other two. The colon is where much of the digestion process is done, so it could be argued you are getting the most important data. Conversely, it could be argued that because we have a hard time measuring the gut lining, you are not getting the most crucial data. The corollary to both of those arguments is this; what you don't have gut, is more important than what you currently do have.

KEY IDEA: Your current microbiome is less relevant than the one you can have in 7 days by simply restoring Akkermansia and Bifidobacteria.

Because the gut bacteria is so rapidly modifiable, your current profile is like today's weather. It's here today, gone tomorrow. You don't need to sample your poop to do that. Focusing not on what you have today, but on loading those 2 bacteria starting today, is far more beneficial and effective. This is a very different way of thinking. It's not only based on research, it's based on thousands of outcomes over 13 years.

There are a few instances where poop testing can be useful. One is in the case of cancer. If you have been diagnosed with cancer then getting poop tested for fusobacteria can help your practitioner with a course of treatment. Since we now know fusobacteria can begin in the mouth, sampling the oral microbiome is a practice I predict will grow to become equal if not bigger than poop testing. You can test for the same cancer causing bacteria and it's more practical to do so.

WHY YOU ONLY NEED TO FOCUS ON TWO BACTERIA

As we age, there is a **distinct shift** in key species of bacteria in the gut. We lose key health promoting species and gain bacteria that correlate with accelerating the aging process! The Peak Human Enterotype is the gut bacteria profile shared by the leanest,

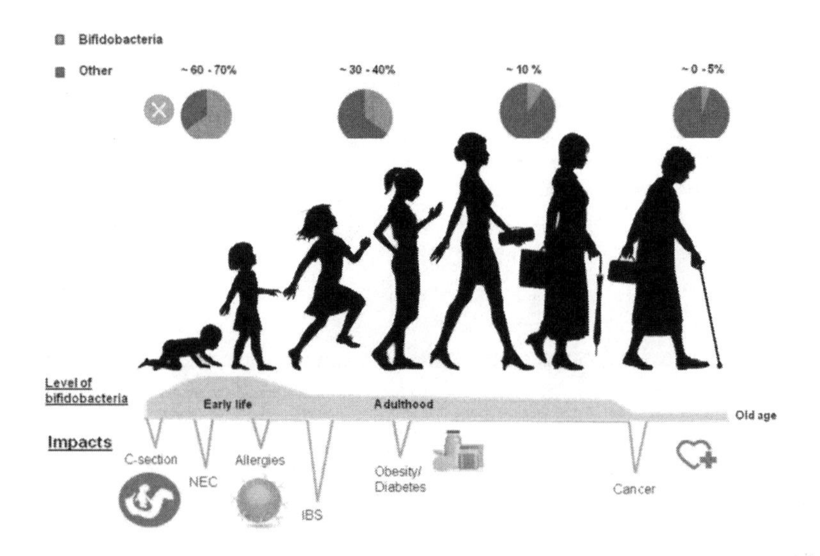

healthiest, and longest lived people in the world. Two particular species are of such incredible value to your health, metabolism, and longevity they are called ***gut symbionts.***

The number one health promoting symbiont bacteria we lose is Bifidobacteria.

Each strain of the bifido family can have unique and powerful effects. Together, they are the workhorse bacteria for human health. As kids, we have about ninety-five percent Bifidobacteria in our gut. As adults the number declines to approximately five percent.

A 2016 science paper on Bifidobacteria and human aging showed how declining levels of Bifido correlate to every major milestone of declining health.

At a high level Bifido helps us digest carbs, protects against pathogens, and helps us make vitamin B and antioxidants. Bifidobacteria is also central to immunity. Here are just a few of the amazing particulars this super bacteria does.

- Oral administration of Bifidobacteria has shown to protect against tumors and melanoma.

- Bifido correlates with decreased inflammation status and improved ability to use blood sugar for energy instead of store it as fat.

- Bifido stimulates production FAIF, the protein from Chapter 1 that *suppresses* fat storage.

- Bifido promotes production of Butyrate, the master molecule governing gut barrier permeability and immunity.

- Bifidobacteria Longum produces a key protein called serpin that sidesteps gluten intolerance.

- Very long lived individuals, over one hundred years old, all have significantly higher levels of bifidobacteria than average lifespan humans in old age.

FEEDING BIFIDO FEEDS EVERYONE ELSE

The reason Bifido strains correlate to gut biome diversity is due to what are called **cross feeding reactions.** In simplest terms, you feed Bifido, and in turn, the metabolites of Bifidobacteria feed other bacteria. What this means in practice is you don't need to feed or supplement for diversity. You just need to feed Bifidobacteria what it needs to ferment. Not ironically, you began this in Chapter 1 with HMO.

HOW HMO FEEDS THE YOUTH BACTERIA

Bifidobacteria Longum is one of the important strains of health promoting Bifidobacteria associated with youth. This strain digests HMO, the carbs you started on in Chapter 1. Conversely, feeding the body HMO helps ferment this bacteria. When HMO is present, it makes anti-inflammatory signal molecules. It also makes proteins that tighten the gut junctions

AGE AND DIVERSITY: ALL YOU NEED IS BIFIDO.

One consistent marker among elderly is a decrease of Bifidobacteria populations. Now here is the point all roads lead to.

KEY IDEA: Decreases in bifidobacteria promote decreases in gut bacteria diversity.

Several studies have clearly linked old age with low bifidobacteria and declining gut diversity. It looks like this.

Aging => Declining Bifidobacteria =>Low diversity

Perhaps the most important bacteria downstream of the cross feeding reactions of Bifidobacteria is Akkermansia Mucinilpha.

AKKERMANSIA: THE OTHER HALF OF THE DREAM TEAM

We began targeting Akkermansia at the end of the introduction for a very good reason. Akkermansia is the master regulator of the gut lining. Akkermansia eats mucins. Mucins are a component of gels that make them, well, gel-like. By feeding on mucins in the gut layer, Akkermansia has been shown to be the primary bacteria thickening the gut mucous layer. A 2017 paper by a team of researchers in the Netherlands were able to identify the exact mechanism by which Akkermansia controls the gut mucus lining.

Akkermansia produces key proteins, called **pill proteins.** Pill proteins have a direct effect on Interleukin-10, which is the primary signal to shut the gut junctions.

Even more fascinating, specific types of mucins seem to shuttle back and forth between the gut mucus barrier and the cells it covers and report back to the immune system regarding potential immunity challenges.

HOW AKKERMANSIA CONTROLS NET CALORIES

Akkermansia has a unique ability. It can contract the surface area of the gut. The first result is the gut junctions seal and tighten. The other result is less food energy gets absorbed. In this sense Akkermansia is like a calorie dial.

KEY IDEA: The more Akkermansia in the gut the fewer calories absorbed.

Akkermansia is positively correlated to being lean, having lower body weight, and reduced weight gain. The leanest people in the world all seem to have plentiful amounts of Akkermansia in the gut. Conversely people who are overweight or struggle with metabolic disease seem to be lacking in Akkermansia. The more we discover about Akkermansia, the more it becomes clear Peak Human metabolic health is impossible without it. Just a few highlights of the power this bacteria wields are.

- Akkermansia wields vast control over immune homeostasis in the gut by influencing immunoglobulins and T-cell responses to antigens.

- Akkermansia controls genes involved in fat storage and blood sugar function.

- Akkermansia also correlates with preventing weight gain.

- Low levels of Akkermansia correlated to inflammatory Bowel disease.

- Akkermansia strains are pivotal in vitamin b-12 synthesis.

- Increasing Akkermansia has been shown to reduce inflammation of your fat tissue.

COLD EXPOSURE & AKKERMANSIA

New science papers have shown a remarkable connection between cold adaption and Akkermansia. Short term cold exposure has been shown to decrease Akkermansia in the gut lining. Prolonged exposure to cold increases the surface area of the gut. This allows the body to take in more energy. The net result is weight gain. Stimulating Akkermansia post cold exposure abolishes the weight gain induced by cold. For this reason, fasting combined with cold exposure together, help offset the negatives of cold exposure. Fasting helps restore the Akkermansia lost to cold.

HACKING AKKERMANSIA 101

THE WHAT: Increase Akkermansia.
THE WHEN: During fasting.
THE HOW: With apple peals, and cranberry juice pre and post fasting.

This is a simple add-on to the 2 day core. You simply add cranberry juice and apple peals.

1. Add cranberry juice and apple peals to breakfast of day one, fiber day.
2. Post fasting on day 2 have cranberry and apple peals.

Short term fasting helps to increase Akkermansia. Both apple peal pectin and cranberry juice feed Akkermansia. Combined with cross feeding reactions from Bifidobacteria this is a hack you can use whenever you like. See Appendix A: The Map of Bacterial Guilds to understand why.

One caution with Akkermansia is if there is a pre-existing condition of MS or family history. MS seems to displace Akkermansia into the blood serum. If you have MS, you would not want to target or administer MS without a doctor.

WHY PRE AND PROBIOTICS CAN NEVER MATCH THE POWER OF FOOD

And now we have come to the end game. The end game is simply what should go on your to-do list to load the peak immune gut. There is a ton of competition for your mind. It can be very confusing. In this chapter we have hopefully gone a long way to wipe out much of it. I want to finish the job by quite literally showing you how and why nothing, and I mean nothing, can match the power of food to rapidly tune the gut towards Peak Human health.

PHYSICAL MASS MATTERS

Dr. Stephen Witherly, one of the great minds in flavor engineering that I was privilege to interface with at Quest Nutrition is famous for saying "The body is essentially a tube." This is particularly true when it comes to the gut. The gut is a tube. Lining the surface of that tube in a 360 degree rotation are the cells of the gut. From the intestines to the colon, all along the tube of the gut, one thing holds constant - physical mass is a key property driving the health of the gut. Mass matters. The reason is simple. Think of a pipe cleaner. If you want the pipes clean, you will need a brush that touches all 360 degrees linking the inside of the tube.

KEY IDEA: Only food touches all 360 degrees of rotation inside the gut.

Food has a **physical property** that cannot be mimicked by probiotics or prebiotics.

Food has bulk.

What I have been able to easily prove with not just myself, but thousands of people, is that the near miraculous is possible when food is used correctly to re-populate the gut. Keyword - *correctly.* The trick involves, not surprisingly, *what, when and how.* Let me give you the broad strokes to recolonize the gut anytime.

RECOLONIZING THE GUT: THE BLUEPRINT

THE WHAT: Recolonizing the gut.
THE WHEN: Every meal over 7 days.
THE HOW: The right foods, in massive amounts of bulk.

Once again, the keyword is **bulk.** When recolonizing the gut the size and bulk of meals is quite shocking. The reason people don't see spectacular, near miraculous results, from food is they left out the "how." **The trick is bulk.** If the gut is a tube the trick is to stretch the tube! The gut must be *stretched* in 360 degrees of rotation, meal after meal. When food is used in this way, it's like a paint brush. The inside lining of the gut is being coated in Butyrate. Done properly, what is possible is simply amazing. Here is my personal witness to what I have seen over thirteen years. This is what is possible when using food to recolonize the gut.

- Totally knock out cravings in 7 days and rewire them to healthy foods.
- Totally knock out Parkinson symptoms in 7 days.
- Drop massive amounts of fat with no exercise in 7 days.
- Knock out the need for medications completely within months and restore perfect blood work.
- Help people get lean who never before could get lean.
- Drive energy to levels comparable to early 20's.

These things are not theory. They are things I have either done myself or been witness to. Let me end this chapter with a very important question.

Do we need "treatments" when food is so powerful?

I'm all for medicine. In fact there are key medicines with vast power for anti-aging applications. But this current era is one where solutions for the gut biome are in their infancy. There has been a rush to capitalize on probiotics, drugs, and therapies. Most of what I have seen are not necessary. I personally **know,** this to be true. For example, entire categories are devoted to knocking out food cravings. I have first hand knowledge how knocking out cravings is

easily and rapidly doable simply by recolonizing the gut with nothing more than food. I have several medical professionals on video attesting to this exact thing who have done VEEP.

This is not to say there may not be very powerful applications to come from these new ventures. What **must happen,** is for **you** to personally experience the power of food to map Peak Human physiology into your body via rapid recolonization of the gut.

The Gut Exosome Respiratory Connection: There is a direct connection between the health of your gut and the immune status of your lungs. In simplest terms, if you have an unhealthy gut, after lung injury the gut secretes exosomes. These cellular jump drives trigger signals from the Red Team macrophages, that promote further immune dysfunction to the lungs. Here is how this works.

When you have an unhealty gut, meaning the immune status of the cells lining your gut is compromised, exosomes from the gut are secreted into the lymph surrounding the gut. These exosomes reprogram macrophages to further deplete other key types of immune cells the lungs need to heal after injury from things like Covid 19. Thus, the health of your gut, can and does directly play into the health of your lungs, mediated by exosomes.

TO-DO: THE DAISY CUTTER
Massive recolonization overnight.

The Daisy Cutter is both an ultra useful tool for many things and a powerful way to prove to yourself how quickly the gut can be totally recolonized. The Daisy Cutter involves three things.

1. Lots of bulk from cellulose foods like raw green beans
2. Lots of protein
3. Little to no fat.

HOW IT WORKS:

The Daisy Cutter acts like a giant pipe cleaner. It floods all 360 degrees of rotation of the gut with foods that drive butyrate from bifidobacteria.

THE WHAT: The Daisy Cutter
THE WHEN: 1-7 Days straight
THE HOW: See below.

CAUTION: This is not for anyone with existing gut issues.

The protocol is only for individuals with normal digestion. The Daisy Cutter is not fun! It works rapidly but It is the hardest protocol in existence. Do it for one day at first. You can add an extra day or two depending on how you do. The longer you do it the more powerful the results. I did it seven days in 2007 when I did my first gut hack.

STEP ONE: Do a one meal test.
Some people may have issues with the amount of bulk in the Daisy Cutter. You must do a small test to see if this is right for you.

TEST MEAL: 1/4 plate of raw green beans. 5 Egg Whites.
Low fat cheese. Salsa. If you handle this meal with no issues proceed to step 2.

STEP TWO: One full day.

BREAKFAST: w Animal Proteins

8-12 Egg whites. 1/2 to 3/4 dinner plate of raw green beans. Can also add onions, capers, very thin layer of pesto for flavor to eggs.

BREAKFAST: Vegan Version
1/2 to 3/4 dinner plate of raw green beans. Raw asparagus, onions, garbanzo's, small mount of olive oil. No more than teaspoon. Mix in capers, very thin layer of pesto.

LUNCH: w Animal Proteins
Giant spinach or kale salad, with raw broccoli, cauliflower, green beans, bok choi, tomatoes, and small amount of feta cheese. Must have large protein source. Either chicken breasts, tuna or turkey. Use fat free vinaigrette. The key is the sheer meal size. This should fill a giant mixing bowl.

Vegan Version:
Substitute garbanzo beans and/or soy for chicken.

DINNER: Repeat breakfast

This is the basic pattern of the Daisy Cutter. It is both extremely effective and extremely difficult. It is best done initially as a proof of the power of food.

POST DAISY CUTTER:
If you do the Daisy Cutter more than three days, transition into the feasting hack from Chapter 17. It's a fantastic way to stimulate muscle growth.

Chapter 21

Fibers & Butyrate

Blake Beckford was the picture of health. On the outside he was a super fit bodybuilder. His cut abs invited questions like "What is your routine?" and "How can I look like you?" On the inside, however, a very different story was playing out. Blake was extremely unhealthy. His plans for entering his next fitness competition slammed to a halt in 2003, with a diagnosis of ulcerative colitis. Ulcerative colitis is a disease where the gut lining becomes worn down and compromised. Blake found out the hard way how health issues not only put looking good on the back burner, they put life itself on hold. Over a ten year period, Blake found himself in and out of hospitals. Ultimately, he wound up needing a colostomy bag. After a decade of treatment he was eventually able to return to fitness. The colostomy patch next to his cut abs is a reminder that looking fit is not the same thing as true health. A foundation for true health begins in the lining of the gut.

Let's summarize the most important things we need to overcome.

The Healthy Immune Macrophage Mix:
We must flip the Red Team to the health promoting Blue team macrophages. The first place to begin is the gut lining. If this is compromised, it throws the entire immune system off.

How do we fix this problem? The answer is **Butyrate.**

Aging As a Problem of Data Loss:
We learned to unsilence genes that go dormant as we age, a process called HDAC inhibition. Doing this keeps the body young.

How do we begin to fix this problem? **Butyrate**

Pre Amplify Fasting:
We are learning to amplify the benefits of fasting to spend less time fasted, which itself is a major disruptor of sleep.

How do we do this? **Butyrate**

Cancer Prevention:
Some of the highest incidence of cancer types are found in the gut and colon. Reducing risk for these cancers is part of keeping the immune system at peak function and keeping the body young.

How do we fix this? **Butyrate**

Tissue Translocation from the Gut Lining
As you learned in the fat loss paradox, we must seal the gut lining and prevent relocation of the Red Team and toxins from the gut to your fat mass. This is a key piece of The Immunity Code and it helps to prevent onset of inflammaging.

How do we fix this problem? **Butyrate.**

As you can see, getting the body to produce Butyrate solves many of the barriers to peak immune function and is essential to keep the body young. But how do we do this? How do we get the body to make Butyrate? One word.

Fiber.

In today's Era of Imbalance, baby talk saturates the marketplace. Entire schools of thought think fiber is bad. Yet, here are three intractable truths that make fiber essential.

1.The gut mucus lining is **ESSENTIAL** for peak human health.

2.Butyrate is **ESSENTIAL** for a healthy gut lining.

3. Fibers and carbs are **ESSENTIAL** to produce Butyrate in the gut.

Simply put, it looks like this:

Fibers and Carbs => Butyrate => Healthy Gut Mucus Lining

There is no getting around these three points. They are what's really true and therefore *drive everything else.*

FACT: Without Butyrate production the gut is eventually destroyed.

Perhaps you doubt that statement. Perhaps you are skeptical. Perhaps you have no opinion. Wherever you sit, understanding how Butyrate works will align you with what is most important.

WHAT IS BUTYRATE:
Butyrate is a fat, specifically a short chain fatty acid. It is made in the large intestine. It's a byproduct of the metabolism of very specific bacteria. Specialized bacteria in your gut make Butyrate when key fibers are fermented. The bacteria excrete Butyrate. In turn, Butyrate drives production of interleukin 10, the opposing immune signal to interluekin 6. This seals and heals the gut lining and directly feeds

the cells of the colon. It's a perfect marriage. We feed the right fibers to the right bacteria and they confer peak immune health on the host.

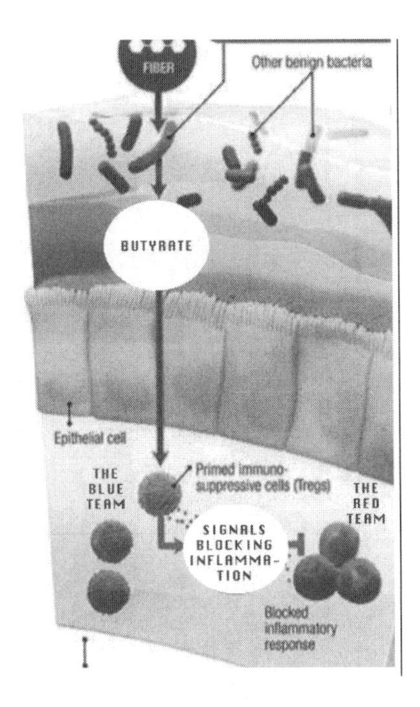

You can see the gut mucous lining. It has two layers. The bottom layer is sterile in a healthy gut. The sterile layer is what separates you from the outside world. The top layer of mucus is colonized by bacteria, principally Akkermansia. You can also see how Butyrate works. Butyrate seals the gut. It spins down immune suppressing signals from things like regulatory T-cells (Tregs). It keeps the outside world, outside. The presence of Butyrate moves key proteins to the outside gut junctions to seal off the gut lining. Butyrate is at the core of the Immunity Code.

BUTYRATE STEERS MACROPHAGES IN THE GUT

Butyrate is **the** mechanism that **"steers"** and directs gut macrophages.

KEY IDEA: Butyrate steers immunity in the gut.

You can see in the image, butyrate steers Macrophages just below the gut lining. Butyrate drives the Blue Team populations. It essentially activates an anti-pathogen "program."

New science papers are loaded with quotes about Butyrate like, "Restoring antimicrobial function via Butyrate in intestinal macrophages may therefore be a **universal mechanism** to prevent or treat IBD." Let me translate that.

KEY IDEA: We can steer macrophages in the gut with Butyrate.

Remember, steering macrophages, and thus immunity itself, is about going tissue by tissue in order of importance. Where is the largest population of macrophages? **In the gut lining.**

Butyrate promotes the Blue Team macrophages via the key signal molecule Interleukin-10 (IL-10). IL-10 steers macrophages toward the Blue Team.

With Butyrate, the Blue Team immune macrophages proliferate in the gut, Blue Team proliferating in the gut lining increases immune function and decreases inflammation across the whole body!

Here is a quick look at some of the things Butyrate does.

- Butyrate stimulates specialized immune cells, called plasma cells, to secrete secratory IgA. This in turn, **limits the growth** of bad bacteria in gut lumen (the lumen is the sloshy aqueous mix in your intestines).

- Clinical studies have shown people with advanced colon cancer all have diminished levels of Butyrate in the colon.

- Butyrate neutralizes cancer promoting micro RNA's packaged into exosomes (The cellular jump drives.)

- Butyrate has been shown to activate genes that protect brain health, a concept called neuroepigenetics, and a perfect example of the three genomes in action. It protects against nearly every known condition, including Alzheimer's, Parkinson's, strokes, autism, Huntington's and others.

- Butyrate regulates key human genes involved in staying young.

- Butyrate activates human genes involved in creating mitochondria, which **mimics the benefits of exercise and fasting** and prolongs lifespan. It enhances oxygen utilization within muscles. By doing so, it can directly effect age related sarcopenia, or loss of muscle.

- Butyrate has been shown to improve learning and memory, especially in the case of dementia, induced by dietary toxins.

- One of the ways you get cancer is signal proteins. They get stuck in the "on" position. One example is a signal pathway controlling cell cycle growth. This pathway, called MAPK, is deactivated by Butyrate. Thus, in colon cancer, **Butyrate directly kills cancer cells** by telling them to switch off growth.

- Butyrate lowers colon Ph and turns up disposal of cellular junk into the trash bin. At the same time, it turns down inflammation.

- Butyrate activates AMPK in the cells of your gut lining by blocking an AMPK inhibitor called Compound C.

WHY Butyrate MATTERS SO MUCH:
Butyrate is so all important for one reason.

Immunity.

Your gut lining is an *interface.* It's where you end. It's where the outside world begins. It's also where immunity begins. The gut lining has to let certain things in while keeping other things out. Food is one thing, bacteria is another. You have trillions of bacteria in the gut. The gut lining must keep the harmful ones out while allowing the beneficial ones to proliferate. Butyrate is what makes all of this possible. It is the rudder steering the ship of the gut. Via an ultra-complex network of sensing and signals, Butyrate mediates the molecules, like Interleukin 10, that keep the gate of the gut shut. Only that which the body needs gets in. Without Butyrate, the gut lining can not do its job. Invaders, like LPS and bad bacteria, can enter the body.

IMMUNE CELL METABOLISM OF THE GUT
In Chapter 14 your learned about ImmunoMetabolism, the idea of how immunity effects metabolism. Conceptually, the idea of taking into account how immunity effects metabolism brings us into entirely new territory. We must now also consider the metabolism of immune cells. Metabolism itself, must expand it ways not previously considered. New research has uncovered how the metabolism of immune cells effects every aspect of your health, aging, and immunity. In the old way of thinking, metabolism is just this idea of how many calories you take in. This view is simply outdated once

we begin to consider the metabolism of immune cells within the gut. Here is why.

KEY IDEA: The metabolism within immune cells drives every aspect of health and aging.

HOW LPS DRIVES IMMUNE CELL METABOLISM:
Immune cells like macrophages are still cells. They have a metabolism. They need to make energy. How they make their energy, it turns out, is a vital mechanism controlling immunity and health across the whole body.

When the gut is penetrated by invaders like LPS, a key shift takes place in the metabolism of immune cell macrophages in the gut lining. In simplest terms, a profound shift takes place in how energy is made. A key metabolite, citrate, begins to accumulate inside these key immune cells. Accumulating citrate drives a number of things, most importantly

- Inflammation.
- Fat storage
- Immune signals

Accumulating citrate within macrophages activates a master molecule, **Itaconate.** This master molecule acts like the brake on a runaway train. It works to slam the brakes on what would otherwise be a signal storm of inflammatory signals acting across the whole body. As the metabolism within the Blue Team macrophages shifts, entire populations of macrophages change. The Blue Team joins the Red Team! As the Red Team grows, your health and immunity goes down.

As you can see, macrophages matter in massive ways. Learning the proper order of operations, i.e., the owners manual for your body, can no longer be thought of apart from how immune cells function. This effects every piece of the equation, from optimal diet, to how you correct things when they go wrong. To understand better, lets employ a simple analogy.

SALAMI AS WOUND DRESSING IS REALLY BAD IDEA
What do you think would happen if a 2x2 inch patch of your skin was removed and the exposed flesh was covered with salami? Not a good idea right? With this analogy you can easily understand when the gut lining is worn down. Your inner body is protected from the outside world by only a 1 millimeter thick layer of mucous. If that layer is compromised, it's like putting salami on your exposed dermis

every time you eat. This crude but accurate analogy illustrates the main point.

Immunity.

Immunity in the gut requires butyrate. Butyrate is the mechanistic driver of immunity in the gut. So why not just supplement for it?

ONLY REAL FOOD GIVES THE PROPER DOSE

Not surprisingly, the dosing of Butyrate matters. The doses of Butyrate from *natural whole food fiber sources* are the sweet spot for the immunity boosting and anti-cancer effects of Butyrate. New research shows when we hyper concentrate Butyrate doses to over 10 times what you food yields, the opposite happens. Even Butyrate can be bad when imbalanced.

KEY IDEA: You **never** want to *supplement* with Butyrate.

At 10 times the dose of real food, cancer cells develop a resistance to Butyrate.

So Butyrate feeds the cells in the gut, it makes them healthy. The result is the tight junctions of the gut seal up. It also feeds the bacteria, principally Akkermansia, that keep the gut mucus layer healthy. The result is the gut makes the specific mucins that control immune responses in the gut.

Hopefully you now understand why sealing the gut mucus layer **is first in the order of operations.** Butyrate production is how you do this. The internet is awash in protocols for your gut. Not a single one has the correct order of operations. Certain things come first. This is called **Luminal Nutrition.**

KEY IDEA: Luminal nutrition refers to feeding the cells lining the gut before you feed anything else.

Luminal nutrition represents the order of operations; feeding the cells of the gut first so they can feed the body and the immune system can work at peak function. It's more than a catchy idea. As you have seen, it's essential. These cells need Butyrate. Here is the Luminal Nutrition formula for overall health and the first order of operations for gut health.

Fiber=>Butyrate=>Gut Lining Cell Health=>Inflammation Inhibition

FIBER IS JUST A WORD. THE REALITY IS FAR MORE

Fiber is just a word. It's a catch all category term. Under the umbrella of "fiber" are literally dozens of unique substances. Each has very specific actions and effects on the body. There are arabinoxylans, inulins, pectins, bran, cellulose, β-glucans, resistant starches, and many others.

FACT: Unique fibers exert unique effects on the body.

The Fantastic 5 Reasons Fiber Works
Despite the many different unique substances under the umbrella of "fiber", they all exert benefits in primarily three ways.

REASON 1: First, fibers resist digestion and drive fermentation. Again, you make **30 grams of bacteria** for every 100 grams of fiber fermented. Fermentation from fiber is how you produce the bacteria you need to achieve peak immune function.

REASON 2: Fibers add bulk and viscosity. Bulk and viscosity reduce the ability of carcinogens to make contact with the cells that line your gut.

REASON 3: Fibers bind cancer causing compounds and bile acids. In effect, they act like detergent for the gut. Bile acids themselves can drive cancer if you imbalance them in the gut. This is very different from how proteins or fats effect the gut.

Proteins and fats drive toxic compounds in the gut.

Like fiber, protein can also ferment in the gut. The difference is protein fermentation produces super toxic byproducts. These byproducts, called adducts, damage DNA. Fats require bile acids. Excess and imbalanced bile acids drive cancer. Fiber is unique in its detergent like effects on the gut.

REASON 4: Fibers yield anti-oxidants that protect the inflamed gut from oxidative stress overload.

REASON 5: Key fibers increase genes involved in many diverse health promoting areas, like carb metabolism, vitamin and enzyme production.

Why does the simple solution, which is just to stay healthy elude the vast majority? More truth. We are not dealing with what is really true about how the gut works. Fiber is essential. And when it comes to fiber, we have been doing baby talk. We need fiber, but we need it in the language of what, when and how. Real truth is real power.

AMINO ACIDS - THE OTHER HALF TO THE EQUATION

"Meat heals" is a catchphrase of the Carnivore and meat eating community. Carnivore advocates swear to the ameliorating nature of meat to sooth and heal gut issues. Ironically, there is a lot of truth to this. The purpose here is to ground you in how things actually work, i.e, the mechanisms. Until we understand the mechanisms at work we are just engaging in fables and narrative. We have spent quite a bit of time on the mechanistic essentiality of butyrate. There is another half to the equation. Collectively, both halves of the equation will form the whole. That whole is defined by the highest truth of the body - balance is essential.

There is good reason for the need for balance in the gut. Returning to **Luminal Nutrition,** we must feed the cells of the gut first in order for the body as a whole to enjoy maximum immunity, energy and health. There are a couple of simple ideas that help you to easily understand the need for balance. The first idea is the intestines vs the colon. Simply put, the cells of the colon are fed by fiber. The cells of the intestines, however, are fed by amino acids. The gut needs *both.*

KEY IDEA: Fiber feeds the colon. Amino's feed the intestines.

Another key idea is innate immunity vs acquired immunity. In the gut, innate immunity means keeping things out. Acquired immunity means letting things in - selectively. We have seen how butyrate is the master controlling mechanism over the gut junctions which keeps things like bacteria from getting in the body. Acquired immunity requires selectively letting things in to sample them, make anti-bodies, and release those anti-bodies back into circulation. An easy way to understand the need for balance in the diet is to understand that innate immunity in the gut requires fiber, but acquired immunity in the gut requires aminos. **You need both.**

KEY IDEA: Fiber feeds innate immunity. Aminos feed acquired immunity.

Are you beginning to see there are two halves to a whole here? Lets look at how selective amino's feed acquired immunity and many other things.

HOW AMINO ACIDS DRIVE IMMUNITY AND HEALTH IN THE GUT

Gut health, and therefore, immunity in the gut, rely to a great degree on specific amino acids. Amino acids act as control checkpoints over essential growth and healing signal pathways in the gut, like AMPK, MAPK and mTor. They also perform critical functions like driving acquired immunity. Here are just a few of the things amino acids do in the gut.

GLUTAMINE:

Glutamine is the primary fuel of the cells that line the small intestine - the enterocytes. Without abundant glutamine, those cells begin to metabolize other fuel sources, usually sugars. When this happens, the gut can become compromised.

Glutamine is also *essential* for immunity. The bodies first line of defense for acquired immunity is Secretory Immunoglobulin, or Secretory IGA. It's the anti-body system that does the initial heavy lifting to null pathogens, viruses and invaders. Glutamine in the diet drives bacteria in the gut to relocate. They move from the sloshy liquid, the lumen, and into gut mucus layer. From there, specialized cells grab antigens, pull them into the lamina propia where macrophages and other immune cells essentially contain them, mature, and then present that specific antigen to T-cells, which mediate production of specific Secratory IGA anti-bodies for that antigen. Voila, immunity for that antigen has been acquired. This is why Glutamine supplementation has been shown to increase Secretory IGA in the gut.

TRYPTOPHAN:

Tryptophan is essential for gut mucus layer defense via the production of key metabolites called indoles. Indoles effect the production of mucins in the gut mucus layer, They are essential for homeostasis of the mucus lining. Tryptophan is also essential for the production of 5HTP to make serotonin, most of which is made in the gut lining via tryptophan activating 5HTP. Experiments have shown that supplementing with tryptophan can ameliorate colitis and other gut inflammatory issues.

METHIONINE:

Methionine is generally considered a growth amino acid. It goes hand it hand with cellular growth as it acts as the word "stop" when assembling amino acids into proteins. In the gut, methionine works to drive the production of glutathione. This lowers oxidative stress in the gut lining. Methionine and its precursors play an important role in maintaining the gut lining. It's important to understand that *growth* is essential for immunity. Growth means the activation of key signal pathways like mTor, and key families of proteins that are essential for the production of Secretory IGA.

ARGININE:
Arginine seems to play two very important roles in the gut lining. Research suggests it helps maintain the gut junctions and integrity of the gut lining, and it also seems to play a powerful role when combined with glutamine in resolving inflammation in the gut. Arginine seems to complement glutamine in the production of Secretory IGA and also helps moderate inflammatory signals in the gut.

GLYCINE:
Glycine seems to exert a number of benefits driving health and balance in the gut. First, glycine inhibits the progression of colon cancer. It also seems to regulate a key gut junction protein that helps seal and heal the gut. Research has shown glycine helps ameliorate colitis. Glycine has a profound effect facilitating key enzymes and signal molecules that resolve inflammation in the gut.

LYSINE:
Lysine plays a very important role with oxidative stress in the gut lining. It drives up the bodies three primary anti-oxidants, glutathione, catalase and Super oxide dismutase, which helps keep viruses and infection from taking hold in the body via the gut.

I could do an entire book just on the functions of amino's in the gut. Unfortunately in a 375 page book with a scope this massive, I needed to devote a lot of space to fiber and butyrate. If you want more on the amino side of the equation, check out my Immunity Crash Course. Even with these few examples, you can readily see how amino's play a very powerful role in gut immunity and integrity.

Now here is the really important question. Where do we most readily find these amino's? The answer? Animal foods! On average, animal foods like meats will have 2x to 3x the amounts of the critical amino acids the gut needs to be healthy. Take Glutamine for example. A recent study showed meat tends to have twice the amount of glutamine per 100 grams of any plant food. Twice the amount of glutamine means more Secretory IGA in the gut which means stronger immunity!

But now consider something. What happens if you get too much meat? One effect of too much meat can be the colon gets excessively alkalized. You might think that's good. Alkalinity is good and acidity is bad right? More baby talk! Experiments have shown that excessive meat intake can push the colon PH above 7. When that happens, cancer promoting DNA adducts form from the excessive alkylation. Excessive alkylation in the colon can be a cancer promoter, and it can be driven by an "acidic" food, i.e., meat! How do you solve this? Those same experiments have shown that the addition of fiber pushed the PH in the colon back down below 7 and the alkylated adducts do not form!

SUMMING IT ALL UP

You have seen how both fibers and aminos play a critical role in immunity and health of the gut. I didn't give you ancestral narratives. We looked at mechanisms. The mechanisms tell us how things actually work. We can sum all of this up in a single word.

Balance.

Immunity in the gut is maximized by a balance of both animal and plant foods. The mechanisms supporting immunity require both.

GUT SOS PROTOCOL

Supplementation with key amino's has been shown to exert very beneficial effects on a number of scenarios where the gut lining is inflamed. The following is a simple protocol you can do any time to help restore and heal the inflamed gut.

THE WHAT: Glutamine, Arginine, Tryptophan, Glycine

THE WHEN:7 days straight at bedtime

THE HOW: Use 500mg of Tryptophan, and between 1 to 2 grams of the other three amino's. An easy way to get in the glycine is no cal jello.

The combination of these amino's may be vastly restorative and soothing in scenarios where inflammation of the gut has manifested into complications.

TO-DO: BUTYRATE PRODUCTION 101

So how do we get the body to make Butyrate?

Fibers and starches. Pure and simple.

This is how things work. We can't make up become down. We can't make clothing from coal. Butyrate gives us a mechanistic drive to substantiate the absolute necessity of fibers and starches.

THE WHAT: Butyrate Production
THE WHEN: The day before the Amplified Fast
THE HOW: Using the modules from day one of The Amplified Fast.

Chapter 22

The New Science of Meal Sequencing

THE BIG PROMISE

We have been building up to a major breakaway in thought and action from everything you know. You are now there, at the point of breakaway.

We are in a new age. Long cycles being at home with long cycles of moving in social circles of work, play and exercise must now co-exist. A new age mandates a new approach. You need a new set of skills. You need skills that were unthinkable just a short while ago.

I want to make you a big promise upfront. Here is what you stand to gain if you will commit to mastering the ideas and techniques for eating I am about to give you.

- You will be healthier. You will age better. You will attain Peak immune health. Learning the 2 Day Immunity Core Pattern, The Amplified Fast, together with the techniques for meal sequencing and offsetting, will allow you to be healthier than ever before.

- You will have real freedom. You will break away from lists. You will be free of avoiding all kinds of foods. You will be free to celebrate life with food. You will be able to offset overeating from long periods at home.

- You will break weight cycling. You will get out of the cycle of "off track/on track". You will break the cycle of unknowingly mimicking famine and feast. You will break out of unwittingly triggering survival mechanisms initiated by the mechanobiology of shrinking fat cells. You will have real power to control your weight.

Healthier. More freedom. Break the cycle. Sounds like a big promise now. Once you get the hang of it, you will see everything you have been doing was baby talk for the body. It was never even based on how your body really works or what people really do. This is.

Learning how to eat is the first power. This chapter will give you the foundation. It's going to free you instead of constrain you. What you will learn is based on working with natural daily and weekly rhythms.

New science papers are using the words **Circadian Nutrition.** For over ten years users of my VEEP system have learned how to use the body's natural daily and weekly rhythms to free themselves from slavery to lists and the paradigm of avoidance. It's the power to eat

Ad Lib while being able to maintain body weight. Here is an overview of how it works.

THE NATURAL DAILY CYCLE

Many times a day your body both stores fat and burns fat. After all, the primary purpose of body fat is to keep you alive between meals.

KEY IDEA: You store fat and burn fat multiple times a day.

In my seminars there is a fun exercise I like to do. I ask participants to think about their day and the process of storing or burning fat. Let's do this now. Fill in the following blanks. Write down your guess for each.

Upon waking in the am - storing or burning fat? ______________

After lunch - storing or burning fat? ________________

It's 5pm and you have not eaten since noon - storing or burning fat? ____________

After dinner -storing or burning fat? ________________

During sleep at 3 am - storing or burning fat?________

You probably filled in a couple of answers with "burning fat" and a few with "storing fat".

The daily rhythm of storing and burning fat can vary dramatically within a single day based on several factors. Upon waking, the body is secreting the hormone glucagon. Glucagon works to raise blood sugar. It also helps to burn fat. After lunch, it's normal to store a bit of fat. Peak hunger is around 6 to 7pm in the daily cycle. Experiencing hunger and burning stored fat for energy often go together. Late afternoon, if you have not eaten for several hours, you may start to burn a bit of fat. After dinner it's normal to store fat. During sleep it's normal to burn a bit of fat.

THE MAIN THING:
What if you could learn to work with this natural daily rhythm? What if you could make it work **for** you? This means two things.

1. Amplify the periods where you burn fat.
2. Minimize the periods where you store fat.

In other words, what if you could make slight improvements in the way your body metabolizes each meal. These improvements in each meal are not a panacea, but over time the cumulative effect mitigates a lot of weight gain. The key is amplifying fat burning and minimizing fat storage wherever they both naturally occur in a given day.

Returning to the Graph of Doom, the goal is to nearly eliminate or drastically reduce the peaks of weight gain when time resources go to zero. We may not 100 percent eliminate all the weight gain from these cycles. There will always be seasons where we focus more time and energy on being in shape. But with the techniques you learn here, we can eliminate the long term upward slope of The Graph of Doom.

Let's begin by understanding the main idea - **you are never really eating a single meal.**

THE SCIENCE OF SEQUENCING

What you eat now will exert a lot of influence over what you eat next. It's easy to prove. Just eat a giant hamburger with fries and a shake right now. At your next meal, what you desire to eat, even how much you eat, will be determined by the hamburger meal. Over the last decade new science has confirmed what everyone already knew. What you eat currently, has a lot to do with you ate previously. The new science of **meal to meal sequencing** has unveiled the amazing impact one meal has on the next. Hunger, metabolism, total food intake, and even gene activation at a given meal, can be influenced by a previous meal. Here are some examples.

- If you have an egg, you will eat less at your next meal and eat less the next day. This is due to suppression of the hunger hormone ghrelin.

- If you have garbanzo beans at lunch, insulin function will be sensitized the rest of the day. After dinner, blood sugar will not go as high. You will also store less fat from dinner.

- A higher protein meal at breakfast will reduce hunger and snacking at dinner.

- Resistant starches and non-digestible carbohydrates, like barley at night, will decrease total food intake the entire following day, via elevating the insulin sensitizing hormone GLP-1.

- Unmilled grains at breakfast, like raw to lightly cooked steel cut oatmeal, will lower your blood sugar levels after lunch.

- Whey protein before a carb meal, slows stomach emptying, and lowers blood sugar after the carb meal.

- Having vegetables or protein, 30 minutes prior to starchy carbs, will lower blood glucose significantly, more than just eating starchy carbs alone.

- Rye bread at night will elevate levels of the fullness hormone PYY in your blood the next morning. This leads to decreased food intake at breakfast. If you have rye at lunch you will have reduced meal intake at dinner.

It's exciting to think. You can learn to subdue the biochemical drivers of weight gain with meal sequencing. Let's look at an example.

EASY HOLIDAY MEAL HACK:
Overeating on Holidays like Christmas and Thanksgiving is common.

1. The day before the holiday, have an egg at breakfast.
2. Next have barley cereal that night.
3. On the day of the holiday, have a protein shake at breakfast. These three, simple adjustments, help you to eat less on big holidays. They also help insulin work better so you store less fat.

I am sure this sounds both exciting and daunting. How can you remember all this? Don't worry. I am going to make this super simple.

EATING IN GROUPS OF THREE

What you are about to learn will change your life. It is the single most powerful concept you will ever learn about eating. It is based on how your body really works. It's also based on how humans really eat. Combined with the 2 Day Immunity Core Pattern, it will enable you to offset *eating whatever.* Let's first go over the basic concepts.

KEY IDEA: You are never really eating a single meal.

Every meal introduces a series of signals to your body. These signals play out across a number of domains.

- Fullness and stomach distention, or lack of.

- Gene activation from food.
- Alterations to the gut bacteria.
- Food pleasure signals.
- Stomach emptying and insulin sensitivity.

Signals from each item above fluctuate with every meal. They will effect the next meal you eat. An easy way to grasp the concept is how eating a big meal will effect the desire to have desert. From this simple example you can understand how the previous meal impacts the next meal. The sequence of what you eat, when you eat, and how, will determine the next meal you eat.

QUICK FAT HACK: Eat one whole avocado and one whole cucumber for your next meal.

Wait two or three hours. Watch what happens at your next meal. It is very likely you will *over eat.* The reason, however, is not for lack of calories. There are plenty of calories in an avocado. It's the way avocados drop insulin secretion via the super sugar manoheptulose. The drop in insulin will drive more food intake at your next meal. This quick hack illustrates a powerful truth. **The next meal is always the product of the previous meal.**

KEY IDEA: The previous meal and the next meal determine your current meal.

The biology of eating works across meal sequences. You are always eating meals in a sequence of three. This is **why meal plans don't work over time.** When you deviate from the plan, the deviation steers and influences the next meal.

What I am speaking to is empirically validated. Hunger, fat metabolism, total food intake, and many other parameters of your next meal are programmed by your current meal. Let's summarize a few concepts we have learned so far.

- Ad Libitum eating can not be avoided over time.

- We store and burn fat multiple times a day.

- Each meal dynamically programs the next. Total food intake, metabolism, insulin function and many other factors at your next meal are "programmed in" at your current meal.

- By controlling meal to meal sequencing you can increase fat burning and decrease fat storage.

Here is an entire meal sequence. Let's break down the mechanics of how each meal influences the next.

OFFSET MEAL SEQUENCE:

BREAKFAST: Egg white omelette =>
LUNCH: Hamburger and fries =>
DINNER: Whey protein shake.

Quite the combination right? Lets see how this works to offset weight gain and amplify fat loss. Your assignment will be to go do it!

FIRST MEAL: Egg white omelette
Six egg whites, chopped onions, hot sauce, mushrooms, a very small amount of cheese, asparagus, and cayenne pepper.

Everything in this meal aids metabolic function. Cayenne pepper and hot sauce increase metabolism. Cheese aids fat oxidation by increasing serum calcium. Onions are loaded with forms of sulfur that lower blood glucose. Egg whites promote fat to burn by stimulate the hormone glucagon. One of the great things about this specific meal is it is very doable on the road at many restaurants. Note: Add onions last and cook minimally. We want them as raw as possible.

This meal serves a basic purpose. It magnifies a period of fat burning. If you wait three to four hours for the next meal, this meal is fantastic at getting the body to burn fat.

CURRENT MEAL: Hamburger and fries
This meal is loaded with calories. You *will* store fat. We are, however, amplifying fat burning before and after this meal. The weight gain will be offset. Instead of worrying about weight gain just **have at it.** Enjoy! It is possible to do a lot to offset this meal as well. We cover the mechanics of offsetting next chapter. For now, here are some very basic hacks to offset weight gain:

- Use mustard and onions but no catsup.
- Have 300mg of Alpha Lipoid Acid twenty minutes prior to this meal. It will help mitigate blood sugar from spiking.
- Let your fries cool down.

Alone, each of these things has a very small impact. Together they effect a slight offset of weight gain. They are additive. The meal sequencing alone will do most of the heavy lifting to offset weight gain.

NEXT MEAL: Whey protein shake with cinnamon and olive oil.

The shake for dinner helps you burn a lot of fat while you sleep. Vegans can sub pea protein or a plant protein. Add olive oil and cinnamon. If you have the shake for breakfast, add crushed ice, which also helps metabolically. Don't add crushed ice at dinner. It could keep you up. Liquid meal replacements have a dark side. If used frequently, they deprive entire hormonal domains, things like fullness, satiety, and stomach distention. Relying on liquid meal replacements long term for weight loss actually drives over eating. Used strategically, however, they can be fantastic tools to offset weight gain.

THE FOUNDATION

- All three meals constitute a single meal.
- Previous meal and subsequent meal offset weight gain of current meal.
- Amplify the fat burning periods and minimize weight gain periods.
- Weight **can be maintained without time intensive workouts or strict dieting.**

TO DO: OFFSET 101

OFFSET HUGE SUNDAY BREAKFAST WITH MEAL SEQUENCING

Elsewhere in the book we hack fat loss by targeting the hormone leptin with huge meals. This to-do is a companion of the fat loss hack. Think of it as hacking the fat loss leptin hack.

KEY IDEA: Use meal sequencing to offset weight gain.

If we want to keep fat off, there is a lot to be done before losing it. The good news is the to-do's are non-time intensive and easy. Before this book was published, I spent several years perfecting the techniques in my seminars and software program.

THE WHAT: Offset huge breakfast
THE WHEN: Sundays
THE HOW: See below

PRIOR MEAL:

1. Whey protein shake w cinnamon and olive oil
2. Add crushed ice and blend.
3. Have 30 minutes prior to weight gain meal.
4. Have 500-1000mg of Berberine

WEIGHT GAIN MEAL:

1.Pancakes, butter, syrup,
2.Have a single egg with pancakes. Slows digestion.
3. Add blueberries.

NEXT MEAL:

1. Hearty vegetable soup. Pho is a good example.

HOW IT WORKS:

You will feel super full from the combination of pancakes and soup at the next meal. Blueberries help increase fat oxidation with high carb meals. Now wait four to five hours. Eat a normal dinner. You can also go super aggressive for fat loss at dinner. You could either do a shake or a daisy cutter meal for aggressive fat loss at dinner.

This to-do combines several techniques presented so far into a sequence.

Chapter 23

The Science Behind Offsetting

OFFSETTING: THE FOUNDATIONAL MOVE

Instead of trying to eliminate ad libitum eating and major groupings of foods, due to fear of weight gain, we have a new way of doing things - ***offsetting.*** The ability to offset food intake isn't just a cool idea. The new reality of seasonal periods at home makes it a real necessity. It's not enough to try and avoid foods. You need a way to offset them.

THE TOOLSETS FOR OFFSETTING

There are six basic ways you can offset weight gain from a meal.

All of these methods effect **net calories.** You can use each of the following six methods alone, or in combination with meal sequences, to dramatically affect the current meal you want to offset. Once more, this is serious science applied in easy to do methods. Some of it may contradict things you have done for years. You may find your self *adding calories* to offset weight gain. Once you understand the mechanisms it will all make sense.

None of these methods by themselves are a panacea. Each of them gives you **a small incremental advantage.**

KEY IDEA: We are using the same pattern of obesity in reverse.

Obesity, or weight gain, is the result of small, positive increases in net calories (energy harvest) from meal to meal.) Meal to meal increases of net calories accrue over a long period of time. The result is obesity and long term weight gain.

What if you did the same thing, but in reverse?

The following methods simply reverse what happens in obesity. These are skills. The skills you gain will help prevent those small, positive energy balances, from accumulating meal to meal. When the six methods are used together, they effect a small difference, that makes a large difference over the long term. Let's start with the rate at which food empties from your stomach.

OFFSET METHOD 1: GASTRIC EMPTYING DELAY:

Normally, the stomach empties at a rate of between one to four calories per minute. This means a four hundred calorie meal takes between an hour and a half to six and a half hours for the contents to empty from your stomach. The rate food empties from your stomach drastically impacts when you should eat next and what you should eat. It also impacts the rate which blood sugar rises after a meal. Thirty to thirty-five percent of the blood sugar response after a meal is **due to the rate of gastric emptying.** Simply by slowing gastric emptying we lower the rate at which your blood sugar rises.

KEY IDEA: Slow gastric emptying = slower rise in blood sugar = less weight gain.

The speed food empties from your stomach has a massive influence on the likelihood of weight gain.

KEY IDEA: One of the simplest ways to slow gastric emptying is with small amounts of fat.

Small Fat Pulses with Carbs:
Adding a small amount of fat when you have carbs or sugars slows gastric emptying. This helps offset weight gain. It also slows how fast blood sugar increases and partially offsets the likelihood of storing fat. One example we have already covered is adding a teaspoon of olive oil to a whey protein shake prior to a carbohydrate meal.

OFFSET HACK: Small fat pulse with carb meals.
THE WHAT: Teaspoon of fat
THE WHEN: With carbs
THE HOW: Amounts of fat must be small.

For example, a small amount of butter with a baked potato is better than the baked potato by itself. Fat from butter delays gastric emptying. The effect depends on the amount of fat. If you add too much fat together with carbs its counterproductive. A way to improve upon this strategy is to introduce the element of timing (when). Lets expand upon the idea of preload meals.

PRELOAD MEALS
A preload meal is a small meal prior to a larger meal. There are several types of preload meals. Once you learn how and when to use them, preload meals yield real power to control weight gain, hunger, and even fat burning. Some examples of preload meals:

- 1/4 avocado.
- A cheese stick.
- Walnuts.
- An egg.

Lets examine each of these examples.

Whey protein has been shown to produce a significant reduction in post meal blood sugar when used as a preload. Here are some others.

Walnuts: Walnuts thirty minutes prior to a meal will increase the hormone adiponectin. Adiponectin makes insulin work more efficiently. The fat from walnuts thirty minutes prior to a carb meal will also help slow gastric emptying. Because walnuts effect adiponectin, they tend to induce hunger. For this reason, use walnuts prior to a satiating carb meal. One example is pasta.

Avocado: Avocado twenty to thirty minutes prior to a meal will not only slow digestive emptying, but also help insulin function, via the sugar manoheptulose. Manoheptulose aids blood sugar function. I first wrote about this over thirteen years ago. It's a concept that has been widely adopted. Avocado is very effective as a preload. Have one quarter of a small avocado prior to high carb meals.

Cheese stick: In the Three Genomes you learned how dairy gets the blame for what is really a problem of missing bacteria. As a functional fat loss tool, dairy has many unique properties *not replicated in any other food.* For example, dairy inhibits the ACE enzyme. You need this enzyme to store fat. The ACE enzyme indirectly acts on receptors of fat cells, telling them to take fat in and store it. The ACE enzyme is also involved with immunity. High expression of the ACE enzyme can drive viral infection to things like SARS CoV 2. Dairy as a preload, prior to sugars or carbs, helps slow gastric emptying and helps inhibit the ACE enzyme.

An Egg: An egg as a preload will stimulate two key hormones. These hormones create what is called "The Incretin Effect." The Incretin Effect is an enhancement of insulin via two key hormones, GIP and GLP-1. Among other things, these two hormones help delay gastric emptying. An egg thirty minutes prior to carbs will help you eat far less. It also yields a nice delay in the rise of blood sugar. I like to do this with the addition of hot sauce to aid thermogenic action. It's easy to do on the go as well.

I know there is a lot of conflicting information about eggs. Let me sum it all up for you. I have read virtually every study ever published on eggs. Some experts like to quote old data. Summarizing the new and old research, eggs have a lot of nutritional benefit. About thirty percent of the population have genetic SNIPS that make them hyper responders to cholesterol. The other seventy percent of the population are not affected by this and eggs in the diet are not the boogeyman some would like them to be. If you are a hyper responder to cholesterol, and you would require testing to know, then eat fewer eggs or avoid them. As with any food, there are grades of quality. Organic pasture raised eggs from chickens that roam freely on grass are ideal. Chickens are not vegan. They eat anything they can catch.

OFFSET METHOD 2: SUBSTRATE TARGETING

Chapter 7 taught you how feeding specific bacteria can lower the energy harvested from food. We can take this a step farther. The way we combine foods together can further lower **energy harvest**. Let's begin with how to feed bacteria to help offset weight gain at a meal.

Substrate Targeting

The *speed* at which bacteria proliferate create an ideal mechanism to offset future meals. You can lower energy harvest at a future meal by targeting specific bacteria at your present meal.

KEY IDEA : Gut communities are rapidly effected by meal to meal sequencing.

Anyone who has ever experienced salmonella poisoning knows how quickly bacteria in your gut proliferate. Bacteria from a single meal work very fast. Bacteria from your current meal can make you sick within hours. The same is true in reverse. Shifts in bacteria from your current meal can improve metabolism or even influence weight gain at your next meal. Gut bacteria dictate net calories. You can literally increase or decrease the amount of calories you absorb meal to meal. This is precisely one mechanism driving obesity. With obesity, bacteria which harvest more energy from food are proliferating meal to meal. Our goal is to do the same in reverse. Here is the basic pattern.

THE BASIC PATTERN

Bacteria Targeted Offset Meal=> Indulgent Meal => Bacteria Targeted Offset Meal

Here is an example.

Lunch: Gut Fermentation 101 from Chapter 7.
Dinner: Mac and cheese.
Breakfast: Grapefruit and semi green banana

This is meal to meal substrate targeting. Each meal is substrate for bacteria. Lunch lowers net calories at dinner. Dinner recolonizes the gut toward weight gain. Breakfast steers the gut back toward lower energy harvest and lower net calories.

OFFSET METHOD 3: ENZYME IMPAIRMENT AND GLYCEMIC CONTROL

Another offset hack is to impair the enzymes required to metabolize sugars and fats. This is a valid and measurable outcome. It has been shown in a number of experiments using foods loaded with key phenol compounds. We have been doing it in my VEEP System since 2009. The big idea is this - ***colors block enzymes.***
Experiments have shown that by *adding calories* to a meal high in sugars, with things like strawberries or raspberries, for example, you actually store less fat than just eating sugars alone.

Color pigments in foods are classified as phenols. From there, we get into very big worlds to describe what are essentially colors. Anthocyanins inhibit the enzyme alpha-glucosidase. Ellagitannins impair the enzyme alpha amylase. One of the ways we can offset weight gain is via the strategic use of foods with these color pigments. Here is an easy meme. Think of fat as yellow.

KEY IDEA: Red blocks yellow.

The same is true for blue, purple and black. The colors in these pigments impair carb enzymes.

Another example is cocoa. Cocoa partially impairs key enzymes needed to digest carbs and fats, most notably the two key fat digesting phospholipase enzymes. The key word here is *partially.* There is no panacea. All of these things give you an incremental improvement. Our goal is a series of incremental improvements. Each small improvement lowers the curve of weight gain and increases fat burning. Combining several of these techniques together is powerful.

By using phenols before, after, or during a meal, you can help offset weight gain. I do it all the time when I need to offset eating whatever. Phenols can be used in a number of forms. All of these things give you an incremental edge in offsetting weight gain. Some examples:

1. Whole berries.
2. Phenol powders like cocoa powder, and red fruit powder.
3. Green tea.

OFFSET METHOD 4: GLUCOSE AND FRUCTOSE DISPOSAL

Through various techniques we can aid the body in disposing of fructose and glucose when we take in too much.

Fruit with Carbs to Offset Glucose

Natural fructose, the kind you find in real fruit, helps to facilitate carb metabolism. Fructose contained in fruit is bound to a natural matrix of fibers, phenols, and other nutrient factors. Have small amounts of fructose from fruit when you have sugar. This helps sugar to not get stored as fat.

KEY IDEA: Fruit with sugar helps offset sugar.

Fructose helps carbs (glucose) to get stored in the liver. Storing carbs in the liver helps carbs to be used for energy instead of stored as fat. The trick is entirely in how you combine the two. Let's look at some examples using the Language of Real Health. I will build on each example, in a good, better, best scenario. Also, notice in each case, we add calories. This is contrary to the old thinking that adding calories is always bad. Quite the opposite, by adding key signals from specific foods, we can redirect metabolic pathways.

FRUIT AND PHENOLS TO REDIRECT METABOLIC PATHWAYS

1.Berries
2.Nopales
3.Cocoa

HACK: OFFSET DONUTS

THE WHAT:1/2 banana or handful of raspberries.
THE WHEN: When you have a donut.
THE HOW: With a few nuts.

HACK: OFFSET CHOCOLATE CAKE

The What: Handful of strawberries.
The When: Thirty minutes prior to chocolate cake.
The How: With a cup coffee, blended with a teaspoon cocoa powder, or cocoa powder sprinkle on the cake.

Glucose and Fructose Disposal Agents.

Perhaps the best known practice of offsetting is via disposal of glucose. A number of agents mimic the action of insulin. In fitness and bodybuilding circles this aspect of offsetting has been around for a long time. Perhaps the bang for the buck winner is the anti-oxidant Alpha Lipoid Acid. Alpha lipoic acid has been shown to mimic the action of insulin. It is particularly effective against fructose. I don't mean fruit. I mean processed foods that contain processed fructose.

GLUCOSE DISPOSAL AGENTS

1. Alpha Lipoic Acid
2. Cinnamon
3. Quercetin
4. Reds powder
5. Berberine

On this list, Berberine is by far the most powerful, but you don't want to use it on a regular basis. Save it for super indulgent meals.

OFFSET METHOD 5: PASS FATS UNDIGESTED AND INCREASE FAT OXIDATION

A very simple and powerful way to offset net calories is by impairing digestion in the gut. Fat digestion varies between individuals. There are several mechanisms involved. These are things like bile acid secretion, fiber content with fat, and the mechanical properties of the foods ingested. One of the simplest techniques is the use of collagen foods at night. The Visceral Fat Hack from Chapter 14 can be repurposed here to help fat oxidation.

FOOD HACK: Take a cup of no-cal jello at night after a meal.

THE WHAT:Jello
THE WHEN: After a fatty meal at night.
THE HOW: With a small amount of low sugar whipped cream.

The glycine in jello helps clear fatty acids from the blood and may increase fat oxidation.

Dairy Helps Fats Pass The Gut Undigested

One of the easiest ways to lower net fat calories is via dairy. Yes dairy, specifically cheese. Why do you think I had you train lactose digestion into the body? Dairy products form "calcium soaps" in the gut. Calcium soaps cause **fats to pass the gut lining undigested**. New research with dairy shows great promise for the functional properties of "bioactive peptides", contained in dairy. Bioactive means that upon digestion, the functional properties of specific dairy proteins become active. Research shows these compounds have health promoting properties, including anti-hypertensive, antimicrobial, anti-oxidative, anti-appetizing, pro-immunity, and pro-lower net calories.

DAIRY OFFSET HACK: A small amount of cheese with or after a meal helps improve fat oxidation and will slightly decrease fat absorption.

While this is not a panacea, the power lies in combining several offset hacks. Each hack give a series of slight improvements to reduce fat calories absorbed. Combined and over time the effect is substantial.

OFFSET METHOD NUMBER 6: FIBER

Different types of fiber have unique properties for offsetting calories. Fiber is particularly effective with fats. Certain types of fiber added to a meal can lower the net calories. This is done in a number of ways. Fiber can speed up gut transit time, lower availably of bile acids, steer bacteria metabolites via fermentation and others. Some examples:

- Butyrate has been shown to inhibit the formation of cholesterol in the gut.
- Fibers found in food like green beans, flaxseed, wheat, and barley help speed up gut transit time. Fats have less time to absorb.
- Fibers found in foods like raw oats reduce bile acid pools. They also bind with fats, reducing net fat absorption.

Insoluble Fiber to Lower Calories in High Fat Meals.

Our goal is to decrease *metabolizable energy.* One of the easiest ways is to add insoluble fiber with high fat meals. If you are having a meal high in fat, like a hamburger, add insoluble fiber. Insoluble fiber helps to bind fats in the gut and pass them undigested.

FAT HACK: Add insoluble fiber to a high fat meal.
THE WHAT: Insoluble fiber
THE WHEN: With a high fat meal.
THE HOW: Usually raw.

Examples:
1. Raw green beans
2. Cooled potatoes
3. Raw Cauliflower
4. Garbanzo beans

5. Oat bran

ON THE GO MEAL SEQUENCE HACK: Garbanzo beans and cabbage

This is a meal you can do on the go. Any Whole Foods or Trader Joe's or similar makes this easy to do. Use the Whole Foods Food Bar

THE WHAT: Garbanzo beans and cabbage.
THE WHEN: Prior to super weight gain dinner.
THE HOW: Raw with mustard or spices sauce. Add chicken or tofu cubes.

This is an on the go fat burning furnace. Garbanzo beans have unique oligosaccharides. These are very long chain carbohydrates. They help blood sugar metabolism and are loaded with protein. Cabbage acts as substrate to drive bacteria that lower energy harvest.

LOWER CALORIES ABSORBED:

1. Green beans
2. Cauliflower
3. Garbanzo beans

LOWER FAT ABSORPTION

1. Raw steel cut oats
2. Locust bean gum
3. Apple skins

LOWER GLYCEMIC LOAD

1. Asparagus
2. Barley
3. Whole grain rye
4. Psyllium

MEAL SEQUENCE FAT HACK: Cheese and raw oats prior to fat.

THE WHAT: Cheese and raw steel cut oats, or raw green beans.
THE WHEN: Prior to high fat meals, ice cream for example.
THE HOW: Add cinnamon to raw steel cut oats.

Do this prior to a very high fat meal, ribs, pizza, Mexican food, etc. You can do a small preload meal or a complete meal 3 hours prior. Raw steel cut oats may sound weird. They are actually addictive. Put them in a bowl. Add water. Microwave for five seconds. Add cinnamon.

Now let's combine all of these. Some of the food combinations will seem strange. Remember, its all for a functional outcome, to offset fat and net calories.

PUTTING IT ALL TOGETHER: OFFSETTING CHEESECAKE

Cheesecake is probably the most calorically dense food imaginable. Now we combine several techniques to offset much of the weight gain and caloric load. Here is the breakdown.

PRE MEAL: 20 grams of whey protein. 300mg alpha lipoic acid. 1000mg berberine. One teaspoon raw steel cut oats.

CURRENT MEAL: Cheesecake

NEXT MEAL: Raw cauliflower, slice of melted cheese, cup of raw green beans, one scoop of red powder, one small cup no-cal jello.

HOW IT WORKS:
The challenge with cheesecake is the energy density. Fat storage is inevitable. There is simply too much combined sugar and fat. However, we can mitigate a lot of fat storage with meal sequencing. The preload lowers blood sugar *significantly.* A teaspoon of raw, cut oats, helps lower the amount of bile acids available in the gut. Jello helps fat oxidation. Green beans and red phenols help offset sugar fermentation in the gut and speed up gut transit time. Each item alone is a small improvement. Combined they make a very big difference.The beauty of using food to offset weight gain is there are literally hundreds of ways to time and combine foods and supplements to aid offsetting meals.

Chapter 24

The 2 Day Immune Core & The Amplified Fast

THE AMPLIFIED FAST

In 2015 I brought a concept to Quest CEO Ron Penna to mainstream starvation by eating. The goal was to engineer foods depleted by 40% of the amino acid methionine. By doing so we could mimic the benefits of fasting without having to fast. It was a tantalizing idea. Could we realize benefits of extended lifespan by reducing a single amino acid? At that time, where no one had gone was dissecting why fasting works to make something very hard to do, not eating, simple and accessible to everyone. Ron loves innovation. What is not generally known is he could have made many millions more than he has. He has sponsored more pure research than anyone in the industry, often with no commercial endgame.

This is precisely what I am about to give you, only much better.

Since 2010 my VEEP system had been using what are called *fasting mimetic meal patterns.* These are sequences and combinations of foods that, for various reasons, mimic the benefits of fasting without having to fast. Beyond mimicking fasting, the next step is to **amplify fasting.** The Amplified Fast takes into account several things; diurnal rhythm, the Genetic Rush hour, signal pathways like AMPK, Butyrate production, and many other things, to amplify the mechanisms of fasting and minimize the negatives. In short, you fast less, benefit more.

FIBER AND FAT: FRIENDS OR FOES?

If you search out doctors having success against cancer with alternative holistic treatments, two patterns quickly emerge. There are doctors who have had success with dietary plant based therapies. There are also doctors who have success with Keto Diets. While neither approach is a panacea, and neither works with all types of cancers, nevertheless, each has their respective inventory of documented success stories.

On the surface these two approaches seem to be opposed. One uses "carbs" while the other uses fats. But once again, carbs and fats are mere words. When we look beyond words and into the mechanisms of action, there is reason to believe these strategies are actually quite **complimentary.**

First, as dietary strategies, both have limitations long term. Alone, each is imbalanced. Each may in fact compromise key aspects of long term health. For example, In Appendix A you learn how Keto diets produce the molecule 4-HNE. Once you understand what 4-HNE is you may rethink very long term Keto diets.

Thus far you have been given clues that each strategy may benefit the other. For example, you learned fiber negates the carcinogenic byproducts of protein fermenting in the gut.

You also learned **fiber is essential.** You need it to make Butyrate. Butyrate feeds the cells lining your colon. It is first key control mechanism over immunity in the gut and is how you steer immunity by controlling macrophages. In turn, macrophages in the gut lining steer whole body immunity. Butyrate made from fiber switches on, or potentiates, all of the beneficial things you want to happen in the gut. These are things like restoring and preserving the gut lining, HDAC inhibition, steering macrophages, restoring NAD+, and many other good things.

FIBER, FAT, FASTING SYNERGY

Could in fact, a fiber centric approach be **combined** with keto protocols **to amplify the benefits** of each while minimizing the downsides? Could the whole be more than the sum of the parts? Could the best aspects of both promote peak immunity in a way neither can?

As we have discovered, fasting is not all positive. The idea that fiber, fasting and keto could be combined so you can fast less, benefit more, and have a balanced and healthy food intake is compelling.

YES AND ITS NOT A DIET

You are going to see how this is clearly **not a diet.** And it is not a theory either. I have been **doing it** since 2008. Thousands of people have benefited from it. The 2 Day Immunity Core Pattern is a functional pattern of food intake. It will become your *core foundation.* It will be how you drive butyrate, which drives immunity in the gut, and in turn effect every network involved in peak immunity.

KEY IDEA: The 2 Day Immunity Core Pattern drives peak immunity.

The pattern laid out in this chapter has been at the heart of producing astounding results. The results produced are seemingly not possible by any other known means, drugs or otherwise, for total body rejuvenation. Most compelling, it's based on what is most true.

Balance rules your biology. Returning balance to your health inputs drives balance back into the body.

What you learn here will form the core foundation of a simple pattern you will do two or three days a week for life. This pattern is simply the **healthiest thing you can possibly do.** Not only that, it takes *everything into account.* The 2 Day Immunity Core Pattern uses immunometabolism and combines it with chronobiology, luminal nutrition, and many other concepts all seamlessly integrated. Best of all, it's designed to be done on the go with no meal prep.

BENEFITS OF THE 2 Day Immunity Core Pattern

- It's perfectly balanced. You take in a wide range healthy foods. You get them in large amounts. Raspberries, blackberries, salmon, asparagus, avocado, oatmeal, garbanzos, lean meats, cheeses, grapefruit, and many other superfoods balance your food intake.

- No baby talk! It is built from the ground up on The Language of Real Health. **What, when, and how** are always at work with every part of it.

- It restores and tunes the gut perfectly for Akkermansia and Bifidobacteria for peak immunity.

- It fine tunes and steers whole body immune macrophages to the Blue Team.

- It drives production of Butyrate prior to fasting.

- It takes into account diurnal rhythm.

- It amplifies the benefits of fasting and minimizes the downside.

- It negates the downside of keto diets while maximizing the positives.

- It can be done 100 percent on the go with **no meal prep!**

- It is modular in nature. You can stack many other protocols on top of it.

- It allows you to eat Ad Libitum **any time you choose.**

WHAT IT IS:
This is a 2 day pattern of using fiber and fats in an exact order of operations to steer immunity toward peak health.

You will utilize "what, when, and how" to maximize immune function, slow aging, prevent disease, keep you lean, keep the gut fine tuned, steer immune macrophages toward the Blue Team and ultimately, to amplify the benefits of fasting without fasting much at all. Best of all it's super easy.

NO MEAL PREP NEEDED
Most amazing, you can do the 2 Day Core Immune Pattern **on the go with no meal prep!** It sounds too good to be true. It's not. Imagine, you get the single healthiest possible pattern of foods, one that extends lifespan, steers macrophages and tunes the gut for Akkermansia and Bifidobacteria, and you do it on the go!

KEY IDEA: The 2 Day Immunity Core Pattern is designed to work on the go. No meal prep needed.

THE TWO DAY CORE NARRATED

I'm going to narrate two full days with the 2 Day Immunity Core Pattern. It's the best way to help you understand how it works. I'm going to narrate this in the plural tense. Let's assume the day begins with breakfast at 8 am. Before we begin understand one key idea.

KEY IDEA: We are not feeding you.

This first day is about feeding bifidobacteria. Feeding bifido is very different from feeding you directly. This pattern is your new core building block. **Learn it well.** We will build many other protocols upon this core pattern to do amazing things otherwise not possible

DAY ONE:

OBJECTIVES:
- Feed Bifidobacteria.
- Spin up Butyrate.
- Burn fat.
- Steer immune macrophages.
- Pre-amplify fasting signals.

HOUR 1: BREAKFAST DAY ONE - DARK FRUITS & KEY FATS

The first meal combines dark fruits with key fats. The goal is to feed bifidobacteria and stimulate the hormone Adiponectin. This potent combo makes insulin work better and fires up b-vitamin production. The trick is the dosing. To make this work requires **bulk.** This is where everyone gets it wrong. I remember showing the folks at Quest a diagram of this in 2013. The response was "that's a lot of carbs!" Depending on your size and weight, you eat between 1/2 to one full 11 inch plate of fruit. For todays meal blackberries with a small amount of walnuts do the trick. Walnuts are key to sensitizing adiponectin which means insulin works better.

HOUR 3:

Your serum is now flooding with *anthocyanins;* the color pigments in blackberries. Loading the blood with anthocyanins at the start of the day *acts as a buffer across the rest of the day.* It helps fat to burn. Contrary to the old carbs/macros paradigm, **fat oxidation is increasing!** Insulin Area Under Curve is actually less than a comparable amount of "carbs" due to the massive influx of phenols into the blood.

Even more important, anthocyanins directly suppress NF-KB, the immune and inflammation master mechanism you learned about in Chapter 4. Suppression of NF-KB is a key component of immune protection from super viruses like SARS- COV2.

Bifidobacteria in the gut is now multiplying. The phenols from blackberries feed **bifidobacteria.** The berries are now starting to ferment in the gut.

Timing is now key. We wait a full 3.5 hours or more before eating again.

HOUR 4:

The trick now is a small snack of fat. We have perfectly waited for "when." Now the key is, "what."

Fat thirty minutes prior to the next meal will slow digestion. Macadamia nuts have very low amounts of the amino acid methionine. In effect they mimic fasting! Fat now also helps insulin work better at the next meal.

Over time, small fat inputs thirty minutes before a meal have a powerful life extending effect. They are actually sensitizing another class of helper hormones - the **incretins.** The incretins help insulin become more efficient. You don't need to make as much. This helps you age slower long term.

Incretin's also have another effect. These fats will hit the duodenum prior to your next meal. Fats in the duodenum stimulate the hormone PYY. This creates a feedback loop to curtail eating. You get fuller, faster at your next meal. Because these fats mimic fasting by restricting methionine, you get the benefits of both fasting and eating at this meal.

HOUR 4.5: LUNCH - RESISTANT STARCHES

This is the main Butyrate producing meal of the day. A lot of different kinds of meals can work here. To illustrate, the optimal foods are **resistant starches.** We have been brainwashed to think starch is bad. That's baby talk. This is "what, when and how" in perfect order of operations. Resistant starches *resist* digestion. They don't really feed us. They feed bifidobacteria. In fact they are the primary source of food for bifidobacteria.

Ideally this meal has things like garbanzo beans, black beans, potatoes, or even oats, but not in the way you are used to having them.

The trick is to have them cold.

KEY IDEA: Cold resistant starches feed bacteria.

Heat breaks the long starch chains into simple sugars. Simple sugars feed you. That's not our goal. Cooling turns the sugars back to starches or fibers that can resist digestion. In this narration I'm going for max functional effect. For this meal we have a burrito bowl with black beans (cooled) chicken (or garbanzo beans for vegans) peppers, lots of mild salsa, small amount of cheese and some hot sauce. *Everything is functional.*

- Cheese drives fullness. It also speeds up fat loss!
- The sheer **bulk** of the meal triggers fullness hormones.
- The low/slow energy yield of the meal will trigger the hormone glucagon later in the day. Glucagon works to raise blood sugar. This helps you burn fat.

- Glucagon also makes you hungry. Cheese now helps offset the hunger later.
- Chicken prolongs fermentation in the gut. This makes more bifidobacteria.
- Peppers, salsa and hot sauce drive heat production in the body.

This meal is a fat loss bomb You can do it on the go with no meal prep! It helps solve the problem of time going to zero over the long haul. You will always have this at your disposal.

VEGAN NOTE: If you are vegan, just use garbanzo beans in place of black beans and leave out the chicken.

We are building the perfect bifidobacteria meal stack. It looks like this.

Breakfast Phenols => Lunch Resistant Starches => Dinner Cruciferous veggies.

HOUR 8

For the last hour the gut has felt like a furnace. All the ingredients of fat loss are at work: glucagon release, heat production, lots of digestive action and fermentation of bifidobacteria. A bit of hunger gnaws up from the belly. How can such a big meal promote hunger? The answer is we have combined **bulk with decreased energy harvest at the same time.**

KEY IDEA: Bulk combined with decreased energy harvest makes you hungry.

Normally with huge meals, the hormone leptin increases. Here the opposite occurs. There is lots of bulk and stomach distention, but not much energy. At the same time a massive shift in energy harvest is taking place. It's not just the bulk. Bacteria is shifting. You are gaining more bacteria that harvest less energy. Consequently the body is trying to raise blood sugar. In turn this drives fat loss. It's an hour or two before the next meal. A small snack here works as a "Pre-load Meal."

PRE-LOAD SNACK: AVOCADO

Pre-load meals give us a lot of power. We can use them for a number of effects. In this case, one goal is to maximize fat loss while sleeping. This helps trigger AMPK. Avocado at this exact time, an hour before the next meal, is perfect. Avocado has a unique effect. It lowers insulin output. It makes our body more insulin sensitive.

Later, you can have tons of choices for foods. This illustration is for maximum functional effect.

HOUR 10: DINNER - BRAZED TUNA, RAW GREEN BEANS, CABBAGE

The last meal of Day One is cruciferous veggies with fibers rich in hemi-cellulose. These fibers are another preferred food for bifidobacteria. This meal will ferment through the deep stretch of the night. We are driving production of Butyrate at the critical hours between 3 and 5 am.

KEY IDEA: We are timing production of Butyrate to peak 24 hour firing of AMPK.

This is signal amplification.

SIGNAL AMPLIFICATION

What you are learning goes so far beyond diet, as to render the idea of diet itself a form of baby talk. Day one has been one big coordinated effort. We are timing maximum Butyrate production to peak AMPK signaling during the Genetic Rush Hour. This is real power to slow aging.

Again, dinner has lots of options. We don't need to eat perfectly. We could even eat Ad Libitum here. Suppose you decided to have pizza and ice cream. The weight gain from such a meal will be totally **offset** by what you did earlier today and what we do tomorrow morning.

Are you starting to see what I promised in Chapter 1, I hope? This is real freedom.

Let's stay on course to amplify AMPK during sleep. The first two meals have done much of the work. For this example, however, we go **aggressive.** Dinner is raw green beans with cabbages and brazed tuna steak. Vegans can substitute their favorite vegan protein option for tuna. It won't work quite as well but it still works.

GLYCINE AT BED

Just prior to bed hunger gnaws up again. We have a cup of no-calorie jello. The glycine in the jello helps hunger and we will burn more fat during sleep from the glycine.

HOUR 20:

It's 4 am in the morning. The Genetic Rush Hour is on. Perfectly timed food inputs - what you ate, when you ate it and how you ate - **amplify** the bodies youth restoring mechanisms. The gut lining has abundant Butyrate from the days meals. Bifidobacteria has proliferated. In cross feeding reactions, other bacteria like Akkermansia and lactate producers that mimic exercise are proliferating. The AMPK pathway is firing. Youth is being restored. Aging has slowed. Autophagy is in full swing. NAD+ is being restored.

Blue Team immune macrophages in the gut lining are proliferating.

The Amplified Fast is well underway. All it took was food in the right sequence of what, when and how.

HOUR 22:
It's around dawn, roughly 6 am. Hunger and AMPK activation wakes our bodies quite easily.

This hour is a key insertion point.

You will learn to stack other "modules" at this exact time, 6am on the morning of the second day. The specific sequence of things you did yesterday primed the body for **this window of time**. Your body is aging much slower right now. Peak Human physiology is loading into your body.

This **exact hour is where other modules can be inserted.** Some of these modules...

- Slow aging,
- Spin down inflammation,
- Steer macrophages in key tissues,
- Amplify fasting signals even further.
- Mitigate disease risk

Two or three times per week you can take your body to this place. In doing so, you will prolong your window of youth.

DAY TWO:

OBJECTIVE:

Amplify fasting while steering fat mass macrophages and targeting pexohpagy.

HOUR 1:
This first meal of day 2 is highly, *highly* functional.

Yesterday primed the body to **steer macrophages in your fat mass with *this* meal.** Remember we steer macrophages *tissue by tissue.* The Blue Team in the gut lining was targeted during sleep. Now we move to your fat.

THE FOUNDATION OF DAY 2:
For today our basic foundation is 4 small fat meals followed by an omega 3 rich dinner.

KEY IDEA: The key is omega 3 fats.

I can not stress this enough for day 2, particularly in the early am. The reason is *pexophagy.*

Omega 3 fats directly target the peroxisomes in your fat mass.

No other food in the entire universe of foods can work as powerfully to target peroxisomes *at this specific time.* There are, however, cautions with Omega 3's. **See Appendix A: Omega 3's and MCT's, friend of foe?**

We could do any number of foods here. Eggs, cheese, avocado, salmon, various nuts, cottage cheese and more can all work. For maximum function, the more Omega 3, particularly Omega 3 rich In EPA, the more we steer macrophages in our fat and spin down inflammation. As an example of maximum function walnuts or an Omega 3 smoothie are perfect for this first meal.

HOUR 4.5
The next meal can be any number of choices. A cheese stick and an egg had from the local Starbucks can work. Let's go for maximum function. A pack of smoked salmon from Trader Joe's is perfect. Vegans go with avocado.

HOUR 7:
We do this on the go. Two small small avocado cups from the local AM/PM do the trick.

HOUR 9.5
A cup of cottage cheese with fat had from the local grocery store.

DINNER
Dinner is a large salmon steak with roasted veggies.

VEGAN MEAL: Vegans can go with a meal high in plant fats. Avocados, olive oil, nuts, garbanzo beans, yogurt, are all good to include.

NOTHING IS HEALTHIER

I want to stress the health aspects the 2 Day Immunity Core Pattern. This is simply the *healthiest thing you can possibly do*. This pattern repeated over a number of years, will drive peak human health in a way not possible via any other approach to food. Here is why.

First, the 2 Day Immunity Core Pattern is extremely balanced. You are not creating long term imbalances from imbalanced healthy foods. Instead there is a wide range of foods.The majority of these foods are considered *superfoods.* Beyond the foods, the "what, when and how" **has a power found nowhere else**.

You are targeting The Genetic Rush Hour and AMPK activation to stay young at the exact hour needed. You are steering macrophages. You are amplifying all the youth promoting mechanisms of the body. You are not provoking the bodies starvation defense with excessive fasting. Pro-aging growth pathways, IIS and mTor, have been balanced with the anti-aging AMPK pathway. And it's something you can do anytime you want the rest of your life. I live around it. Far from being restrictive, it allows me to eat anything I want, whenever I want. The best part about it is **you don't have to do well to do amazing.** You can get fantastic results just by doing parts of it. You can get off track any time, at any meal, and the negatives are already offset by everything else in the 2 day pattern.

Chapter 25

Blueprint For The 2 Day Core

MY ORIGINAL PROMISE

In the Introduction, I said something that sounded quite impossible. I said at my age, I don't take steroids or any physique enhancing substances, I eat anything, anytime, and I do it mostly on the go with healthy fast food. I said you would learn to do the same thing. Most likely you immediately thought I was full of it.

This chapter we come full circle. My goal is for you to come away with the following.

- The power to hack into Peak Human Health.
- The power to eat whatever and offset it.
- The power to do it all on the go with no meal prep.

The power to do all of this is contained in the 2 Day Immunity Core Pattern. Study this chapter well. Learn the modules. They are simple and powerful. They give you a power many seek and so few find.

THE 2 DAY CORE BLUEPRINT

Here is a visual overview of a possible iteration of the 2 Day Core. There are many, many, possible iterations. In this chapter we lay the blueprint and give you several examples and variations. The visual is helpful to get an idea of the patterns and sheer size of some of these meals.

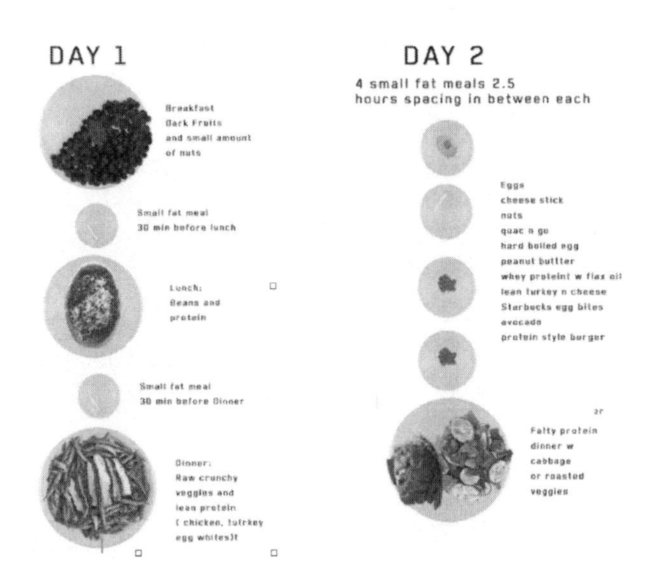

Vegans have plenty of non meat options. This visual is just for illustration.

DAY ONE OBJECTIVE:

The goal of the entire day is to drive Butyrate production while sleeping.

THE BASIC PATTERN OF DAY ONE:

Mornings on day one are generally specific fruits. Afternoons are resistant starches. Evenings are more cellulose, hemi-cellulose and cruciferous veggies. It looks like this.

DAY ONE: Fruits => Resistant starches => Veggies

Think legos. Each meal is a module, like a lego. You can swap it out. Any meal in the 2 day sequence can be swapped with other modules listed in this section.

KEY IDEA: Each meal is a module. You can swap other modules in or out.

MODULES OF THE 2 DAY CORE PROGRAM

DAY ONE	DAY TWO
Berry module	Amplified Fast Module
Starch module	Fat Module
Veggie Module	Dinner Meal
Pre Bed Module	Pre Bed Module

NOTES:

PROTEIN:

Dense fibrous protein is a vital component in all of these sequences. This kind of protein helps to park fibers in the secum of the gut. This aids fermentation. Fermentation produces more bifidobacteria.

RAW FIBER:

Most fibers are consumed raw.

The exception being things like beans, which are cooked, but cooled down. Generally, the harder fibers are, meaning characteristics like crunchy or dense, the more you have to chew them and the more energy you spend on digestion. The closer fibers are to sugar, the faster they absorb.

KEY IDEA: Mushy feeds you. Hard feeds bacteria.

MEAL SIZE:

The meals often seem shockingly large.

PRE-LOADS:

We use pre-load meals 30 minutes prior to lunch and an hour prior to dinner. They are very strategic. It is the exact foods and sequences, timed prior to each meal that gives pre-loads utility and function.

YOU DON'T HAVE TO EAT PERFECT:

Offsetting is built into the 2 day pattern. You can quite literally eat anything at any meal. The pattern offsets much of weight gain.

If initially, you do breakfast, lunch and dinner following the pattern, it works very fast and you feel it. Later, you may choose only to do one or two meals, say breakfast and lunch, as a maintenance pattern. It still works very well. You can follow the pattern any time you need to lean up a bit or amplify a fast.

CONDITIONS:

One caution, if you have an existing gut condition like IBS, Colitis or similar, do not start on this. You need to first restore the gut. Begin with HMO, Red phenols, carb training and the other protocols in the first few chapters. Do not avoid medical help for a serious medical condition. Work with a skilled practitioner who understand how to restore the gut.

DAY ONE FOODS: In order of preference

BREAKFAST:

BERRY MODULE: Bifido promoters
Blackberries, raspberries, blueberries, pomegranate seeds, cranberry juice, semi-green banana, strawberries, dark grapes, black currants, acai, bilberry.

FUNCTIONAL FRUITS MODULE
Grapefruit, pineapple, kiwi, apples, apple peels, oranges.

FUNCTIONAL FOODS MODULE
Yogurt, honey, organic maple syrup, barley cereal, steel cut oats, cheeses.

LUNCH:

STARCH MODULE: Bifido promoters
Garbanzo beans, black beans, potatoes, white beans, pinto beans, brown rice, potatoes, lentils, barley cereal, repeat of any meal from morning.

FUNCTIONAL FERMENTERS MODULE:
Cabbages, red onion, broccoli, cauliflower, saurkraut, green beans, purple corn, black soybeans, black carrots, purple sweet potato, cheese, ricotta cheese, chili, corn, cucumber.

DINNER:

VEGGIES MODULE **:** Bifido promoters
Green beans, cabbage, asparagus, broccoli, cauliflower, Brussel sprouts (These are an exception in that you have to stream them), garbanzo beans, onions, chili, brown rice.

FUNCTIONAL DINNER FOODS MODULE:
Barley cereal, spaghetti squash, mushrooms, cheese, cucumber, artichokes, lentil soups, onion, garlic, tomatoes, celery.

Preferred Proteins:
Animal:
Chicken, Turkey, lean steak, tuna, egg white, whey protein, cod, orange roughy, salmon, roast beef, sardines, protein bars.

Vegan:
Garbanzo beans, mushrooms, brussel sprouts, soy, green peas, seitan, quinoa, spelt.

Preferred Preload Meals:
Walnuts, avocado, macadamia nuts, olive oil. cheese, olive tapenade, whey protein, plant protein, nuts.

HOW MODULARITY GIVES FREEDOM

Here are four examples of day one. You can see how modularity gives you total freedom. Not only can you swap modules out, **you can eat whatever, whenever you want!** This example shows breakfast lunch and dinner on day one.

PERFECT	IMPROVISE	IMPROVISE
Berry module	Berry Module	Functional Fruits
Starch module	Berry Module	Starch Module
Veggie Module	Eat whatever	Eat whatever
Pre Bed Module	Pre Bed Module	Pre Bed Module

You can see in these three examples quite a bit of variety. You can swap other modules or just eat whatever. Now we will look at both days of the 2 Day Immunity Core Pattern. Notice how the basic pattern naturally offsets eating whatever.

HOW THE 2 DAY CORE NATURALLY OFFSETS EATING WHATEVER

DAY ONE:	DAY TWO:
Breakfast: Berry module	Fasting Module
Lunch: Eating whatever	Fat Module
Dinner: Eating whatever	Fat dinner
Pre Bed Module	Pre Bed Module

The first meal was the normal berry module. The next 2 meals were eating ad lib. We just ate whatever: pizza for lunch, mac and cheese for dinner. You are probably thinking of the weight gain from those meals. Not so fast. Look at Day Two.

Day Two goes right into the Amplified fast. Most if not all of the weight gain from lunch and dinner is naturally offset on Day Two. On top of the base pattern, you have all of the offsetting techniques of the prior chapter at your disposal.

I made the point we must allow eating whatever, whenever. Now you can begin to see how its possible.

2 Day Immunity Core Pattern + Offsetting Techniques => Eating whatever

Here are several examples.

EXAMPLES

SUPER AGGRESSIVE FOR FAT LOSS EXAMPLE:

This first example is extremely aggressive for fat loss at dinner time. It promotes rapid gut recolonization.

Breakfast: 3/4 plate of blackberries, 3 oz macadamia nuts
Snack: 5 oz walnuts
Lunch: Tex mex bowl: cold black beans, onions and salsa, chicken, peppers, cheese
Snack: 100 cal avocado
Dinner:Cabbage wraps with garbanzo's, chicken and asparagus.

MODERATE EXAMPLE

This example uses the three modules but the foods are less aggressive.

Breakfast: 2 scoops whey protein, 1/2-3/4 plate blueberries, 5 oz walnuts
Snack: Starbucks avocado cup
Lunch: Baked potato cooled down w cheese.
Snack: 2 Cheese sticks
Dinner: Lean steak with raw green beans

ON THE GO EXAMPLE

This example is done all on the go.

Breakfast: 2 semi-green bananas and 1/2 grapefruit
Snack: Starbucks cheese stick
Lunch: Chipolte bowl with : cold black beans, onions and salsa, chicken, peppers, cheese
Snack: 2 Starbucks avocado cups
Dinner: Chicken breast with asparagus

EATING WHATEVER EXAMPLE

Here is another example of how the 2 Day Core allows for eating whatever.

Breakfast: 3/4 plate of blackberries, 3 oz macadamia nuts
Snack: Starbucks cheese stick
Lunch: Lean steak
Snack: 2 Starbucks avocado cups
Dinner Pizza and ice cream

In this example, dinner is almost totally offset by the meals earlier in the day. Day Two will finish the job of offsetting dinner from day one.

DAY TWO OBJECTIVE:

- Amplify fasting
- Slow aging
- Steer macrophages
- Lower inflammation
- Reducing long term risk of disease states.

THE BASIC PATTERN OF DAY TWO:

- 4 small fat meals
- Space 2.5 hours between
- Large fatty dinner rich in omega 3 fats.

PREFERRED FATS:
Eggs, cheese, avocado, cottage cheese, walnuts, high EPA omega 3 oil, macadamias, olives, salmon, omega 3 smoothie, extra virgin olive oil, peanut butter, nut butter, heavy cream, pistachios, pine nuts, sesame seed oil, butter, ghee, ground flax, pecans, pistachios.

Vegans have lots of choices in this list. There are some things not on this list like bacon, for example. Bacon and ham are loaded with purines and pyrmidamines which work contrary to getting inflammation down during The Amplified Fast.

ANIMAL PROTEIN EXAMPLE

Meal 1:
2 Omega 3 enriched eggs.

Meal 2;
Avocado

Meal 3:
Smoked salmon

Meal 4:
Walnuts

Dinner
Salmon and cabbage.

VEGAN EXAMPLE

Meal 1:
1/2 Avocado

Meal 2:
Olives

Meal 3:
Sunflower seeds

Meal 4:
Walnuts

Dinner:
Soy chorizo with garbanzo beans and salsa.

LIST OF MODULES

A word on supplements. This at first glance could seem rather supplement heavy. I want to stress the foundation of this is food! Food is where the horsepower lies. Supplements here are additive in nature. Just using a single supplement from any of the modules is very powerful. You can do just a few things, or everything or somewhere in between. Before we start, late me give you good, better, best. Just realize good is amazing. Anything beyond that is gravy.

GOOD:
All inexpensive and powerful.
Vitamin D, melatonin, chelated minerals, rutin

BETTER:
All the above + high EPA Omega 3 oil, ketones, pterostilbene, apigenin. niacin

BEST:
All the above + berberine, molecular hydrogen, nicotinamide mononucleotide or nicotinamide riboside.

THE AMPLIFIED FAST MODULE

The Amplified Fast module can be inserted on Day Two. The fasting module consists of three parts.

THE WHAT: Small molecules + Omega fats
THE WHEN: Morning of the second day.
THE HOW: With the fiber day precursor.

Here is the basic formula for the Amplified fast

Day One Fibers => Amplified Fast Module => Day Two Fats

1. Upon waking take the small molecules module.
2. Fast until hungry.
3. Do the Omega fats module the rest of the day.

As a bonus, add molecular hydrogen in the form of hydrogen water.

SUPPLEMENTAL MODULES

1. Evening Pre Bed Module
2. Inflammation Small Molecule Module
3. Cold Induction Module
4. Omega Centric Meals
5. Oleate Centric Meals Module
6. Feast Module

INFLAMMATION SMALL MOLECULE MODULE

1. Fisetin +
2. Exogenous Ketones
3. Niacin
4. NAC
5. Vitamin D

AMPLIFIED FAST MODULE:

1. 2 Day Immunity Core Pattern
2. Small molecules
3. Omega fats
4. Molecular Hydrogen

FULL SMALL MOLECULES MODULE:

You can get these separately. My Amped Keto product has them all in one except Berberine, which is a great addition.

- Apigenin*
- Nicotinamide Riboside or Nicotinamide Mononucleotide
- Berberine
- Ketones
- Pterostilbene

OMEGA 3 FATS:

You want a good omega 3 fat supplement high in EPA. Omega 3 fats target the peroxisomes and pexophagy in unique ways.

MOLECULAR HYDROGEN:

Molecular hydrogen can be obtained as Hydrogen Infused water. Several products are on the market. Molecular hydrogen is a unique antioxidant. It selectively targets a key signal cascade involved in membrane permeability called the RhoA/ROCK signaling pathway. Molecular hydrogen inhibits excessive housekeeping and directly targets activation of peroxisomes and enhances metabolism of fats.

* Several studies suggest Apigenin has a anti-tumor effect on breast cancers. 2 studies showed it may promote breast cancers. More recent studies seem to exonerate Apigenin showing a health supportive role suppressing breast cancers. Most recently, a December 2019 study comparing apigenin with another compound for breast cancers stated "...may explain the differential effect of these compounds on the phenotype of the breast cancer cell. Together, our results confirmed the potential health benefit effect of apigenin." I mention both sides so women can be informed. Women may wish to leave Apigenin out of this stack or consult your doctor.

BEDTIME MODULES MASTER MAP

Can also combine with

EVENING PRE BED MODULE
1. Melatonin
2. Vitamin D (if more than 4 weeks straight at high dose leave out)
3. Rutin
4. Pterostilbene

DEEP SLEEP BEDTIME MODULE
1. Oleamide
2. GABA

Rotate in 2-3 times per week.

1. Nicotinamide Riboside or Nicotinamide Mononucleotide

Ad this in during periods of feasting

BEDTIME HORMONE MODULE
1. ZMA
2. Chelated minerals

FOOD MODULES:

BERRY MODULE:

Blackberries, raspberries, blueberries, pomegranate seeds, cranberry juice, semi-green banana, strawberries, dark grapes, black currants, acai, bilberry.

STARCH MODULE:

Garbanzo beans, black beans, potatoes, white beans, pinto beans, brown rice, potatoes, lentils, barley cereal, repeat of any meal from morning.

VEGGIE MODULE:

Green beans, cabbage (steamed or raw), asparagus, broccoli, cauliflower, Brussel sprouts (steamed), garbanzo beans, onions, chili, brown rice, cabbages, red onion, broccoli, cauliflower, saurkraut, green beans, purple corn, black soybeans, black carrots, purple sweet potato, corn, cucumber,

FAT MODULE

Eggs, cheese, avocado, cottage cheese, walnuts, high EPA omega 3 oil, macadamias, olives, salmon, omega 3 smoothie, extra virgin olive oil, peanut butter, nut butter, heavy cream, pistachios, pine nuts, sesame seed oil, butter, ghee, ground flax, pecans, pistachios.

HIGH OMEGA FATS MODULE:

Avocado, salmon, walnuts, cheese, omega 3 smoothie, Omega 3 enriched eggs, chia seeds, hemp seeds, flax seeds, endamame, tuna, sardines, cod, mackerel, sea bass, macadamia nuts, hazelnuts, pecans, cottage cheese, olive oil, olives peanut butter, tofu, pumpkin seeds.

HIGH OLEATE FATS MODULE:

Olive oil, avocado, avocado oil, peanuts, cheese, cashews, Almond oil, almond butter, cocoa butter, coconut oil.

Chapter 26

The Inflammation Spin Down

In Chapter 2 we learned how spinning down inflammation is the most powerful factor effecting your rate of aging. It is also the factor most realistic for you to control. The new science speaks to the power that inflammation and inflammaging wields over keeping your body young.

This chapter gives you a key life skill. The Inflammation Spin Down is a power. It will be with you the rest of your life. You will acquire the ability to rewire inflammatory signals in the body. The inflammation Spin Down is based on the Core 2 Day Program. It simply ads a few more modules. It also takes place over 4 days. Here is the basic pattern

Let's break down the new modules.

MORNING COLD MODULE:
Cold induction is a powerful technique for controlling cells from the outside in. It helps induce peroxisomes to multiply via a protein called Fibroblast Growth Factor 21, or FGF21. FGF21 helps the body adapt to fat loss. It basically induces a state of fat feeding upon itself. Morning cold also activates AMPK. This is the hardest module to do**. *It's optional.*** Some ways to get cold

- Cold water immersion
- Access to a large refrigerator
- Cold shower.

INFLAMMATION SMALL MOLECULE MODULE
Fisetin + Niacin + Regular Small Molecules

FISETIN:
Fiesetin is phenol like Quercetin. Fisetin flushes non dividing cells in your fat. It is one of the ways we remove old fat from the body. It has even been shown to extend maximum lifespan. Its main use here is to flushes senolytic non dividing cells in your fat to magnify anti-inflammatory signals.

NIACIN:
Niacin here reprograms the Red Team macrophages into the Blue Team. Steering macrophages to the Blue Team over these 4 days is effectively swiping the off toggle on your phone for inflammation.

OMEGA CENTRIC MEALS MODULE
DAY TWO-THREE:
1. Wake.
2. Inflammation Small Molecules

3. Fast until hungry
4. 3 Omega fat meals

THE INFLAMMATION SPIN DOWN

THE WHAT: The Inflammation Spin Down
THE WHEN: Over 4 days
THE HOW: See below

In addition to what you have learned in the 2 Day Core, there are 5 modules to insert over 4 days.

1. Evening Pre Bed Module
2. Inflammation Small Molecule Module
3. Cold Induction Module
4. Omega Centric Meals
5. Feast Module

Day One:
The Fiber Pattern + Evening Pre Bed Module

Day Two-Three:
Inflammation Small molecules + Cold Induction + High Omega Food Module + Evening Heat + Evening Pre Bed Module

DAY 4:
Feast Module

HIGH OMEGA FATS MODULE:
Avocado, salmon, walnuts, cheese, omega 3 smoothie, Omega 3 enriched eggs, chia seeds, hemp seeds, flax seeds, endamame, tuna, sardines, cod, mackerel, sea bass, macadamia nuts, hazelnuts, pecans, cottage cheese, olive oil, olives peanut butter, tofu, pumpkin seeds

KEY IDEA: The first 2 meals are small 200 calorie meals and dinner is very large.

EXAMPLE 1:
First Meal: Omega 3 eggs
Second Meal: Avocado and cheese
Third Meal: Salmon steak and veggies of choice.

EXAMPLE 2:
First Meal: Cheese sticks and avocado
Second Meal: Macadamia nuts
Third Meal: Sea bass and asparagus

EXAMPLE 3 VEGAN:
First Meal: Walnut, flax seed peanut butter mash.
Second Meal: Avocado and macadamia nuts
Third Meal: Dinner spinach salad with avocado, hemp seeds, pumpkin seeds, tomatoes, olives and olive oil.

HEAT MODULE

In the evening any one of the following

- 20 minutes in a sauna or jacuzzi
- Hot yoga

DAY FOUR: FEAST MODULE

Too much autophagy is not good. It can actually drive inflammation. This day is a checkpoint to the last two days. You will 2x your calories for one day. This helps the body to stimulate growth and healing. You can repeat the Day One Fiber Pattern and just increase the portions by 50 percent and add the following. The main thing is to get 1.5 to 2x what you normally eat in non-inflammatory whole foods.

GUIDELINES
1. 2x your calories.
2. Repeat the Day One Fruit/Fiber Pattern.
3. Add additional items to get calories up.

Breakfast Additions:
1. Bowl of oatmeal w/ cinnamon and honey.
2. or 2 slices of Ezekial bread.
3. 1- 2 scoops of your favorite plant or whey protein.

Snacks:
Swap out nuts for cheese sticks or whole eggs.
Vegans can use peanuts or figs.

Lunch:
In addition to the regular pattern of starches here at lunch, you have a lot of freedom to ad lib. The idea is to 2x your calories. You need at least 40 percent protein at this meal. Stay away from inflammatory foods like pork, fried food or high sugars. Good suggestions are hamburgers, wraps, large salads, healthy burritos, chicken, salmon or steak, harvest bowls quinoa or greek bowls, chili, half chicken, tuna melts, fajita platter, kabob meals, sushi meals.steak and potatoes and others. Once again, the idea is today is a feast of large, fairly healthy non-inflammatory meals.

Dinner:
Still following the Day One pattern at dinner. Bigger portions and feasting are the rule. Meal suggestions.

Salmon with zucchini pasta.
Roasted Brussels sprouts and balsamic chicken.
Garbanzo curry.
Turkey chili and avocado.
Seared ahi poke and veggies.
Roast chicken w fennel and turmeric.
Stuffed peppers.
Eggs Benedict pizza.
Steak and veggies.
Lamb chops.
Rib eye and potatoes w asparagus.

VARIATION ON THE INFLAMMATION SPIN DOWN
Targeting Pexophagy and Membrane Function

This is a variation you can do to target Pexophagy. There is only one difference. You can rotate between this version and the standard inflammation spin down. You can also substitute the High Oleate Food Module once in a while on Day 2 of the 2 Day Core.

1. The high omega foods are swapped out with the High Oleate Food Module - see below.

Day One:
The Fiber Pattern + Evening Pre Bed Module.

Day Two-Three:

Inflammation Small molecules + Cold Induction + **Oleate Fats Module** + Evening Heat + Evening Pre Bed Module.

DAY 4:
Feast Module

HIGH OLEATE FATS MODULE:
Olive oil, avocado, avocado oil, peanuts, cheese, cashews, almond oil, almond butter, cocoa butter, coconut oil.

Here is a sample day using the High Oleate Fats Module. This is would be either Day two, or Day three.

MEAL 1: 1/2 Avocado

MEAL 2: Two tablespoons almond butter

MEAL 3: Coconut butter bar

DINNER: Large salad with Olive Oil

Day four is the feast day once again. The large amount of glucose slamming into the body after high oleate feeding is a powerful signal that effects the peroxisomes and helps them shift into pexophagy.

Chapter 27

The Master To-Do List

HACKING A YOUNG BODY: THE NEW TO-DO LIST

Here is your master to-do list. As I said in Chapter 2, you don't have to do well to do amazing. You may only do one or two things on this list. Just one or two can powerfully impact your life.

MY PICKS

If I just had to do 3 of the things on this list, it would be the 2 Day Immunity Core Pattern, The Integrated Interval and The Amplified Fast. Those 3 things alone, with their particulars, powerfully and radically impact your body long term for the better. They effect the body in dozens of ways. They bring balance and across the years, I have done those three continually no matter what. I don't always do them perfect, but even done at 50% they are remarkably powerful to keep the body young.

FOR IMPULSE READERS

A caution. **The impulse reader** will skip the book and go right to the list. Make sure you read Chapter 4 and 5 first. If you do not understand **what, when and how,** for anything and everything, you stay in the baby talk of this era. The items on this list were presented in the perfect timing and execution within the book contents.

MOBILITY & FLEXIBILITY & DAILY EXERTION

- [ ] Bedtime Yoga Flows
- [ ] The Integrated Interval
- [ ] Ancestral Squat

PEAK HUMAN SLEEP

- [ ] Breath rights
- [ ] Mouth tape
- [ ] Darkness
- [ ] EM Smog Protocols
- [ ] Restore Hard Chewing Interval
- [ ] Deep Sleep Bedtime Module
    - [ ] Melatonin
    - [ ] Vitamin D
    - [ ] Oleamide
    - [ ] GABA

Additional Sleep Hacks When Needed

- [ ] Ancestral Sleep Cycle
- [ ] Carb pulse meal before bed
- [ ] Slow breathing
- [ ] Soak hands and feet

PEAK HUMAN GUT

- [ ] HMO Cycle
- [ ] Red Phenol Cycle
- [ ] Apple Peels Cycle
- [ ] Carb Training
- [ ] 2 Day Immunity Core Pattern

Additional When Needed

- [ ] Bacteria Fermentation 101 Hack
- [ ] Hunger Signal Amplification Hack
- [ ] Gut Lining Orange Juice and Fasting Hack
- [ ] Daisy Cutter Hack

SLOWING AGING

- [ ] 2 Day Immunity Core Pattern
    - [ ] Fiber module
    - [ ] Starch Module
    - [ ] Veggies module
    - [ ] Fat module
    - [ ] Bedtime Inflammation Module

- [ ] Amplified fast module
    - [ ] Small molecules module
    - [ ] Cold module
    - [ ] exercise

- [ ] Inflammation Spin Down
    - [ ] Day 1
    - [ ] Day 2
    - [ ] Day 3
    - [ ] Day 4

PEAK HUMAN HEALTH

- [ ] Hif-1 Bedtime Clear Protocol
- [ ] Hif-1 Workout Hack
- [ ] Gum Cleaning Every 3 Months
- [ ] Endothelium Hack

- [ ] Omega 3 Hif-1 Hack
- [ ] NAD+ Repletion Hack
- [ ] Bedtime Hormone Module
- [ ] Signal Amplification Muscle Growth Hack
- [ ] ERK Massage Hack
- [ ] Pexophagy Targeting Hack
    - [ ] Day 1
    - [ ] Day 2
    - [ ] Day 3

FOOD OFFSET HACKS

- [ ] 3 Meal Sequences
- [ ] Whey, cinnamon, olive oil preload
- [ ] Berry preload
- [ ] Berberine, alpha lipoic acid
- [ ] Asparagus, onions, olive oil, vinegar post load
- [ ] Cheese with Meal
- [ ] Cheese and Raw Oats Preload
- [ ] Cooled Starches
- [ ] Walnut Pre Load
- [ ] Cheese Pre Load
- [ ] Egg Pre Load
- [ ] Jello Post Meal Hack

ANTI-OXIDANTS

- [ ] With Omega fats
- [ ] With Large meals
- [ ] When Sleep Deprived

CONTROL OF FAT

- [ ] Intermittent Fat Browning
- [ ] Rutin Body Prep Hack
- [ ] Post Fat Loss Biome Intervention
- [ ] Leptin Intervention

APPENDIX A

What Are Genes Really?

The word "gene" to most people, despite its commonplace use, is shrouded in mystery. Most of us don't exactly understand what genes are or what they actually do on a daily basis. A better understanding of what genes are helps you to understand how your body really works. To understand what genes are we need to begin with the idea, that in one sense, cells are quite literally computers.

CELLS ARE ESSENTIALLY COMPUTERS

These things we call cells are in one sense literally, *computers.* It sounds far fetched. In reality, cells do many of the things computers do.

- **FACT:** Cells read and process **digitally encoded** instructions.
- **FACT:** Cells **make decisions** based on inputs of information.
- **FACT:** Cells process signal from "noise." Scientists call it "stochastic decision making." It means they can make decisions from random bits of information in the environment.
- **FACT:** Cells do "networking." They exchange information and programs just like we do between computers with a thumb drive. They use what amounts to a cellular thumb drive. It's basically a micro cell within a cell. Scientists call them **exosomes.** These traveling mini-cells store small programs called micro RNA's and "download" them into other cells.
- **FACT:** Based on decisions, cells activate "programs." We call these programs ***genes.***

Simply put, cells *compute.*

But cells are more like computers we will build in the future. They merge things like energy production, 3D printing, information processing, and structural support together and it all works as a single thing. If cells are essentially computers then can they be programmed?

Yes!

New science papers deal exactly that. Scientists call it **cellular reprogramming.** Cellular reprogramming is exactly what it sounds like. We can program cells for different outcomes, things like killing tumors, clearing non-dividing cells, and even aging slower.

In 2018, the Department of Neurology at Louisiana State, published a paper highlighting the power of both cellular programming and the three genomes. The paper described the potential interaction between the human and bacterial genome. Over 1000 strains of bacteria add over four million micro RNA's into our body! This creates millions of possible interactions between the bacterial and human genome for good or bad. We can't ignore the reality or power of the three genomes any longer.

3D printers atom by atom make solid objects. Your body has something like a 3D printer in every cell. It "prints" proteins. Just like a 3D printer needs a blueprint of the thing it's making, your body needs a "blueprint" of the proteins it makes. The 3D printer uses a **computer program** as the blueprint. The computer program is just a set of instructions in a digitally encoded format. Your body does the same thing. To "print" proteins, it uses a set of instructions in a digitally encoded format. We call those instructions genes.

KEY IDEA: The word "gene" refers to what is essentially a computer program for a biological 3D printer.

A gene is a set of instructions. Those instructions are contained within a kind of digital computer code. Where computers use a two character code called binary, genes use a four character code called quaternary. Every minute of every day inside your cells, genes are used as the blueprints to **"print"** proteins. We tend to think proteins are just nutrients. The reality, however, is **"proteins"** are very complex. For example, enzymes are proteins, but many enzymes are essentially molecular machines.

On a daily basis our bodies "print" thousands of different molecular machines. These machines, or proteins, run the various functions that keep us living. It's like your car. Your car requires special tools and machines to maintain it. Your body works the same way. Instead of storing the tools and machines it needs, it's just easier to make them when you need them and recycle the parts for energy when you don't need them.

The word "genome" in reality, is referring to something like a **library** of programs. Our human genome is the library of blueprints for making the proteins that run our body.

Could Sustained Keto Diets Promote Cancer?

A lot of people, even with seemingly great credentials, are saying a lot of ridiculous things for shock value in this age when it comes to nutrition and food. This is not one of them. What follows is a reveal of the mechanisms at work when a long term intake of fats takes place. All that follows here is an examination of an imbalance of fats to its mechanistic outcome. The purpose of this example is to illustrate how biological duality can effect virtually everything. Generally, we think of Keto Diets as healthy.

The point of this section is that even healthy things can drive disease when imbalanced. We can not expect long term health from a course of action opposing what is true about health. I'm not anti-keto. I use keto-protocols in my nutrition system and have done so since 2009. Keto diets are extremely useful for a number of objectives. They are fantastic protocols. A protocol, however, is not the same thing as a way to eat for life.

KETO DIETS: THE GOOD

The Keto diet has been shown to slow the growth of many cancers. As a result, it has gained a lot of popularity as a diet. Many have made it a way of life. For some cancer patients, the Keto diet is a life saver.

But what if you don't have cancer to begin with?

This is where things get interesting.

We have seen how free radical stress can work both ways, for good or bad. This is especially true in the mitochondria. Free radical stress in the mitochondria can be both good and bad, or even apocalyptic. At low levels free radical stress in the mitochondria is highly beneficial. However, at higher levels and for longer sustained durations, free radical stress in the mitochondria can be highly damaging. Elevated free radical stress in the mitochondria is one of the most powerful drivers of aging, disease and cancer when it gets elevated.

Now here is the point on which everything turns. Free radical stress works **differently in normal vs cancer cells.**

In normal cells you get one set of effects from free radical stress. In cancer cells you can get an **entirely different set of effects** from free radical stress. If a cell doesn't have cancer to begin with, sustained imbalance of free radical stress beyond any debate *promotes* cancer in many tissues. Things often work the opposite way in many cancer cells. At super high levels, free radical stress will kill some cancers. But even then, not all cancers.

FACT: Some cancers actually thrive on high levels of free radical stress.

The effects of oxidative stress depend on the tissue, the duration, concentration, the type of free radical, and **if there is currently cancer present or not.**

Now here is the main point.

Keto diets drive oxidative stress.

When you first go on a Keto diet, free radical stress from oxidized lipids goes up. Then there is a compensation reaction. Free radical stress then goes down. But not indefinitely. Over the very long term, free radical stress from Keto diets begins to go up again. I'll explain how and why. First we need to consider an all important question.

Is free radical stress induced from Keto diets always good?

The answer; oxidative stress from Keto diets has biological duality. Oxidative stress from Keto diets can and does work both ways. It can be beneficial and it can be harmful when (key word) *imbalanced.*

THE MECHANISM AT WORK

There is a primary underlying mechanism driving free radical stress from oxidized lipids from Keto diets. This mechanism is how we can readily see that Keto diets are **not** exempt from biological duality. That mechanism is a very special molecule called 4-HNE.

4-HNE is a huge word but fear not. It's easy to say when we break it up. Broken up, 4-HNE stands for

- 4
- hydroxy
- no
- nenal

Run together its 4-hydroxynonenal, or 4-HNE.

4-HNE IF GODZILLA WERE A MOLECULE

4-HNE can be formed inside the mitochondria. 4-HNE belongs to a special class of molecules called electrophiles. An electrophile is a highly, highly reactive molecule. 4-HNE is highly damaging when it is produced in anything other than small amounts.

FACT: 4-HNE can and does promote direct cancer onset.

One way 4-HNE is formed is when you drink alcohol, which is why heavy drinkers look so aged. The really important thing you need to understand is this.

FACT: 4-HNE is also formed when you eat fats.

4-HNE is a key mechanism behind the beneficial effects on oxidatlve stress in the short term from Keto diets. In the short term, it's the hero of the story. Keto diets produce 4-HNE, which initially causes causes free radical stress. The body responds by making more glutathione. Overall free radical stress then improves The key is small amounts of free radical stress and the short term.

In higher amounts and longer durations, 4-HNE can damage your DNA, tissues and cells in a number of ways. 4-HNE is an oxidized phospholipid. Phospholipids are special fats that make up cellular membranes. We have a chapter called *Young Membranes* because damage to cellular membranes has a lot to do with aging and disease. 4-HNE can be formed in several ways. One way 4-HNE is formed is when very specific fats lining the inside of the mitochondria become oxidized. This very special fat, called *cardiolipin*, is a very big deal. Cardiolipin gives the mitochondria their ability to bend. When cardiolipin becomes oxidized you get 4-HNE. 4-HNE a bit like Godzilla in Tokyo. If it hangs around too long it wrecks total havoc. Damage from 4-HNE makes the mitochondria lose their shape, and in essence, burst. A 2015 paper in the *Journal of Redox Biology* stated, "Evidence provided thus far clearly demonstrated that 4-HNE played an important role in cancer through mitochondria. 4-HNE at low concentrations can protect cancer cells against further damage"

4-HNE BIOLOGICAL DUALITY: The Good , The Bad, The Ugly.
4-HNE exhibits biological duality, but it's not equal. The bad is very bad.

The Good:

- At low levels, for short durations. 4-HNE is good. It promotes antioxidant defenses.
- At medium high levels in some cancer cells it's also good. It induces cell death. 4-HNE is a principal mechanism by which Keto diets kill certain cancers.

The Bad:

- Sustained 4-HNE production in non cancer cells is very, very bad.
- The reason is **4-HNE accumulates** over time.
- As 4-HNE accumulates it ***promotes direct cancer onset in many tissues.***
- 4-HNE can diffuse through membranes. Some cancer cells have the ability to push it next door. Experiments have observed 4-HNE can diffuse from cancer cells and move to non-cancer cells where it can damages cardiolipin in non-cancer cells.

The Ugly:

- At high levels 4-HNE basically makes cells explode, a process called necrosis.

THE PROBLEM

The main problem with 4-HNE is that it *accumulates over time.*

As 4-HNE accumulates biological duality comes into play. The more 4-HNE that accumulates it stops being beneficial at low levels and becomes highly damaging as it accrues. Sustained 4-HNE production in the mitochondria can cause glutathione, the bodies main defense against 4-HNE, to become depleted. As glutathione depletes 4-HNE can then accumulate which in turn causes damaged and mis-folded proteins to accumulate. In particular, as we age and senescent cells accumulate, 4-HNE may be profoundly more damaging with age.

This is the mechanism by which prolonged production of 4-HNE promotes cancer in many cell types.

Once again we see the truth of biological duality. In non cancerous cells at low amounts and for short durations 4-HNE is beneficial. Over time, however, with sustained production, as 4-HNE accumulates it overwhelms the bodies defense mechanisms. **4-HNE works both ways.**

4-HNE is clearly implicated in onset of many cancers by causing mitochondria dysfunction. It can directly promote colon cancer onset by causing pre-cancer cells in the colon to spread. Kidney cancers show high levels of 4-HNE compared to surrounding non cancer cells. Finally, 4-HNE can even promote cancer by inhibiting the repair of DNA.

A number of science papers implicate 4-HNE as central in onset of many kinds of cancer.

- 4-HNE switches off a key protein that inhibits breast cancer.
- 4-HNE is implicated in many gastric cancers
- 4-HNE is known to drive prostate cancer

Summing it up, a little 4-HNE is good. Sustained production of 4-HNE is disastrous for non cancer cells. Now here are three crucial, incontrovertible facts to consider.

FACT: Keto diets drive production of 4-HNE
FACT: 4-HNE has biological duality.
FACT: Sustained production of 4-HNE drives cancer onset.

ADDING IT ALL UP
Keto diets imbalance fats. The science literature has already established that high fat diets can promote cancer. A number of papers in the scientific literature link high fat diets with cancer.

A 2017 paper in the *Journal of Free Radical Biology* noted "...4-hydroxynonenal ..can be produced in big quantities...Notably, an important source of these two compounds is represented by a high fat diet, which is undoubtedly a risk factor for inflammation and Colo Rectal Cancer development." But Keto diets are not necessarily the same thing as high fat diets are they? It depends. Some research papers define high fat diets in a way consistent with Keto diets. Other define high fat diets more in line with the SAD diet.

Can imbalanced Keto Diets promote cancer? Perhaps unlike everything else that shows biological duality, Keto diets get a pass and are only good. That could be a tenable concept if not for one thing - Keto diets produce 4-HNE. Sustained production of 4-HNE is a problem. The scientific evidence suggests that 4-HNE has a dual nature wherever it is produced, by whatever means. The dual nature of 4-HNE is inherit to the molecule. Biological duality of 4-HNE does not simply shut off and go away because you label the thing producing 4-HNE a Keto diet.

In low amounts and short durations 4-HNE helps explain the beneficial effects of Keto diets on free radical stress. For sustained durations, however, 4-HNE accumulates. The effects could become damaging, perhaps even cancer promoting. The course it takes depends on how much, how long and non-cancer versus cancer cells.

The early evidence with animals actually supports biological duality at work in Keto diets. Animal studies show that at the 8 month mark Keto diets inflict mitochondrial damage from oxidative stress.

The thinking of this era is Keto diets are only good and everyone should do them. Let me give you an updated way of thinking about them consistent with the known mechanism of 4-HNE.

- Keto diets **are very effective** against certain kinds of cancers.

- Short term Keto protocols (under one year) in non-cancerous humans are no doubt ***highly beneficial.***

- Long term sustained Keto diets represent a sustained imbalance of fats. Sustained high fat diets can drive imbalanced oxidative stress via 4-HNE production.

As I mentioned earlier, I have had Keto protocols in my VEEP system since 2009. The key is they are balanced with other protocols and we don't do them long term. It's been this way for 10 years. The reason? Balance **is** health. Imbalance **is** disease.

Top 3 Stupidest Things You Can Do While On Keto Diet

4-HNE requires may of the same enzymes needed to detoxify alcohol. In a sense, continued 4-HNE production is like drinking alcohol. The effects in terms of glutathione depletion and mitochondrial damage are very similar. The worst thing you can do is sustained Keto diets with alcohol, and even worse, God help you, fried food.

- Keto diet during week, drink on weekends and eat fried food
- Keto diet during week and drink on weekends
- Keto diet during week with glass of wine every night.

The Map of Bacterial Guilds

This chapter was originally the 5th of the New Foundations. In editing, this chapter took away from the easy flow of readability. **Nevertheless, the contents of this section are among the most important of the entire book.** This idea of bacterial guilds is the 5th foundation. It is essential knowledge. My hope is you will give it a very focused read.

I want to introduce you to a new concept. This is not the 10 year trickle down. What follows is today's real cutting edge. If you are into the gut biome pay maximum attention to what follows. It's going to give you a compass that will allow you to orient what you are doing at any given time and how it will impact the long term. It's going to eliminate confusion and explain how things work.

Welcome to the reality of the Bacterial Guild.

BACTERIAL GUILDS: THE MACRO NUTRIENT COMPASS

There have been a very few landmark scientific papers published regarding the gut biome and our ability to influence it for health. Two of those became the foundation of my VEEP Nutrition System; Dr. Jeffrey Gordon's original study in 2006 and another in 2009 by the Fred Hutchinson Cancer Research Center entitled "Human Gut Bacterial Communities Are Altered by Addition of Cruciferous Vegetables."

In 2017 while researching and writing this book, another was published in the *Journal of Cell Metabolism*, entitled "Diet-Microbiome Interactions in Health Are Controlled by Intestinal Nitrogen. " I believe this particular paper ultimately may be one of the most, important papers ever published in the whole of research on the gut. The reason this paper was/is so important, is that for the first time every, it provides a master framework to create repeatable predictions. It gives us a power to map the long term outcome of any given diet strategy on the gut in a predictive manner. Let me summarize the big ideas in a simple way.

MACRO RATIOS DRIVE GUT MACRO CHEMISTRY

At its core eating is really about giving the body basic elements on the periodic chart. The basic chemistry of life needs a steady supply of things like oxygen, hydrogen, carbon and nitrogen. It's easy to prove. Deprive yourself of any one of these things long enough and you die.

For example, carbohydrates are at the foundation really just ***carbon.*** Carbs bind carbon with water, but essentially they are a source of carbon. Protein is essentially nitrogen. Fats are really just long strings of carbon bound to hydrogen (both of which are absolutely essential to life). If you substitute the word "food", with "elements", it gives you a way to understand how eating is really about getting in the basic elements of biochemistry. I'm not saying that food is just chemistry. It's also signaling and many other things, but viewing food as chemistry is useful. It allows us to make **predictions.** What's powerful is the predictions are not based on narrative (which is what mostly we deal in these days).

The predictions are instead based on **chemistry.**

Chemistry is your friend. It's based on math. The math never lies.

For example, if you get too much nitrogen on a regular basis there are some known outcomes. The chemistry tells us one outcome of too much nitrogen is excess ammonia in the body. Excess ammonia in the body is not good. It interferes with lots of things like cell metabolism, promotes inflammation, and can predispose you to weight gain and colon cancer.

WHY HIGH PROTEIN DIETS DON'T WORK WITH OBESITY

If you suffer from obesity you want to stay away from high protein diets. The reason is obesity or being highly overweight impairs nitrogen disposal Moderate protein intake is suggested during active fat loss until weight is normalized and stable.

THE DAWN OF BACTERIAL GUILDS

A bacteria guild is like a club. Like a lot of clubs, the members can be of different races, backgrounds, preferences, but they all share something in common. Think of a Porsche owners club, for example. You have people from all over the world united by love for Porsches.

What the members of a bacterial guild have in common is they respond in similar ways to **macro nutrient ratio's.** Even though the individual members are totally different species, categories and taxa, they all have the same needs chemically. The Fats guild favors nitrogen, but only from internal nitrogen production. The Carb Guild favors carbon from external sources. favors fats. The Protein Guild favors nitrogen from external sources. You want todays real cutting edge; here it is.

THE REAL CUTTING EDGE

KEY IDEA: Guilds allow health outcome predictions from macro imbalances.

The big idea here has to do with imbalances of raw materials. Long term imbalances of carbon, or in particular, nitrogen, allow reliable predictions regarding disease.

HOW IT WORKS:
The bacteria in your gut are in one sense a giant chemistry plant. Food goes in, chemistry comes out. You eat and breath. Things like Co2, nitrogen, carbon, and nitric oxide get moved around or produced.

KEY IDEA: The end product of bacterial chemistry are chemicals and signals.

What this means is at. the most basic level there are **simple chemical mechanisms driving interactions** between you and the bacteria in your gut.

Why should you care? Because bacterial guilds show us a way to control youth! Specifically, the give us a way to steer **immunity and metabolism via eating!**

Steering immunity and metabolism is one of the principal ways we keep your body young. Now you should care.

THE MAP OF BACTERIAL GUILDS

What bacteria guilds give us is a map - **the Map of Bacterial Guilds**.

The map allows us to make long term predictions, based on the chemistry of basic elements, for macro nutrient imbalances. The key is **nitrogen partitioning.**

NITROGEN PARTITIONING

Nitrogen partitioning just means where do you get your nitrogen from? You can get nitrogen from the diet. You can also manufacture it internally. How nitrogen is produced is very big deal long term. In a process called ***quorum sensing,*** entirely different species of bacteria in your gut work together. They essentially cooperate for availability of nitrogen.

The Map of Bacterial Guilds also tells us what/why will happen in the **absence of food**, such as fasting or time restricted feeding. It unifies both eating and not eating. It gives predictions and explanations.

THE 3 FUNDAMENTAL FORCES STEERING THE GUT

The Map of Guilds tells us how three totally different things drive the gut bacteria composition.

1. Eating: How the sheer ***amounts*** of food impact the gut.
2. Not Eating: How lack of food impacts the gut.
3. Macro Composition: How combinations of macro's impact the gut.

This is big.

Until now, there wasn't a way to explain the disparity of why, in the absence of food, the gut bacteria seem to improve in the short term. This view goes beyond the *properties of foods.* Properties of foods is what I began with in my gut biome career starting in 2006. The main stream marketplace of solutions still has not really figured out how diverse properties of foods and how unique combinations of foods can impact the gut, even though all that is really 10 years old.

KEY IDEA: Properties of food drive individual species.

For example the starches in banana or the dark phenols is blackberries can drive certain strains of bifidobacteria.

The power to drive individual species of bacteria by knowing *what, when and how,* is a big focus in this book. That power alone is many years ahead of the marketplace. But much, much farther ahead still, is **the ability to steer entire guilds.** There are 2 previously unconsidered variables other than properties of foods. These 2 variables are how large amounts of food impact the gut and how lack of food at all impacts the gut.

KEY IDEA: Macro ratio's effect entire guilds.

For example, carbs do not supply nitrogen the way protein does. When carbs are high nitrogen will be generated *somewhat* from diet, but to a great degree **nitrogen will be made internally**. If you eat a lot of carbs or fiber, bacteria that get nitrogen from the diet are at a *disadvantage.* Do you see how macro imbalances can very, very significant consequences.

Protein does the exact opposite. **Protein drives nitrogen from the diet.** At the upper end of very high protein intakes, the limiting resource becomes carbon (carbs = carbon). With high carb ratio's bacteria that get carbon from the diet are disadvantaged. Species of bacteria that get nitrogen from the diet will dominate. This also has very significant consequences.

How your body gets nitrogen will drive entire entire guilds of bacteria in the gut to be either advantaged or disadvantaged. One guild will prosper. Another will wither. The concept of Bacterial Guilds makes if clear that imbalanced macro's disadvantage entire guilds of bacteria. The consequences of this can range from signifiant to catastrophic. Ironically, we live in the Era of Imbalance. This era is all about sustaining long term imbalances from macro ratio's.

KEY IDEA: Deriving nitrogen internally drives health.
From a long term health and immune system perspective, getting nitrogen internally verses from the diet has several advantages for keeping the body young.

INTERNAL NITROGEN DRIVES HEALTH
The immune system is aided and enhanced from bacteria that get nitrogen internally. When nitrogen is derived internally, entire guilds of bacteria that maintain gut lining integrity and optimal immune and

macrophage function are **advantaged.** This is one of the principle benefits of fasting.

KEY IDEA: In the absence of food the body secretes nitrogen internally instead of getting it from the diet.

For example, in Chapter 1 you began spinning up Akkermansia Mucinilpha.

Akkermansia exists inversely with disease.

Wherever we find lots of Akkermansia we find health. Akkermansia needs nitrogen and carbon to live. Akkermansia gets nitrogen and carbon not from diet but from **mucin** (think mucus) **in the gut lining.** Large amounts of dietary nitrogen disadvantage bacteria that get nitrogen from the diet. As a consequence bacteria that rely on internal nitrogen, like Akkermansia, *starve.* When Akkermansia starves the gut mucous layer dies and the immune system becomes compromised.

KEY IDEA: Sustained long term feeding of the Protein Guild starves Akkermansia.

Brock's Colitis From Nitrogen Excess

In 2008 Brock Lesnar was the next big thing in mixed martial arts. His combination of size and power seemed unstoppable. Ironically, the first thing to stop Brock was not another opponent. Brock was taken out by too much protein in the diet. Brock developed severe gut issues that ultimately sidelined him from performing at his peak. His gut issues even threatened his general health. The culprit, according to Brock, himself?

Sustained high protein.

Sustained high protein drives dietary nitrogen. The Protein Guild is advantaged. The Fats Guild is disadvantaged. Akkermansia, specifically, begins to starve. The result? Long term gut and health issues. Mechanistically, high protein diets activate key immune receptors, CD4 and CD8, more than any other diet. Over activation of these receptor drives very important inflammatory responses across the body. Caution, **do not** automatically jump on the time restricted feeding and fasting all the time bandwagon. **You will create more problems than you solve**.

The 2 Day Immunity Core Pattern is designed to perfectly balance out all the needs of the gut by creating cross feeding reactions and the perfect marriage of key fibers to fasting.

The Map of Bacteria Guilds explains why/how different diets and protocols (Keto, carnivore, vegan, fasting, low carb, high protein, high fiber, time restricted feeding) impact the gut biome and tells us the long term inevitable result.

Because the Map of Bacteria Guilds is not based on narrative or story telling (much of what passes for science in nutrition these days is simply narrative or story telling) but chemistry, it's going to win the long game. Its going to win because the math and chemistry always win. There is one huge problem. Reason is dead. It's true.The age of reason has passed. We live in an era where people only want to hear things that make their current position more comfortable.

That's not reason. That's tribalism.

In general we do not want to hear things that, no matter how reasonable, make our position uncomfortable. But reason is the mechanism to learn new things. Without it, we can't learn and grow. So we must suspend tribalism. If you want to grow put back on the armor of reason. Reason gives you the power to acquire new and better ideas based on how things really work.

THE MAP TELLS US THE LONG TERM

Let's see the general overview of the Map of Bacterial Guilds. One thing critical to understand is I am not advocating a Zone type diet.

KEY IDEA: You **do not** need to have balanced macros every meal!

This is not about the four food groups every meal. Quite the opposite.

KEY IDEA: Season of imbalance are normal.

Seasons of imbalance are normal and natural. Our ancestors ate differently j winter versus summer. The problem is not seasons of imbalance. **The problem is sustained long term imbalance.** What the Map of Bacterial Guilds speaks to are sustained imbalances. You can drive short term imbalances without issue. Often short term imbalances can even be for months on end.

THE MAP OF GUILDS

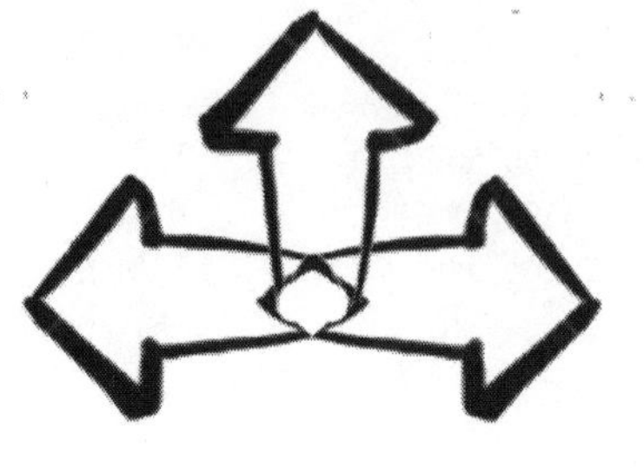

THE PROTEIN GUILD
Nitrogen from diet
Shortest life span
Lower total caloric intake
Poorest long term immunity
Loss of species that maintain intestinal barrier
Lower bacterial diversity

THE CARB GUILD
Nitrogen split between diet and internal
Highest likelihood of obesity & adiposity
Highest bacterial diversity
Paradox - greatest long term health.

THE FAT GUILD
Shortened life span
Increased adiposity
Improved intestinal function

TRIGGERED BY THE MAP

There is a very good chance the map has possibly got you triggered. Some things may seem outrageous or counter-intuitive. For example, The Carb Guild has the greatest long term health? How is that possible? If I use the word vegan in the same statement your mind can now accept it. And it's true, vegan diets are proven to extend lifespan. And yet, vegan diets can also drive obesity and adiposity. Obesity is after all, a plant based disease. Try to see past the labels.

What the Map of Guilds illustrates are extremes.

The map shows the predictable outcome from long term sustained imbalances of each macro group. Seasons and balance are your takeaway ideas. Far from exclusionary, these ideas are inclusive. **They allow all things.** For a season.

KEY IDEA: The bacteria advantaged by each guild drive the predicted health outcomes.

WHEN YOU IMBALANCE FAT

Top 3 Reasons Sustained High Fat Diets (even Keto) Promote Disease

1. **4-HNE:** Sustained high fat diets imbalance 4-HNE. Imbalanced 4-HNE promotes cancer and many other disease states.

2. **Bacterial Guilds:** Sustained high fat diets imbalance bacterial guilds. Long term they advantage guilds that favor obesity.

3. **BIle Acid Residues:** Sustained high fat diets promote non digestible residues of bile acids in the gut. These are called **secondary residues of bile acids.** Sustained accumulation of these secondary residues drive both inflammatory signals and cancer promoting effects.

WHEN YOU IMBALANCE PROTEIN:

Top 3 Reasons Sustained High Protein diets promote diseases.

1. **Cancer Promoting Protein Residues**: Sustained high protein diets leave protein residues in the gut from protein fermenting. These residues drive cancer promotion. You learned about one of these in Chapter .22: Fibers and Butyrate.

2. **Toxic Nitrogen and Sulfer compounds:** When protein ferments in the gut the metabolites are ammonia, amines, nitrates, and hydrogen sulfide, all toxic. Excess ammonia from sustained high protein intake interacts with nitrate compounds. Other bacteria can metabolize these into nitrosamines, one of the most powerful cancer promoters known

3. **Low Butyrate Production:** The metabolite Butyrate is essential for human health. Without it the gut lining is destroyed. Butyrate production from protein has a very limited repertoire of pathways to make Butyrate. When protein is used to make Butyrate it differs dramatically from using fiber. All the pathways to make Butyrate from protein drive the residues listed above while providing lowering total Butyrate production as opposed to fiber.

WHEN YOU IMBALANCE CARBS OR FIBER

Top 3 Reasons Sustained High Carb diets promote diseases.

1. **Excessive Fermentation:** Balance also applies to fermentation, the process by which your body makes bacteria. Too much fermentation can result in intestinal injury along with bloating and diarrhea.

2. **Excessive Insulin Production:** The single most powerful factor aging you after age 45 is insulin production.

3. **Dietary Nitrogen:** Sustained high carb diets, even from healthy carbs, shift the gut towards species that rely on dietary nitrogen. Species that reduce energy harvest from the diet get crowded out. You harvest more energy from food. This promotes weight gain, metabolic syndrome and diabetes. You already know this. What happens when you eat mostly carbs as a way of life?

KEY IDEA: Sustained anything goes against how your body is designed to work.

The ability to utilize various nutritional techniques at the right time in the right way for *functional outcomes is the future.* **Functional outcomes** means you harness and unlock the power of food for various effects. You are learning to do it here. You have learned in this book to use food for functional outcomes like these.

- Slow aging
- Restore the gut lining
- Increase energy
- Burn fat
- Mitigate weight regain from fat loss
- Reduce cancer risk

The best part is you can still have you preferences. Plant based folks can still be plant based. Keto people can still be keto. The shift is you know now seasons of balance are essential. More importantly, you have gained the power to use various foods for function when you ***need to***.

Rethinking Mitochondrial Anti-Aging Strategies

Most of the book I worked very hard to eliminate science jargon and use relatable analogies. This section is not written in the same style. It needs to go right at the science jargon to make the point.

You don't need to read this section to get benefit from the book.

This section is purely supplemental. It is meant to provoke thought and discussion amongst solution providers about the optimal strategies to keep the body young.

The last several years have seen an explosion of products and therapies targeted at the mitochondria to slow aging. At first glance there is very good reason to think this is a solid idea. Age related loss of mitochondria function correlates nearly one to one with aging. To that end we have specialized anti-oxidants, drugs, small molecules and many other things. All promise better health and longer life by targeting the mitochondria.

We may want to rethink that one.

There are a growing number of researchers who support and espouse the view that the peroxisomes are in essence co-organs with the mitochondria. Mechanistically, this view is probably on very safe ground.

Peroxisomes are critical. New research has clearly shown decreased peroxisome function is catastrophic for the body as a whole. In terms of maintaining the cellular redox state, peroxisomes are equal to the mitochondria in importance. Peroxisomes turn hydrogen peroxide into oxygen and water. Low levels of H202 drive anti-aging. When imbalanced from age, excess hydrogen peroxide in the cell damages fats, proteins and DNA via oxidation, slows metabolism and destroys mitochondria function. Perhaps the most pervasive consequence is the activation of what several researchers call a "pro-aging program."

Peroxisomes seem to be at the center of control over cell function, or at the very least, equal to the mitochondria in terms of driving loss of cell function when not functioning optimally. In particular, loss of function in peroxisomes drives loss of function in the mitochondria. Imbalanced redox function with peroxisomes, impairs mitochondria membrane function, redox balance and energy production.

Conversely, when peroxisome redox balance is restored mitochondria function is restored. Markers of mitochondria senesce also improve. A recent paper in the *World Journal of Biologic*

Chemistry noted " We suggest enhancing peroxisome function and maintaining the organelle's redox balance by all means possible."

The majority of current thinking is that cell aging is the result of impaired mitochondria function, damaged DNA, redox stress, glycation, loss or excess of autophagy, and impaired proteasome function. Many researchers are now commenting how profound it is that peroxisomes have been largely ignored until now. It's actually quite shocking to think peroxisomes wield so much power and have been mostly ignored.

REASONS TO RECONSIDER WHAT TO TARGET

Aging of the mitochondria is much more complex that previously believed. It's not as simple as you get old, and have fewer mitochondria. With age, we lose total mitochondria, but not the OXPHOS subunits. The OXPHOS subunits are proteins in the inner mitochondrial membrane. There are five of them and 2 electron carriers. The numbers of these sub units stay consistent.

What seems to drive the decline of mitochondria function with age is a loss of nuclear NAD+ in the mitochondria. What drives this? Pseudo hypoxia via our friend HIF-1. It's mediated by peroxisomes via a unique PGC1/a/b pathway.

All of this brings us to PGC1a.
Activation of signal pathways to enhance mitochondrial function have converged at a single point in recent years, PGC-1a. The transcriptional activator PGC 1a, together with the peroxisome receptor PPAR gamma, serve as the master peroxisome control mechanisms. When activated peroxisomes, proliferate. PGC 1a and PPARg peroxisome proliferator seem to function as a master regulator of the mitochondria. AMPK, the SIRT proteins, all converge on PGC1a. All of the newer modalities of longevity target PGC1a. The long neglected role of peroxisomes as a cellular master regulator merits a rethink of the way we go about doing things to stay young.

We Don't Totally Understand The Mitochondria
The first thing to consider is that how the mitochondria work is not fully known. And while this is also true of peroxisomes, the consequences for tinkering with the mitochondria may have far greater liabilities long term. Strategies like flooding the mitochondria with anti-oxidants could easily do more harm than good. There are simply too many unknowns.

Targeting Peroxisomes May Be The Best of All Worlds
What do peroxisomes do? They metabolize long chain fats. What happens when we either burn fat or feed the body long chain fats? Peroxisomes proliferate. What happens then? The bodies youth pathways activate.

KEY IDEA: The way to get the anti-aging action we want is via targeting peroxisomes not the mitochondria.

Targeting peroxisomes also means rethinking a lot of things. When peroxisomes proliferate there is a greater need to clean up the ones that malfunction. Old cells accumulate malfunctioning peroxisomes which damage the cell. This is Pexophagy. How do we initiate Pexophagy? At this time the optimal way seems to be by feeding the body carbs! Switching substrate from fat to carbs initiates Pexophagy in peroxisomes. This merits a serious rethink of dietary strategies popular today. The Pexophagy unit here in the book does exactly that. Long term, targeting peroxisomes for longevity along with Pexophagy may be the best and safest route to get what we all want.

Why Do Fit People Get Cancer?

WHY DO FIT PEOPLE GET CANCER?

We have all seen or heard of someone fit who came down with cancer - perhaps a bodybuilder, or a trainer you know. There seems to be a paradox. Exercise and diet modifications have been shown to be protective against cancer risk. Yet the modern paradigm of fitness doesn't seem to totally protect against cancer. The key is to understand exercise and the modern paradigm of fitness have diverged. Even as daily exertion is not the same thing as working out, in many ways the modern incarnation of "doing fitness" has veered into many practices that could create a "perfect storm" for cancer onset. It isn't any one thing. It is the presence of many things together at once. Here is a short list.

- Chronic weight cycling.
- High protein intakes and high nitrogen retention.
- High nitric oxide imbalance from pre-workout drinks
- Extreme growth signaling and the practice of spiking insulin

While all of these topics are a book unto themselves, I want to focus on a few of them to illustrate how the effects in theory could work synergistically to increase the probability of cancer onset.

REPEATED WEIGHT CYCLING

Fat cells and cancer cells are **remarkably similar** in how they grow! Cancer cells utilize what is known as the Warburg effect, meaning a high reliance on glycolysis to grow. Fat cells utilize a **Warburg like effect** to facilitate remodeling of the ECM. People who reduce fat repeatedly for a living may be messing with consequences that reach far beyond just being fit. Here is how this works.

Stiffer, more resilient, types of collagen fibers can deposit into the ECM during ECM remodeling. These fibers in turn, emit signals that direct and control immune cell populations. In turn, these populations, like the Red team and the Blue team can control whole body health. Here are just a few things collagen fibers can do.

- They can direct baby fat cells to mature into other types of cells like macrophages.
- They can direct fat cells to make stiffer fibers for the ECM.
- They can even promote cancer onset!

Reshaping the ECM after fat loss takes a **lot** of energy. In fact, the process of growth for any tissue, collagen fibers or otherwise, takes a lot of energy. In one sense, energy consumption and tissue growth are two sides of the same coin. Without a lot of energy, it's very hard for any tissue to grow. When you lose fat, the ECM needs to remodel. To do this fat cells need enormous amounts of glucose and drives a Warburg effect in fat cells. Most surprising is this Warburg like effect in fat cells **can actually feed cancer cells!** We see this a lot in breast cancer. A type of fat cell can develop as a result of ECM signals called a Cancer Adjacent Adipocyte. A Cancer Adjacent Adipocyte is a fat cell that feeds cancer cells the energy they need to grow! Another area where the Warburg like effect of fat cells can feed cancer is obesity. Whether breast cancer, or cancer from obesity, the mechanism is the same.

ECM Stress =>Warburg Like Effect=> ECM remodeling=> Inflammatory immune signaling = > Cancer.

There is clear evidence in the science that repeated weight cycling correlates to all cause mortality. Does it increase cancer risk? The mechanisms of ECM remodeling support the idea. It is an area that remains to be studied.

HIGH PROTEIN INTAKES AND NITROGEN RETENTION

You have so far seen via the Map of Guilds and other chapters that high protein intakes by themselves can promote cancer promoting compounds in the gut. Fiber can neutralizes these compounds. The principle risk would be high protein and low to no fiber. There are other issues related to high protein intakes and cancer.

A 2014 paper in the *Journal of Gerontology* reported individuals in the age bracket of 50-65 with high protein intake had a 4x greater increase of cancer death risk. Conversely, after 65, higher protein intakes actually decrease all cause mortality. A 2019 study of aged men over 65, aligned with the 2014 paper, showing Chinese men over 65 showed protective effects of high protein intake. The principle issues seems to be the **age range of high protein intake.**

KEY IDEA: Lower protein in middle age may protect against cancer. Higher protein intake in old age helps you live longer.

ENERGY DRINKS AND MACROPHAGE POLARITY:

With age most individuals need more stimulation of nitric oxide. It may be that heavy consumption of pre-workout energy drinks in the fitness ecosystem drives the opposite effect. It's possible to have too much nitric oxide.

THE MACROPHAGE NITRIC OXIDE CONNECTION

The presence of excess nitric oxide can dramatically **shift and steer macrophage populations.** The Red Team and the Blue Team compete for arginine. The Blue team converts arginine into ornithine and urea. The Red Team makes nitric oxide. Nitric oxide produces citrulline. Over time the Red Team will be imbalanced. This means inflammatory macrophages become imbalanced. There are two principle reasons. First, citrulline is recycled to make more nitric oxide. Second, most pre-workout drinks ad lots of citrulline. The added citrulline and recycling of citrulline eventually will imbalance the equation and steer macrophages toward the Red Team. Excess nitric oxide drives peroxinitrate formation which is extremely damaging. A pre-wokout drink here and there is not a problem. But daily consumption of pre-workout drinks combined with other nitric oxide enhancing supplements clearly have the potential to **steer macrophages toward the Red Team.**

Now lets ad things up. Sustained high protein intakes, chronic weight cycling, nitric oxide over production, inflammatory macrophages, sustained high growth signaling. Over short periods these things, even combined, **are probably a good thing.** We need growth. We even needs periods of short, intense bursts of growth. It helps us heal up and prevent age related muscle loss. The sustained practice of these things over the long term, however, likely drives the opposite of health.

Omega 3's & MCT's: Friend or Foe?

MCT's are Medium Chain Triglycerides. They are a kind of fat that is currently very popular. I first began using and studying MCT's in the late 80's. A company called Champion Nutrition used them in a product. The label said they were "the fatless fat", a fat that could not be stored as fat. I was fascinated. Fat was the enemy in those days. Everything was "no fat" and "fat free." I began studying them and how they work. Notice something.

I did not make use of MCT's in the 2 Day Immunity Core Pattern.

Why?

The first reason is MCT's do not target fat mass in the way omega 3's do. There are some very important differences. They may even overload the liver with fatty acids, which drives upper body fat storage over the long term.

Also, our objective is to target peroxisomes.

Omega 3's target peroxisomes better than any other food. The peroxisomes exist specifically to handle long chain fats. The idea of peroxisomes and the mitochondria being co-partners changes how we get the things we want: mitochondria biogenesis, extended health span and many other things. Targeting peroxisomes is probably much safer. We need omega 3's to do this. Worse, many forms of MCT break down into palmitic acid. Palmitic acid down-regulates genes that make adiponectin. It also nullifies adiponectin in the blood stream. This is quite detrimental long term. I first wrote on this in 2013 and the market is only now waking up to the long term effects of MCT's. In moderation they are fine. You have a to-do in Young Muscle using them.

OMEGA THREE DUALITY

Just when you thought I was hailing Omega fats as the hero of the story, duality rears its head yet again. Sustained high levels of serum omega **3's shorten lifespan.** The reason is they oxidize. Research with super long lived humans shows they are able to prevent oxidation of long chain fats in the blood. Generally speaking, continual dosing of Omega fats in the diet may drive up serum levels of these fats and oxidation along with them. Sustained lipid peroxidation of long chain fats shortens your life.

KEY IDEA: Sustained high levels of Omega fats in your blood may shorten lifespan.

If this sounds confusing don't worry. The answer is so simple.

Balance.

With the 2 Day Core you have a perfect balance. You get small doses of Omega fats. You don't do them all the time. They are balanced out with high levels of phenols in your serum from the day before. You get the best of both worlds. The serum phenols help offset oxidation of fats in the blood. Key takeaways here are **balance and duality.**

Over Reduction and Aging

What happens if you have too many anti-oxidants? This is a very important question. Today's marketplace seems to convey the idea there is nothing bad to lots of anti-oxidants. Many products try to outcompete one another based on measures of "ORAC Value." ORAC value is a measure of how many anti-oxidants a product has.

TOO MUCH OF A GOOD THING?

Several studies have shown too many anti-oxidants can be harmful.

- Studies have shown high dose vitamin E may increase all cause mortality.
- Excessive anti-oxidants can interfere with critical immune function like cancer suppression.
- Too much vitamin C has been shown to be pro-oxidative.
- One mechanisms of DNA repair is oxidative stress. Excess reduction may actually hurt repair of DNA.
- One researcher, Dr. Barry Halliwell, contends the best defense against free radicals is mild free radical stress. This up regulates the bodies own defenses. As you learned with Keto Diets and 4-HNE, this is exactly why Keto Diets lower oxidative stress in the short term.

IMMUNE SYSTEM OVER REDUCTION

One of the important consequences of over reduction happens with T-cells as we age. Aged T-cells lose the ability to use sugar. The journal Frontiers in Immunology, published a 2017 paper demonstrating how the first step of energy production in the cell, glycolysis, becomes compromised. Instead of using glucose, T-cells push glucose into another cell pathway that makes anti-oxidants called the pentose phosphate pathway. In this state t-cells make too many reducing agents. The result is t-cells become energy starved and can't do their job.

KEY IDEA: Too many anti-oxidants are not good.

Anti oxidants at the wrong time, or too many can drive over reduction. As we age over reduction can be almost as bad as oxidative stress. Here are a few key instances where small amounts of anti-oxidants can be beneficial.

WHEN DO WE NEED ANTI-OXIDANTS:

While the over use of anti-oxidants is probably not good. There are times when anti-oxidants can be very important. Here are some of the safe bets.

1. After large energy dense meals.
2. When taking omega fats.
3. When eating fried food.
4. When sleep deprived.
5. When losing fat.
6. When eating sugar
7. When overexposed to the sun
8. During sleep when chronically inflamed.

How Fibers Offset Cancer Risk of Red Meat

Study after study has shown red meat intake increases risk of colorectal cancer. The culprit? Fermentation of animal protein residues in the gut. Animal Protein residues are metabolized by gut bacteria. They metabolize into compounds that can be mutagenic, that is, they can cause mutations in DNA.

KEY IDEA: Meat feeds bacteria.

Anyone who has ever left a steak out overnight knows that bacteria can grow on meat. Fast. The same is true inside your gut. Meat can ferment in the gut. The residues of this fermentation can be cancer causing. The worst of them is (wait for it)

0-
6-
Methyl-
2-
de-
oxy-
guanosine.

Run together the word is O(6)-methyl-2-deoxyguanosine, a carcinogenic compound. It does absolutely nothing good. It binds with your DNA and can promote cancer promoting mutations. So how do you offset it?

Fiber.

Study after study has shown that resistant starches, things like corn or beans, spin up Butyrate production and **shift fermentation away from protein** to fermentation of starches. The result?

Carcinogenic protein residues from meat do not form.

Once again the highest truth of biology, balance shows itself. When you balance meat out with fibers and starches, the toxic elements of meat are ameliorated.

BIBLIOGRAPHY

AMPK and SIRT:
Mitochondrial sirtuins: regulators of protein acylation and metabolism
AMPK at the Nexus of Energetics and Aging.
AMPK as a Pro-longevity Target.
AMPK activation protects cells from oxidative stress-induced senescence via autophagic flux restoration and intracellular NAD(+) elevation
AMPK at the Nexus of Energetics and Aging Comparing and Contrasting the Roles of AMPK and SIRT1 in Metabolic Tissues
Comparing and Contrasting the Roles of AMPK and SIRT1 in Metabolic Tissues: Marcella Fulco and Sartorel
β-Hydroxybutyrate suppresses inflammasome formation by ameliorating endoplasmic reticulum stress *via* AMPK activation
AMPK activation protects cells from oxidative stress-induced senescence via autophagic flux restoration and intracellular NAD(+) elevation
Adipose tissue and liver expression of SIRT1, 3, and 6 increase after extensive weight loss in morbid obesity.
Enhances Mitochondrial Function in Models of Human Liver.
SIRT5 is under the control of PGC-1α and AMPK and is... [FASEB J. 2014
Mitochondrial energy production correlates with the age-related BMI.[Pediatr Res. 2009]
The role of mitochondria in mTOR-regulated longevity [Biol Rev Camb Philos Soc. 2014]
Inadequate mito-biogenesis in primary dermal fibroblasts from old humans is associated with impairment of PGC1A-independent stimulation [Exp Gerontol. 2014]
AMPK as a Pro-longevity Target.
AMPK and HIF signaling pathways regulate both longevity and cancer growth: the good news and the bad news about survival mechanisms.
SIRT1-AMPK crosstalk is involved in high glucose-dependent impairment of insulin responsiveness in primary rat podocytes.
Effects of Eicosapentaenoic Acid and Docosahexaenoic Acid on Uncoupling Protein 3 Gene Expression in c2c12 Muscle Cells
AMPK and Cancer

MICROBIOME
Cross-feeding between bifidobacteria and butyrate-producing colon bacteria explains bifdobacterial competitiveness, butyrate production, and gas production.
Metabolic activities and probiotic potential of bifidobacteria.
Crosstalk between the gut microbiota and the endocannabinoid system: impact on the gut barrier function and the adipose tissue.
Oral supplementation of healthy adults with 2'-O-fucosyllactose and lacto-N-neotetraose is well tolerated and shifts the intestinal microbiota
Genomic Microdiversity of Bifidobacterium pseudocatenulatum Underlying Differential Strain-Level Responses to Dietary Carbohydrate Intervention.
Microbiota-mitochondria inter-talk: consequence for microbiota-host interaction.
Embracing the gut microbiota: the new frontier for inflammatory and infectious diseases.
Gut Microbiota Promotes Obesity-Associated Liver Cancer through PGE2-Mediated Suppression of Antitumor Immunity.
In vitro modulation of gut microbiota by whey protein to preserve intestinal health.
Prebiotic effects: metabolic and health benefits.
Autoimmunity and the Gut Transkingdom control of microbiota diurnal oscillations promotes metabolic homeostasis
Microbial reprogramming inhibits Western diet-associated obesity.
Diet-Induced Dysbiosis of the Intestinal Microbiota and the Effects on Immunity and Disease
Diet and specific microbial exposure trigger features of environmental enteropathy in a novel murine model.
High-protein diet modifies colonic microbiota and luminal environment but not colonocyte metabolism in the rat model: the increased luminal bulk connection.
Hypothesis: bacteria control host appetites
Changes of the human gut microbiome induced by a fermented milk product.
Gut microbiota fermentation of prebiotics increases satietogenic and incretin gut peptide production with consequences for appetite sensation and glucose response after a meal
Fructose: A Dietary Sugar in Crosstalk with Microbiota Contributing to the Development and Progression of Non-Alcoholic Liver Disease.
Obesity and the gastrointestinal microbiota: a review of associations and mechanisms.
Benefits of polyphenols on gut microbiota and implications in human health - Journal of Nutritional Biochemistry
Gut Microbiota, Short-Chain Fatty Acids, and Herbal Medicines.
Gut Microbiota Orchestrates Energy Homeostasis during Cold
Gut microbiota directs PPARγ-driven reprogramming of the liver circadian clock by nutritional challenge.
Flavonoid metabolism: the interaction of metabolites and gut microbiota
Human milk oligosaccharides and infant gut bifidobacteria: Molecular strategies for their utilization.
Gut Microbiota and Extreme Longevity.
Effect of Lipopolysaccharide on Inflammation and Insulin Action in Human Muscle
Emerging significance of NLRs in inflammatory bowel disease

Dietary red raspberries attenuate dextran sulfate sodium-induced acute colitis
Intestinal Flora and Aging
Effects of diet on gut microbiota profile and the implications for health and disease.
The type and quantity of dietary fat and carbohydrate alter faecal microbiome and short-chain fatty acid excretion in a metabolic syndrome 'at-risk' population.
Differential modulation by Akkermansia muciniphila and Faecalibacterium prausnitzii of host peripheral lipid metabolism and histone acetylation in mouse gut organoids
Combined effects of oligofructose and Bifidobacterium animalis on gut microbiota and glycemia in obese rats.
Glucosinolates and the Human Gut Microbiome
Barley β-glucans-containing food enhances probiotic performances of beneficial bacteria.
Changes in abundance of oral microbiota associated with oral cancer.
Efficacy of Bifidobacterium infantis 35624 in patients with irritable bowel syndrome: a meta-analysis.
The Gut Microbiome and the Brain
Rethinking the bile acid/gut microbiome axis in cancer
The influence of endotoxemia on the molecular mechanisms of insulin resistance.
Gut Bifidobacteria Populations in Human Health and Aging.
Human Gut Bacterial Communities Are Altered by Addition of Cruciferous Vegetables to a Controlled Fruit- and Vegetable-Free Diet
High-protein diet modifies colonic microbiota and luminal environment but not colonocyte metabolism in the rat model: the increased luminal bulk connection.
The NAD dependent deacetylase, Bifidobacterium longum Sir2 in response to oxidative stressThe role of *Escherichia coli* in inflammatory bowel disease
Common gut microbial metabolites of dietary flavonoids exert potent protective activities in β-cells and skeletal muscle cells.
Dietary fructooligosaccharides and potential benefits on health.
Dietary fiber constituents of selected fruits and vegetables.
Health benefits of non-digestible oligosaccharides.
The Microbiome and Butyrate Regulate Energy Metabolism and Autophagy in the Mammalian Colon
Inflammation-Induced Downregulation of Butyrate Uptake and Oxidation Is Not Caused by a Reduced Gene Expression
The bacterial fermentation product butyrate influences epithelial signaling via reactive oxygen species-mediated changes in cullin-1 neddylation.
Combined effects of starvation and butyrate on autophagy-dependent gingival epithelial cell death.
The neuropharmacology of butyrate: The bread and butter of the microbiota-gut-brain axis?
Potential Synergies of *β*-Hydroxybutyrate and Butyrate on the Modulation of Metabolism, Inflammation, Cognition, and General Health
β-Hydroxybutyrate suppresses inflammasome formation by ameliorating endoplasmic reticulum stress via AMPK activation.
Evidence for greater production of colonic short-chain fatty acids in overweight than lean humans.
Butyrate Enhances the Intestinal Barrier by Facilitating Tight Junction Assembly via Activation of AMP-Activated The ketone metabolite β-hydroxybutyrate blocks NLRP3 inflammasome-mediated inflammatory disease.
Butyrate, neuroepigenetics and the gut microbiome: Can a high fiber diet improve brain health?
Protein Kinase in Caco-2 Cell Monolayer

OFFSETTING:

Consumption of blueberries with a high-carbohydrate, low-fat breakfast decreases postprandial serum markers of oxidation
Relationships Between Gastric Emptying, Postprandial Glycemia, and Incretin Hormones.
Blackberry Feeding Increases Fat Oxidation and Improves Insulin Sensitivity in Overweight and Obese Males.
Berries modify the postprandial plasma glucose response to sucrose in healthy subjects.
Postprandial glucose, insulin and glucagon-like peptide 1 responses to sucrose ingested with berries in healthy subjects.
Differential roles of breakfast only (one meal per day) and a bigger breakfast with a small dinner (two meals per day) in mice fed a high-fat diet with regard to induced obesity and lipid metabolism
Lipid Lowering with Soluble Dietary Fiber
Effects of a Protein Preload on Gastric Emptying, Glycemia, and Gut Hormones After a Carbohydrate Meal
Inhibition of Key Digestive Enzymes by Cocoa Extracts 1 and Procyanidins.
Long-term consumption of a raw food diet is associated with favorable serum LDL cholesterol and triglycerides but also with elevated plasma homocysteine and low serum HDL cholesterol in humans
Rebelling against the (Insulin) Resistance: A Review of the Proposed Insulin-Sensitizing Actions of Soybeans, Chickpea Lectin Inhibits Human Breast Cancer Cell Proliferation and Induces Apoptosis Through Cell Cycle Arrest
ACE-inhibitory activity of enzymatic protein hydrolysates from lupin and other legumes.
Chickpeas, and Their Bioactive Compounds.
Sucralose Promotes Food Intake through NPY and a Neuronal Fasting Response.
An afternoon snack of berries reduces subsequent energy intake compared to an isoenergetic confectionary snack.

KETO DIETS:

Ketogenic Diets Enhance Oxidative Stress and Radio- Chemo-Therapy Responses in Lung Cancer
4-hydroxy-2-nonenal metabolism in heart disease
A long-term high-fat diet increases oxidative stress, mitochondrial damage and apoptosis in the inner ear of D-galactose-induced aging rats.
Inflammation and Oxidative Stress in Neurological Disorders
4-Hydroxynonenal metabolites and adducts in pre-carcinogenic conditions and cancer
Ketogenic diet in cancer therapy
Long-term ketogenic diet contributes to glycemic control but promotes lipid accumulation and hepatic steatosis in type 2 diabetic mice

Induced and controlled dietary ketosis as a regulator of obesity and metabolic syndrome pathologies
A high-fat, ketogenic diet causes hepatic insulin resistance in mice, despite increasing energy expenditure and preventing weight gain
Low-carbohydrate ketogenic diets, glucose homeostasis, and nonalcoholic fatty liver disease
Ketogenic Diet Impairs FGF21 Signaling and Promotes Differential Inflammatory Responses in the Liver and White Adipose Tissue.
The Mechanisms by Which the Ketone Body D-β-Hydroxybutyrate May Improve the Multiple Cellular Pathologies of Parkinson's Disease
Ketogenic diet regulates the antioxidant catalase via the transcription factor PPARγ2.
Acute oxidative stress and systemic Nrf2 activation by the ketogenic diet
Indispensable Amino Acid–Deficient Diets Induce Seizures in Ketogenic Diet–Fed Rodents
Disordered mineral metabolism produced by ketogenic diet therapyThe Gut Microbiota Mediates the Anti-Seizure Effects of the Ketogenic Diet
Cancer growth regulation by 4-hydroxynonena.

SLEEP:
Human Behavior: Sleep in Hunter–Gatherer Societies
The arrival of circadian medicine
Rhythmic Oxygen Levels Reset Circadian Clocks through HIF1α
Mitochondrial bioenergetics decay in aging: beneficial effect of melatonin
How does diurnal intermittent fasting impact sleep, daytime sleepiness, and markers of the biological clock? Current insights.
High-glycaemic index and -glycaemic load meals increase the availability of tryptophan in healthy volunteers.
The physiological effects of slow breathing in the healthy human.
Carbon monoxide and nitric oxide: interacting messengers in muscarinic signaling to the brain's circadian clock
Relationship between obstructive sleep apnea and endogenous carbon monoxide.
The coupling between peripheral microcirculation and slow breathing.
A Pilot Study on the Effects of Slow Paced Breathing on Current Food Craving.
The putative role of oxidative stress and inflammation in the pathophysiology of sleep dysfunction across neuropsychiatric disorders: Focus on chronic fatigue syndrome, bipolar disorder and multiple sclerosis
Fasting Induces a Large, Leptin-Dependent Increase in the Intrinsic Action Potential Frequency of Orexigenic Circadian Reprogramming in the Liver Identifies Metabolic Pathways of Aging.
Functional central rhythmicity and light entrainment, but not liver and muscle rhythmicity, are Clock independent. - Nutrition in the spotlight: metabolic effects of environmental light
The circadian clock regulates inflammatory arthritis.
Metabolism and the Circadian Clock Converge
Publications | National Institute on Alcohol Abuse and Alcoholism
The association of pineal gland volume and body mass in obese and normal weight individuals: a pilot study.
The adipocyte clock controls brown adipogenesis through the TGF-β and BMP signaling pathways.
Molecular clock integration of brown adipose tissue formation and function.
24-hour rhythms of DNA methylation and their relation with rhythms of RNA expression in the human dorsolateral prefrontal cortex.
Effects of aging on circadian patterns of gene expression in the human prefrontal cortex.
The transcriptional regulators, the immune system and the the circadian clock.
Diurnal Variations of Human Circulating Cell-Free Micro-RNA.
The association among chronotype, timing of food intake and food preferences depends on body mass status. - Sleep restriction increases free fatty acids in healthy men.
A single night of partial sleep deprivation induces insulin resistance in multiple metabolic pathways in healthy subjects.
Role of the clock gene Rev-erbα in metabolism and in the endocrine pancreas.
A high-fat diet has a tissue-specific effect on adiponectin and related enzyme expression.
Aged Stem Cells Reprogram Their Daily Rhythmic Functions to Adapt to Stress.
Analysis of circadian properties and healthy levels of blue light from smartphones at night
Unique aspects of competitive weightlifting: performance, training and physiology.
Circadian nutritional behaviours and cancer risk: New insights from the NutriNet-Santé prospective cohort study. - Arcuate Nucleus Neuropeptide Y/Agouti-Related Protein Neurons
How Breath-Control Can Change Your Life: A Systematic Review on Psycho-Physiological Correlates of Slow Breathing.
Ketone bodies mimic the life span extending properties of caloric restriction
Human gut bacteria as potent class I histone deacetylase inhibitors in vitro through production of butyric acid and valeric acid
Histone deacetylase inhibitors: Understanding a new wave of anticancer agents

AGING:
Longevity and diet in Okinawa, Japan: the past, present and future.
Microbial Genetic Composition Tunes Host Longevity
Cellular Decision-Making and Biological Noise: From Microbes to Mammal
New data on programmed aging - slow phenoptosis.
NAD+ metabolism: Bioenergetics, signaling and manipulation for therapy.
The power to reduce: pyridine nucleotides – small molecules with a
multitude of functions
The NAD World: a new systemic regulatory network for metabolism and aging--Sirt1, systemic NAD biosynthesis, and their importance.
Exploiting methionine restriction for cancer treatment.
Dietary methionine restriction regulated energy and protein homeostasis by improving thyroid function in high fat diet mice
Prevention of Senescence in Vasculature Through Quiescence.

Rejuvenation: It's in our blood
Small Molecule–Mediated Activation of the Integrin CD11b/CD18 Reduces Inflammatory Disease
Profiling IgG N-glycans as potential biomarker of chronological and biological ages: A community-based study in a Han Chinese population.
Oxidative stress and vascular inflammation in aging.
PI3K / Akt Signaling Resources
Changes in serotonin (5-HT) and brain-derived neurotrophic factor (BDFN) expression in frontal cortex and hippocampus of aged rat treated with high
Nutritional strategies to optimise cognitive function in the aging brain.
Targeting mTOR signaling by polyphenols: a new therapeutic target for ageing.
Polyphenols control and reduce inflammation through a series.
Chrono-nutrition: a review of current evidence from observational studies on global trends in time-of-day of energy intake and its association with.
Glycans are a novel biomarker of chronological and biological ages
Dietary methionine restriction regulated energy and protein homeostasis by improving thyroid function in high fat diet mice
Inflammaging and 'Garb-aging
The mechanism of phenoptosis:. Hayflick limit is caused by the programmed attenuation of bioenergetics]
Inflammaging: disturbed interplay between autophagy and inflammasomes.
Preferential PPAR-α activation reduces neuroinflammation, and blocks neurodegeneration in vivo.
New data on programmed aging - slow phenoptosis.
What has passed is prolog: new cellular and physiological roles of G6PD
Regulation of Copper and Iron Homeostasis by Metal Chelators: A Possible Chemotherapy for Alzheimer's Disease.
Aging: progressive decline in fitness due to the rising deleteriome adjusted by genetic, environmental, and stochastic processes
IL-10 prevents aging-associated inflammation and insulin resistance in skeletal muscle.
rBTI extends Caenorhabditis elegans lifespan by mimicking calorie restriction.
The pif1 helicase, a negative regulator of telomerase, acts preferentially at long telomeres.
Intranasal Insulin Improves Age-Related Cognitive Deficits and Reverses Electrophysiological Correlates of Brain Aging.
Aging as an Evolvability-Increasing Program Which can be Switched Off by Organism to Mobilize Additional Resources for Survival.
Combined effects of starvation and butyrate on autophagy-dependent gingival epithelial cell death.
Insulin, Aging, and the Brain: Mechanisms and Implications
Vitamin C Treatment Restores TET2 Deficiency and Confers Sensitivity to PARP Inhibition
Clinical applications of fucoidan in translational medicine for adjuvant cancer therapy
Discovery of IDO1 inhibitors: from bench to bedside
Glucose Restriction Plus Refeeding in Vitro Induce Changes of the Human Adipocyte Secretome with an Impact on Complement Factors and Cathepsins.
Dietary Strategies for Weight Loss Maintenance.
Weight loss-induced stress in subcutaneous adipose tissue is related to weight regain.
Changes in the blood antioxidant defense of advanced age people
An Update on Inflamm-Aging: Mechanisms, Prevention, and Treatment
DNA methylation-based estimator of telomere length
N-glycomic biomarkers of biological aging and longevity: a link with inflammaging.
A role for leukocyte integrins and extracellular matrix remodeling of adipose tissue in the risk of weight regain after weight loss.
Matrix metalloproteinase interactions with collagen and elastin
Incorporation of Omega-3 Fatty Acids Into Human Skeletal Muscle Sarcolemmal and Mitochondrial Membranes Following 12 Weeks of Fish Oil Supplementation
The cardiometabolic benefits of glycine: Is glycine an 'antidote' to dietary fructose?
Mechanisms of hypoxia signalling: new implications for nephrology.
Molecular mechanism and physiological role of pexophagy
Exploring the molecular interface between hypoxia-inducible factor signalling and mitochondria
Ketosis may promote brain macroautophagy by activating Sirt1 and hypoxia-inducible factor-1
Phosphatidylethanolamine Is a Key Regulator of Membrane Fluidity in Eukaryotic Cells
Sarcopenia: Molecular, Cellular, and Nutritional Aspects
Deletion of Pofut1 in Mouse Skeletal Myofibers Induces Muscle Aging-Related Phenotypes in cis and in trans
Fisetin is a senotherapeutic that extends health and lifespan.
Molecular hydrogen stimulates the gene expression of transcriptional coactivator PGC-1α to enhance fatty acid metabolism
Recent Advances in Studies of Molecular Hydrogen against Sepsis
Peroxisomes and Cellular Oxidant/Antioxidant Balance: Protein Redox Modifications and Impact on Inter-organelle Communication.
Redox Regulation of Homeostasis and Proteostasis in Peroxisomes.
Anthocyanidins and anthocyanins: colored pigments as food, pharmaceutical ingredients, and the potential health benefits
Targeting the ROS-HIF-1-endothelin axis as a therapeutic approach for the treatment of obstructive sleep apnea-related cardiovascular complications
A New Proposal for the Pathogenic Mechanism of Non-Coeliac/Non-Allergic Gluten/Wheat Sensitivity: Piecing Together the Puzzle of Recent Scientific .
Understanding the physicochemical properties and degradation kinetics of nicotinamide riboside, a promising vitamin B3nutritional supplement.
Molecular hydrogen suppresses superoxide generation in the mitochondrial complex I and reduced mitochondrial membrane potential.
Akkermansia muciniphila reduces Porphyromonas gingivalis-induced inflammation and periodontal bone destruction.

Oral microbiota-induced periodontitis: a new risk factor of metabolic diseases.
Bacterial CpG-DNA Triggers Activation and Maturation of Human CD11c−, CD123+ Dendritic Cells
Muscle-Derived Extracellular Signal-Regulated Kinases 1 and 2 Are Required for the Maintenance of Adult Myofibers and their Neuromuscular Junctions
MicroRNA-425-5p promotes breast cancer cell growth by inducing PI3K/AKT signaling.
Sleep patterns in Amazon rubber tappers with and without electric light at home
Alternate day fasting for weight loss in normal weight and overweight subjects: a randomized controlled trial-
Nutrition and the Circadian System
Effects of whole grain rye, with and without resistant starch type 2 supplementation, on glucose tolerance, gut hormones, inflammation and appetite regulation in an 11–14.5 hour perspective; a randomized controlled study
Whole Fruits and Fruit Fiber Emerging Health Effects
Arabinogalactan-Proteins: Key Regulators at the Cell Surface]
Dietary lignans: physiology and potential for cardiovascular disease risk reduction
The Metabolic Signature of Macrophage Responses
Nitric Oxide Produced by Macrophages Inhibits Adipocyte Differentiation and Promotes Profibrogenic Responses in Preadipocytes to Induce Adipose Tissue...
Attenuating Cholinergic Transmission Increases the Number of Satellite Cells and Preserves Muscle Mass in Old Age.
Angiotensin-II Drives Human Satellite Cells Toward Hypertrophy and Myofibroblast Trans-Differentiation by Two Independent
Age-dependent effects of caloric restriction on mTOR and ubiquitin-proteasome pathways in skeletal muscles.
ENOX2 target for the anticancer isoflavone ME-143.
IL-1β- and IL-4-polarized macrophages have opposite effects on adipogenesis of intramuscular fibro-adipogenic progenitors in humans.
Ketogenic diet in cancer therapy
Inducible Brown Adipose Tissue, or Beige Fat, Is Anabolic for the Skeleton
Effect of body fat distribution on the transcription response to dietary fat interventions
Vitamin D deficiency changes the intestinal microbiome reducing B vitamin production in the gut.
A Closer Look at Hypoglossal Nerve Stimulation for Obstructive Sleep Apnea
The Impact of Aging on Adipose Function and Adipokine Synthesis
Inflammation, But Not Telomere Length, Predicts Successful Ageing at Extreme Old Age: A Longitudinal Study of Semi-supercentenarians.
Inflamm-aging. An evolutionary perspective on immunosenescence.
Immunosenescence and Inflamm-Aging As Two Sides of the Same Coin: Friends or Foes?
DNA damage and transcription stress cause ATP-mediated redesign of metabolism and potentiation of anti-oxidant buffering.
Thermodynamics in Neurodegenerative Diseases: Interplay Between Canonical WNT/Beta-Catenin Pathway-PPAR Gamma, Energy Metabolism and Circadian Rhythms.
Eicosapentaenoic acid and arachidonic acid differentially regulate adipogenesis, acquisition of a brite phenotype and mitochondrial function in primary human adipocytes.
Eicosapentaenoic Acid Reduces Adiposity, Glucose Intolerance and Increases Oxygen Consumption Independently of Uncoupling Protein 1.
Angiotensin II revisited: new roles in inflammation, immunology and aging
A metabolic profile of all-cause mortality risk identified in an observational study of 44,168 individuals
Sweetening the Pot: Adding Glycosylation to the Biomarker Discovery Equation
Hemostasis and ageing
Young blood products: emerging treatment for Alzheimer's disease?
The Possible Mechanisms Underlying the Impairment of HIF-1α Pathway Signaling in Hyperglycemia and the Beneficial Effects of Certain Therapies
Red blood cell oxidative stress impairs oxygen delivery and induces red blood cell aging.
Modulatory influence of sex hormones on vascular aging.
Parabiosis Incompletely Reverses Aging-Induced Metabolic Changes and Oxidant Stress in Mouse Red Blood Cells.
Omega-3 fatty acids and adipose tissue biology.
Chronic Inflammation as a Link between Periodontitis and Carcinogenesis
Exosomes derived from M1 macrophages aggravate neointimal hyperplasia following carotid artery injuries in mice through miR-222/CDKN1B/CDKN1C pathway.
Antibiotics promote inflammation through the translocation of native commensal colonic bacteria.
Periodontitis and breast cancer: A case-control study.
Earliest evidence of the cooking and eating of starch
Insulin signaling in the arterial wall
Nitric Oxide and Peroxynitrite in Health and Disease
High glucose induces DNA damage in cultured human endothelial cells.
Hydroxytyrosol Ameliorates Endothelial Function under Inflammatory Conditions by Preventing Mitochondrial Dysfunction.
Zinc Downregulates HIF-1α and Inhibits Its Activity in Tumor Cells In Vitro and In Vivo
Exogenous Ketone Bodies as Promising Neuroprotective Agents for Developmental Brain Injury Neuroscience 2018,
Action of nicotinic acid on the reversion of hypoxic-inflammatory link on 3T3-L1 adipocytes | Lipids in Health and Disease |
Interacting NAD+ and Cell Senescence Pathways Complicate Antiaging Therapies.
Metabolic Dysregulation and Adipose Tissue Fibrosis: Role of Collagen VI | Molecular and Cellular Biology
Selective and membrane-permeable small molecule inhibitors of nicotinamide N-methyltransferase reverse high fat diet-induced obesity in mice
Small molecule nicotinamide N-methyltransferase inhibitor activates senescent muscle stem cells and improves regenerative capacity of aged skeletal muscle.
Covalent targeting of the vacuolar H+-ATPase activates autophagy via mTORC1 inhibition
Cellular senescence in aging and age-related disease: from mechanisms to therapy

Substantial fat mass loss reduces low-grade inflammation and induces positive alteration in cardiometabolic factors in normal-weight individuals.
CD4+ T cells memorize obesity and promote weight regain
Adipocyte abundances of CES1, CRYAB, ENO1 and GANAB are modified in-vitro by glucose restriction and are associated with cellular remodelling during weight regain
Combined Analysis of Stress- and ECM-Related Genes in Their Effect on Weight Regain
Extracellular matrix remodeling and matrix metalloproteinase inhibition in visceral adipose during weight cycling in mice. -
Macrophage polarization and Metainflammation
On the role of macrophages in the control of adipocyte energy metabolism
Hyperoxygenation revitalizes Alzheimer's disease pathology through the upregulation of neurotrophic factors.
Hesperetin, a Citrus Flavonoid, Attenuates LPS-Induced Neuroinflammation, Apoptosis and Memory Impairments by Modulating TLR4/NF-κB Signaling.
Dietary Intervention Modifies DNA Methylation Age Assessed by the Epigenetic Clock.
Oral Lactobacillus Counts Predict Weight Gain Susceptibility: A 6-Year Follow-Up Study
Is Obesity an Oral Bacterial Disease?
Dietary Alteration of the Gut Microbiome and Its Impact on Weight and Fat Mass: A Systematic Review and Meta-Analysis
Dietary n-6/n-3 FA Ratio, but Not Total Content of n-3 PUFA, Regulates Diet-induced Obesity, Insulin Resistance, and Metabolic Dysfunction
Dairy consumption and insulin sensitivity: a systematic review of short- and long-term intervention studies.
Targeting glucose metabolism for healthy aging
A Multi-omics Approach to Unraveling the Microbiome-Mediated Effects of Arabinoxylan Oligosaccharides in Overweight Humans
Effects of Dietary Fiber and Its Components on Metabolic Health
Diet, microorganisms and their metabolites, and colon cancer
Colonocyte metabolism shapes the gut microbiota
Alpha-Ketoglutarate and intestinal function.
Metabolic Adaptation of the Small Intestine to Short- and Medium-Term High-Fat Diet Exposure.
High-dose ascorbic acid increases intercourse frequency and improves mood: a randomized controlled clinical trial
Aging of the mammalian gastrointestinal tract: a complex organ system
Macrophage-derived IL-10 mediates mucosal repair by epithelial WISP-1 signaling
Orange juice neutralizes the proinflammatory effect of a high-fat, high-carbohydrate meal and prevents endotoxin increase and Toll-like receptor expression.
Altered ascorbic acid status in the mucosa from inflammatory bowel disease patients.
Tumor necrosis factor alpha reduces butyrate oxidation in vitro in human colonic mucosa: a link from inflammatory process to mucosal damage?
Diurnal transcriptome atlas of a primate across major neural and peripheral tissues
A circadian gene expression atlas in mammals: Implications for biology and medicine
Pterostilbene alleviates hydrogen peroxide-induced oxidative stress via nuclear factor erythroid 2 like 2 pathway in mouse preimplantation embryos.
Chronobiology of Aging: A Mini-Review.
Natural Products for Antithrombosis.
The Gut Microbiota Mediates the Anti-Seizure Effects of the Ketogenic Diet.
From the Cover: The microbial metabolite butyrate regulates intestinal macrophage function via histone deacetylase inhibition
Association of dietary folate and vitamin B-12 intake with genome-wide DNA methylation in blood: CCL11, a novel mediator of inflammatory bone resorption.
Young Blood Rejuvenates Old Bodies: A Call for Reflection when Moving from Mice to Men
Dietary bioactive peptides: Human studies.
Three Natural Inhibitors of Coagulation - Laboratory Continuing Education
FGF stimulation of the Erk1/2 signalling cascade triggers transition of pluripotent embryonic stem cells from self-renewal to lineage commitment
Lactate administration activates the ERK1/2, mTORC1, and AMPK pathways differentially according to skeletal muscle type in mouse - Cerda-Kohler - 2018 - Physiological Reports
Aging impairs contraction-induced human skeletal muscle mTORC1 signaling and protein synthesis
Redox signaling in skeletal muscle: role of aging and exercise
Solstice Pod Guide
ERK1/2 MAP kinases: structure, function, and regulation.
Validation of USP30 as a Therapeutic Target for Parkinson's Disease Modification | Parkinson's Disease
Chronobiology of the Immune System
Seven-day human biological rhythms: An expedition in search of their origin, synchronization, functional advantage, adaptive value and clinical relevance
Acute effects of resistance exercise and intermittent intense aerobic exercise on blood cell count and oxidative stress in trained middle-aged women
Circadian and circaseptan rhythms in implant-based thoracic impedance
Adipose Tissue Inflammation in Aging
Role of microRNA-mediated MMP regulation in the treatment and diagnosis of malignant tumors
Systematic review of the association between dietary acid load, alkaline water and cancer.
The Relationship Between the Human Genome and Microbiome Comes into View.
The Crosstalk between the Gut Microbiota and Mitochondria during Exercise
Vitamin D receptor genotype is associated with Addison's disease.
Aging is associated with an increase in T cells and inflammatory macrophages in visceral adipose tissue.
Nitric Oxide Synthase 2 Induction Promotes Right Ventricular Fibrosis.
Oral Microbiome and Nitric Oxide: the Missing Link in the Management of Blood Pressure.

The role for adipose tissue in weight regain after weight loss
Dieting and restrained eating as prospective predictors of weight gain
Long-term ketogenic diet contributes to glycemic control but promotes lipid accumulation and hepatic steatosis in type 2 diabetic mice.
A Common Allele in FGF21 Associated with Sugar Intake Is Associated with Body Shape, Lower Total Body-Fat Percentage, and Higher Blood Pressure.
Matrix metalloproteinase 11 protects from diabesity and promotes metabolic switch.
Unsolved mysteries: How does lipid peroxidation cause ferroptosis?
Diet, microorganisms and their metabolites, and colon cancer.
Gut microbiota, metabolome and immune signatures in patients with uncomplicated diverticular disease.
Abstract
Sirtuin 1 (SIRT1): the misunderstood HDAC.
NAD+ metabolism and the control of energy homeostasis - a balancing act between mitochondria and the nucleus
Activation of Gpr109a, receptor for niacin and the commensal metabolite butyrate, suppresses colonic inflammation and carcinogenesis.
α-Tocopherol succinate enhances pterostilbene anti-tumor activity in human breast cancer cells in vivo and in vitro.
L-Arginine supplementation inhibits the growth of breast cancer by enhancing innate and adaptive immune responses mediated by suppression of MDSCs in vivo
Poly(ADP-ribose) polymerase-1 modulation of in vivo response of brain hypoxia-inducible factor-1 to hypoxia/reoxygenation is mediated by nitric oxide.
Lipopolysaccharide Stimulates p62-Dependent Autophagy-Like Aggregate Clearance in Hepatocytes
Pexophagy: Molecular Mechanisms and Implications for Health and Diseases
The Gut Microbiome Alterations and Inflammation-Driven Pathogenesis of Alzheimer's Disease-a Critical Review.
Role of Physiological Levels of 4-Hydroxynonenal on Adipocyte Biology: Implications for Obesity and Metabolic Syndrome
4-Hydroxy-2(E)-nonenal (HNE) catabolism and formation of HNE adducts are modulated by β oxidation of fatty acids in the isolated rat heart
Acute oxidative stress and systemic Nrf2 activation by the ketogenic diet
Mitochondria and Cancer: Cell
Senescence-Inflammatory Regulation of Reparative Cellular Reprogramming in Aging and Cancer
NAD+ ameliorates inflammation-induced epithelial barrier dysfunction in cultured enterocytes and mouse ileal mucosa.
NAD(P)H Oxidase Activity in the Small Intestine Is Predominantly Found in Enterocytes, Not Professional Phagocytes.
Sulfide, the first inorganic substrate for human cells. - -
Oxidation of hydrogen sulfide remains a priority in mammalian cells and causes reverse electron transfer in colonocytes.
Characterization of the Pro-Inflammatory Cytokine IL-1β on Butyrate Oxidation in Colorectal Cancer Cells.
Why NAD+ Declines during Aging: It's Destroyed: Cell Metabolism
Palmitate-induced IL6 expression ameliorated by chicoric acid through AMPK and SIRT1-mediated pathway in the PBMCs of newly diagnosed type 2 diabetes
The Time of Metabolism: NAD+, SIRT1, and the Circadian Clock
Flavonoid apigenin is an inhibitor of the NAD+ ase CD38: implications for cellular NAD+ metabolism, protein acetylation, and treatment of metabolic
Mechanism and cell signaling pathways of 4-HNE-induced pathophysiology variability in duodenal peptic ul
4-Hydroxynonenal metabolites and adducts in pre-carcinogenic conditions and cancer
Cancer growth regulation by 4-hydroxynonenal.
Diet, Gut Microbiota, and Vitamins D + A in Multiple Sclerosis.
The Effect of High Dose Isoflavone Supplementation on Serum Reverse T3 in Euthyroid Men With Type 2 Diabetes and Post-menopausal Women.
Relationships Between Gastric Emptying, Postprandial Glycemia, and Incretin Hormones | Diabetes Care
Circadian toxicity of environmental pollution. Inhalation of polluted air to give a precedent
The role of hypoxia-inducible factors in carotid body (patho) physiology.
Effects of hypoxia on the brain: neuroimaging and neuropsychological findings following carbon monoxide poisoning and obstructive sleep apnea.
Reactive oxygen radicals and gaseous transmitters in carotid body activation by intermittent hypoxia.
Relationship between obstructive sleep apnea and endogenous carbon monoxide.
Carbon Monoxide Exposures to Los Angeles Area Commuters: Journal of the Air Pollution Control Association:
The coupling between peripheral microcirculation and slow breathing.
A Pilot Study on the Effects of Slow Paced Breathing on Current Food Craving.
How Breath-Control Can Change Your Life: A Systematic Review on Psycho-Physiological Correlates of Slow Breathing.
Frontiers | Gut Microbiota, Short-Chain Fatty Acids, and Herbal Medicines | Pharmacology
Fluoride deposition in the aged human pineal gland.
Nasal high flow therapy: a novel treatment rather than a more expensive oxygen device
Pineal Calcification, Melatonin Production, Aging, Associated Health Consequences and Rejuvenation of the Pineal Gland
Daily ingestion of alkaline electrolyzed water containing hydrogen influences human health, including gastrointestinal symptoms.
Flavonoid metabolism: the interaction of metabolites and gut microbiota.
Common gut microbial metabolites of dietary flavonoids exert potent protective activities in β-cells and skeletal muscle cells.
Cocoa procyanidins with different degrees of polymerization possess distinct activities in models of colonic inflammation. -
Role of Apigenin in Cancer Prevention via the Induction of Apoptosis and Autophagy
PPAR Agonists and Metabolic Syndrome: An Established Role?
Berberine is a potential therapeutic agent for metabolic syndrome via brown adipose tissue activation and metabolism regulation.
Berberine reversed the epithelial-mesenchymal transition of normal colonic epithelial cells induced by SW480 cells through regulating the important.

An afternoon snack of berries reduces subsequent energy intake compared to an isoenergetic confectionary snack.
Effects of a Protein Preload on Gastric Emptying, Glycemia, and Gut Hormones After a Carbohydrate Meal in Diet-Controlled Type 2 Diabetes
Exercise Increases 24-h Fat Oxidation Only When It Is Performed Before Breakfast.
Berries modify the postprandial plasma glucose response to sucrose in healthy subjects.
Postprandial glucose, insulin and glucagon-like peptide 1 responses to sucrose ingested with berries in healthy subjects.
Blackberry Feeding Increases Fat Oxidation and Improves Insulin Sensitivity in Overweight and Obese Males.
The Fibrillin-1 RGD Integrin Binding Site Regulates Gene Expression and Cell Function through microRNAs
The arrival of circadian medicine
Capsaicin increases sensation of fullness in energy balance, and decreases desire to eat after dinner in negative energy balance.
Human Behavior: Sleep in Hunter–Gatherer Societies: Current Biology
Differential roles of breakfast only (one meal per day) and a bigger breakfast with a small dinner (two meals per day) in mice fed a high-fat diet with regard to induced obesity and lipid metabolism
How does diurnal intermittent fasting impact sleep, daytime sleepiness, and markers of the biological clock? Current insights.
Mitochondrial bioenergetics decay in aging: beneficial effect of melatonin.
Histone deacetylase inhibitors: Understanding a new wave of anticancer agents - Villar-Garea - 2004 - International Journal of
Calcium and electrical signaling in arterial endothelial tubes: New insights into cellular physiology and cardiovascular function.
Insulin, Aging, and the Brain: Mechanisms and Implications
Mitochondrial sirtuins: regulators of protein acylation and metabolism
Human HMGCS2 Regulates Mitochondrial Fatty Acid Oxidation and FGF21 Expression in HepG2 Cell Line
Repairing the Damaged Plasma Membrane of the Cell and the Membrane-Bound Organelles
Omega-3 Fatty Acids and PPARγ in Cancer
Ascorbate induces autophagy in pancreatic cancer.
Consumption of blueberries with a high-carbohydrate, low-fat breakfast decreases postprandial serum markers of oxidation.
Human skeletal muscle ascorbate is highly responsive to changes in vitamin C intake and plasma concentrations.
Retinol palmitate and ascorbic acid: Role in oncological prevention and therapy.
Peroxisomes, oxidative stress, and inflammation
Ascorbic acid, but not dehydroascorbic acid increases intracellular vitamin C content to decrease Hypoxia Inducible Factor -1
Mammalian glutamine metabolism controls circadian rhythm through regulation of reactive oxygen species | Cancer Research
Circadian Regulation of Glutamate Transporters
Hypoxic insomnia: effects of carbon monoxide and acclimatization.
Long-term consumption of a raw food diet is associated with favorable serum LDL cholesterol and triglycerides but also with elevated plasma homocystein
The putative role of oxidative stress and inflammation in the pathophysiology of sleep dysfunction across neuropsychiatric disorders:
Skeptical approaches concerning the effect of exposure to electromagnetic fields on brain hormones and enzyme activities.
Carbon monoxide and nitric oxide: interacting messengers in muscarinic signaling to the brain's circadian clock.
Potential Crosstalk between Fructose and Melatonin: A New Role of Melatonin-Inhibiting the Metabolic Effects of Fructose.
Gut microbiota directs PPARγ-driven reprogramming of the liver circadian clock by nutritional challenge.
The neuronal and endocrine roles of RCAN1 in health and disease.
The Use of a Stem and Leaf Aqueous Extract of Cissus Quadrangularis (CQR-300) to Reduce Body Fat and Other
A new role for ATM in selective autophagy of peroxisomes (pexophagy).
Pexophagy is responsible for 65% of cases of peroxisome biogenesis disorders.
Lipid Lowering with Soluble Dietary Fiber
Biochemistry of peroxisomes in health and disease
Longevity and diet in Okinawa, Japan: the past, present and future.
A reduced M1-like/M2-like ratio of macrophages in healthy adipose tissue expansion during SGLT2 inhibition | Scientific
Best Rated in Diet Kits & Systems & Helpful Customer Reviews - Amazon.com
Recent advances in understanding body weight homeostasis in humans
Switch from stress response to homeobox transcription factors in adipose tissue after profound fat loss. - -
Rhythmic Oxygen Levels Reset Circadian Clocks through HIF1α: Cell Metabolism
New data on programmed aging - slow phenoptosis.
Nitric oxide mediated redox regulation of protein homeostasis.
Ketone bodies mimic the life span extending properties of caloric restriction.
Prevention of Senescence in Vasculature Through Quiescence.
Exploiting methionine restriction for cancer treatment.
Dietary methionine restriction regulated energy and protein homeostasis by improving thyroid function in high fat diet mice.
Methionine Restriction Extends Lifespan in Progeroid Mice and Alters Lipid and Bile Acid Metabolism.
Sarcosine Is Uniquely Modulated by Aging and Dietary Restriction in Rodents and Humans.
Methionine restriction for improving progeria: another autophagy-inducing anti-aging strategy?
Methionine coordinates a hierarchically organized anabolic program enabling proliferation.
Hypocholesterolaemic and antioxidant activities of chickpea (Cicer arietinum L.) protein hydrolysates.
ACE-inhibitory activity of enzymatic protein hydrolysates from lupin and other legumes.
Butyrate Enhances the Intestinal Barrier by Facilitating Tight Junction Assembly via Activation of AMP-Activated Protein Kinase in Caco-2 Cell Monolayers
Human milk oligosaccharides and infant gut bifidobacteria: Molecular strategies for their utilization.

BODY FAT:

Switch from stress response to homeobox transcription factors in adipose tissue after profound fat loss.
Chronic l-menthol-induced browning of white adipose tissue hypothesis: A putative therapeutic regime for combating obesity and improving metabolic health

HDAC3 is a molecular brake of the metabolic switch supporting white adipose tissue browning.
Matrix Metalloproteinase Inhibitors as Investigative Tools in the Pathogenesis and Management of Vascular Disease
Circulating Adipose Fatty Acid Binding Protein Is a New Link Underlying Obesity-Associated Breast/Mammary Tumor Development
Adipocyte-Macrophage Cross-Talk in Obesity
Gamma-tocotrienol attenuates high-fat diet-induced obesity and insulin resistance by inhibiting adipose inflammation and M1 macrophage recruitment.
Gut microbiota controls adipose tissue expansion, gut barrier and glucose metabolism: novel insights into molecular targets and interventions using prebiotics.
Fish oil as a potential activator of brown and beige fat thermogenesis
Crosstalk between the gut microbiota and the endocannabinoid system: impact on the gut barrier function and the adipose tissue.
The effects of polyphenol supplementation on adipose tissue morphology and gene expression in overweight and obese humans
Supra-Additive Effects of Combining Fat and Carbohydrate on Food Reward
White-to-brite conversion in human adipocytes promotes metabolic reprogramming towards fatty acid anabolic and catabolic pathways
Stimulation of mitochondrial oxidative capacity in white fat independent of UCP1: a key to lean phenotype
M1-M2 balancing act in white adipose tissue browning - a new role for RIP140
Phytochemicals as modulators of M1-M2 macrophages in inflammation
Impact of body composition during weight change on resting energy expenditure and homeostasis model assessment index in overweight nonsmoking adults.
Appetite regulation and weight control: the role of gut hormones
A Mathematical Model of the Human Metabolic S
Emerging role of protein kinase C in energy. CBI
Protein kinase C-beta:
Macronutrients and obesity: revisiting the calories in, calories out
Effect of weight loss and regain on adipose tissue distribution.
Weight cycling of athletes and subsequent weight gain in middleage
Weight regain after a diet-induced loss is predicted by higher base.
Insulin resistance and inflammation predict kinetic body weight change
Insights on Adipose Tissue Extracellular Matrix Remodeling: Models of Diet-Induced Obesity and Weight Loss A reduced M1-like/M2-like ratio of macrophages in healthy adipose tissue expansion during SGLT2 inhibition

PEROXISOMES:
Omega-3 Fatty Acids and PPARγ in Cancer
Biochemistry of peroxisomes in health and disease
PGC-1 alpha regulates HO-1 expression, mitochondrial dynamics and biogenesis: Role of epoxyeicosatrienoic acid.
A new role for ATM in selective autophagy of peroxisomes (pexophagy)
Peroxisome Metabolism and Cellular Aging
Library Peroxisomes, oxidative stress, and inflammation

HIF-1
The role of hypoxia-inducible factors in carotid body (patho) physiology.
Rhythmic Oxygen Levels Reset Circadian Clocks through HIF1α
Effects of hypoxia on the brain: neuroimaging and neuropsychological findings following carbon monoxide poisoning and obstructive sleep apnea.
Selective Inhibition of Collagen Prolyl 4-Hydroxylase in Human Cells
Reactive oxygen radicals and gaseous transmitters in carotid body activation by intermittent hypoxia.
Effects of continuous and intermittent aerobic exercise upon mRNA expression of metabolic genes in human skeletal muscle [J Sports Med Phys Fitness. 2014]

BERBERINE:
Berberine reverts hepatic mitochondrial dysfun... [Mitochondrion. 2013]
Berberine and its more biologically available deriv... [Diabetes. 2008
Berberine increases adipose triglyceride lipase in 3T3-L1 adipocytes through the AMPK pathway.
Berberine attenuates arthritis in adjuvant-induced arthritic rats associated with regulating polarization of macrophages through AMPK/NF-κB pathway.
Inhibition of M1 macrophage activation in adipose tissue by berberine improves insulin resistance.
Berberine is a potential therapeutic agent for metabolic syndrome via brown adipose tissue activation and metabolism regulation.
Berberine reversed the epithelial-mesenchymal transition of normal colonic epithelial cells induced by SW480 cells through regulating the important components in the TGF-β pathway.

RUTIN:
Troxerutin improves hepatic lipid homeostasis by restoring NAD(+)-depletion-mediated dysfunction of lipin 1 signaling in high-fat diet-treated mice.

APIGENIN:
Flavonoid apigenin is an inhibitor of the NAD+ ase CD38: implications for cellular NAD+ metabolism, protein acetylation, and treatment of metabolic syndrome.
Role of Apigenin in Cancer Prevention via the Induction of Apoptosis and Autophagy

Made in the USA
Columbia, SC
12 December 2020